Management of GI and Pancreatic Neuroendocrine Tumors

Editor

JAMES R. HOWE

SURGICAL ONCOLOGY CLINICS OF NORTH AMERICA

www.surgonc.theclinics.com

Consulting Editor
TIMOTHY M. PAWLIK

April 2020 • Volume 29 • Number 2

ELSEVIER

1600 John F. Kennedy Boulevard • Suite 1800 • Philadelphia, Pennsylvania, 19103-2899

http://www.theclinics.com

SURGICAL ONCOLOGY CLINICS OF NORTH AMERICA Volume 29, Number 2
April 2020 ISSN 1055-3207, ISBN-13: 978-0-323-69601-2

Editor: John Vassallo (j.vassallo@elsevier.com)
Developmental Editor: Laura Kavanaugh

Surgical Oncology Clinics of North America (ISSN 1055-3207) is published quarterly by Elsevier Inc., 360 Park Avenue South, New York, NY 10010-1710. Months of publication are January, April, July, and October. Business and Editorial Offices: 1600 John F. Kennedy Blvd., Ste. 1800, Philadelphia, PA 19103-2899. Customer Service Office: 3251 Riverport Lane, Maryland Heights, MO 63043. Periodicals postage paid at New York, NY and additional mailing offices. Subscription prices are $309.00 per year (US individuals), $562.00 (US institutions) $100.00 (US student/resident), $352.00 (Canadian individuals), $711.00 (Canadian institutions), $100.00 (Canadian student/resident), $422.00 (foreign individuals), $711.00 (foreign institutions), and $205.00 (foreign student/resident). Foreign air speed delivery is included in all *Clinics* subscription prices. All prices are subject to change without notice. **POSTMASTER**: Send address changes to *Surgical Oncology Clinics of North America*, Elsevier Health Science Division, Subscription Customer Service, 3251 Riverport Lane, Maryland Heights, MO 63043. **Customer Service: 1-800-654-2452 (US and Canada). 314-447-8871 (outside US and Canada). Fax: 314-447-8029. E-mail: journalscustomerservice-usa@elsevier.com (for print support); journalsonline support-usa@elsevier.com (for online support)**.

Reprints. For copies of 100 or more, of articles in this publication, please contact the Commercial Reprints Department, Elsevier Inc., 360 Park Avenue South, New York, New York 10010-1710. Tel. 212-633-3874; Fax: 212-633-3820; E-mail: reprints@elsevier.com.

Surgical Oncology Clinics of North America is covered in *MEDLINE/PubMed (Index Medicus)* and *EMBASE/ Excerpta Medica, Current Contents/Clinical Medicine, and ISI/BIOMED.*

Contributors

CONSULTING EDITOR

TIMOTHY M. PAWLIK, MD, MPH, MTS PhD, FACS, FRACS (Hon.)
Professor and Chair, Department of Surgery, The Urban Meyer III and Shelley Meyer Chair
for Cancer Research, Professor of Surgery, Oncology, Health Services Management and
Policy, The Ohio State University, Wexner Medical Center, Columbus, Ohio

EDITOR

JAMES R. HOWE, MD
Director, Division of Surgical Oncology and Endocrine Surgery, Professor, Department of
Surgery, Roy J. and Lucille A. Carver College of Medicine, University of Iowa, Iowa City,
Iowa

AUTHORS

ANDREW M. BELLIZZI, MD
Clinical Associate Professor, Department of Pathology, University of Iowa Hospitals and
Clinics, Iowa City, Iowa

KELLIE L. BODEKER, MSHS, CCRC
Clinical Trials Specialist, Department of Radiation Oncology, University of Iowa Hospitals
and Clinics, Iowa City, Iowa

DAVID L. BUSHNELL, MD
Professor, Department of Radiology, University of Iowa Hospital and Clinics, Iowa City
Veterans Administration Health Care System, Iowa City, Iowa

CHANDRIKHA CHANDRASEKHARAN, MBBS
Clinical Assistant Professor, Department of Oncology, University of Iowa, Iowa City, Iowa

JOSEPH S. DILLON, MB, BCh, BAO
Associate Professor, Division of Endocrinology, University of Iowa, Iowa City, Iowa

ALAN G. HARRIS, MD, PhD
Adjunct Professor of Medicine, Department of Medicine, Division of Endocrinology and
Metabolism, New York University Langone School of Medicine, New York, New York

JAMES R. HOWE, MD
Director, Division of Surgical Oncology and Endocrine Surgery, Professor, Department of
Surgery, Roy J. and Lucille A. Carver College of Medicine, University of Iowa, Iowa City,
Iowa

JENNIFER HRABE, MD
Clinical Assistant Professor, Colorectal Surgery, University of Iowa Hospitals and Clinics,
Iowa City, Iowa

XAVIER M. KEUTGEN, MD, FACS
Assistant Professor, Department of Surgery, Division of General Surgery and Surgical Oncology, Endocrine Research Program, The University of Chicago Medicine, Chicago, Illinois

AMANDA M. LAIRD, MD, FACS
Chief, Section of Endocrine Surgery, Rutgers Cancer Institute of New Jersey, Associate Professor of Surgery, Rutgers Robert Wood Johnson Medical School, New Brunswick, New Jersey

STEVEN K. LIBUTTI, MD, FACS
Director, Rutgers Cancer Institute of New Jersey, Professor of Surgery, Rutgers Robert Wood Johnson Medical School, New Brunswick, New Jersey

KRISTEN E. LIMBACH, MD
Resident, General Surgery, Department of Surgery, Oregon Health & Science University, Portland, Oregon

PARREN McNEELY, MD
Clinical Assistant Professor, Department of Radiology, Roy J. and Lucille A. Carver College of Medicine, University of Iowa, Iowa City, Iowa

YUSUF MENDA, MD
Professor, Department of Radiology, Roy J. and Lucille A. Carver College of Medicine, University of Iowa, Iowa City, Iowa

M SUE O'DORISIO, MD, PhD
Professor of Pediatrics, Division of Pediatric Oncology, University of Iowa Hospitals and Clinics, Iowa City, Iowa, USA

THOMAS M. O'DORISIO, MD
Professor of Medicine, Division of Endocrinology, University of Iowa Hospitals and Clinics, Iowa City, Iowa, USA

JANET POLLARD, MD
Clinical Assistant Professor, Department of Radiology, Roy J. and Lucille A. Carver College of Medicine, University of Iowa, Iowa City Veterans Healthcare System, Iowa City, Iowa

RODNEY F. POMMIER, MD
Professor of Surgery, Division of Surgical Oncology, Department of Surgery, Oregon Health & Science University, Portland, Oregon

AARON T. SCOTT, MD
Resident in Surgery, Roy J. and Lucille A. Carver College of Medicine, University of Iowa, Iowa City, Iowa

TANAZ VAGHAIWALLA, MD
Fellow, Department of Surgery, Division of General Surgery and Surgical Oncology, Endocrine Research Program, The University of Chicago Medicine, Chicago, Illinois

Contents

Erratum   xi

Foreword: Management of Gastrointestinal and Pancreatic Neuroendocrine Tumors   xiii
Timothy M. Pawlik

Preface: Neuroendocrine Tumors   xv
James R. Howe

Evolution of Neuroendocrine Tumor Therapy   145
Thomas M. O'Dorisio, Alan G. Harris, and M Sue O'Dorisio

To better understand developments in treatment of neuroendocrine tumors of the gastroenteropancreatic system, and the pivotal roles of native somatostatin and its long-acting analogues play in normal peptide regulation and neuropeptide excess associated with neuroendocrine tumors (NETs), this article delineates and defines distinct eras in the history and discovery of gastrointestinal endocrinology. We highlight the collaboration between academia and industry in basic science and the clinical research that advanced Lu-177-DOTATATE to approval as standard of care therapy for low-grade NETs. Examples of new radioisotopes and therapy compounds currently in development for diagnosis and therapy for high-grade NETs are also discussed.

Workup of Gastroenteropancreatic Neuroendocrine Tumors   165
Joseph S. Dillon

Neuroendocrine tumors of the gastrointestinal tract or pancreas are rare. Their presentation overlaps with other intra-abdominal neoplasms, but can have unique features. The workup involves recognition of unusual clinical features associated with the tumors, imaging, analysis of blood or urine concentrations, and biopsy. Functional imaging takes advantage of the neuroendocrine tumor-specific expression of somatostatin receptors. There are characteristic features supporting the diagnosis on contrast-enhanced cross-sectional imaging. The use of tumor markers for biochemical diagnosis requires an understanding of the confounding variables affecting these assays. There are unique and specific immunohistochemical staining and grading requirements for appropriate diagnosis of these tumors.

Pathologic Considerations in Gastroenteropancreatic Neuroendocrine Tumors   185
Andrew M. Bellizzi

This review serves as a primer on contemporary neuroendocrine neoplasm classification, with an emphasis on gastroenteropancreatic well-differentiated neuroendocrine tumors. Topics discussed include general features of neuroendocrine neoplasms, general neuroendocrine marker immunohistochemistry, the distinction of well-differentiated neuroendocrine tumor from pheochromocytoma/paraganglioma and other diagnostic mimics and poorly differentiated neuroendocrine carcinoma from diagnostic mimics, the concepts of differentiation and grade and the application of Ki-67 immunohistochemistry to determine the latter, the various WHO classifications of neuroendocrine neoplasms including the 2019 WHO classification of gastroenteropancreatic tumors, organ-specific considerations for gastroenteropancreatic well-differentiated neuroendocrine tumors, immunohistochemistry to determine site of origin in metastatic well-differentiated neuroendocrine tumor of occult origin, immunohistochemistry in the distinction of well-differentiated neuroendocrine tumor G3 from large cell neuroendocrine carcinoma, and, finally, required and recommended reporting elements for biopsies and resections of gastroenteropancreatic neuroendocrine epithelial neoplasms.

Nuclear Imaging of Neuroendocrine Tumors   209

Janet Pollard, Parren McNeely, and Yusuf Menda

Consensus guidelines acknowledge the role of gallium Ga-68 (^{68}Ga) 1,4,7,10-tetraazacyclododecane-N,N',N'',N'''-tetraacetic (DOTA) somatostatin receptor (SSTR) positron emission tomography/computed tomography (PET/CT) in management of neuroendocrine tumor (NET) patients. ^{68}Ga-DOTA-SSTR PET/CT demonstrates superior performance to conventional imaging in initial detection, staging, detection of recurrent tumor, and detection of unknown primary in known metastatic disease. ^{68}Ga-DOTA-SSTR PET/CT is low yield for NET detection in the setting of symptoms or elevated biomarkers when conventional imaging is negative, but may still guide management. The role of ^{68}Ga-DOTA-SSTR PET/CT is not established in monitoring response to systemic therapy but may identify progression through detection of new metastases.

Management of Small Bowel Neuroendocrine Tumors   223

Aaron T. Scott and James R. Howe

Small bowel neuroendocrine tumors (SBNETS) are slow-growing neoplasms with a noted propensity toward metastasis and comparatively favorable prognosis. The presentation of SBNETs is varied, although abdominal pain and obstructive symptoms are the most common presenting symptoms. In patients with metastases, hypersecretion of serotonin and other bioactive amines results in diarrhea, flushing, valvular heart disease, and bronchospasm, termed carcinoid syndrome. The treatment of SBNETs is multimodal and includes surgery, liver-directed therapy, somatostatin analogues, targeted therapy, and peptide receptor radionuclide therapy.

Surgical Management of Pancreatic Neuroendocrine Tumors   243

Tanaz Vaghaiwalla and Xavier M. Keutgen

Surgical management of pancreatic neuroendocrine tumors (PNETS) is steadily evolving and is influenced by multiple factors. Sporadic PNETs are generally managed more aggressively than those occurring in the background of hereditary syndromes, and functioning PNETs are almost always resected if they are not metastatic. Localized nonfunctioning PNETs less than 2 cm can often be observed. Surgical resection for localized PNET greater than 2 cm comprises parenchymal sparing pancreas resections, such as enucleations, or formal anatomic resection, such as distal pancreatectomy or pancreaticoduodenectomy. PNETs commonly metastasize to the liver, and several systemic and liver-directed options to treat hepatic metastases are available.

Management of Other Gastric and Duodenal Neuroendocrine Tumors   253

Amanda M. Laird and Steven K. Libutti

Gastric and duodenal neuroendocrine tumors (NETs) are increasing in incidence as a result of increased detection and awareness of neuroendocrine tumors as distinct tumor types. The three types of gastric NETs and duodenal NETs have different etiologies and tumor-specific factors, such as grade, location, and hormone-production, and the clinical settings influence management. Options for treatment include removal by local endoscopic resection and surgical resection. Medical therapy is used to treat the inciting condition or as systemic therapy in advanced disease. Although the overall prognosis for most is good, higher grade tumors behave aggressively and have reduced survival.

Neuroendocrine Tumors of the Appendix, Colon, and Rectum   267

Jennifer Hrabe

Neuroendocrine neoplasms of the colon and rectum are rare, although surgeons are likely to encounter appendiceal neuroendocrine tumors while caring for patients with appendicitis. Surgery remains the primary treatment, provided disease is resectable, although for small rectal lesions endoscopic resection is often sufficient. Metastastic disease has a variety of treatment options. Poorly differentiated neuroendocrine carcinomas continue to have a poor prognosis.

Management of Metastatic GEPNETs   281

Kristen E. Limbach and Rodney F. Pommier

The chief causes of death of patients with GEPNETs are liver failure from hepatic replacement by tumor in the majority and bowel obstruction in the remainder. Many patients are with liver metastases are actually eligible for hepatic cytoreductive operations, even if they have numerous bilobar metastases and extra-hepatic disease, provided that greater than 70% of the liver tumor volume can be removed. This can often be done by combinations of parenchyma-sparing enucleations, wedge resections and radio frequency ablations. Patients with higher liver tumor burden can be treated with intra-arterial therapies, such as embolization and chemoembolization. Patients with peritoneal carcinomatosis are recommended to undergo cytoreductive operations including peritoneal stripping and bowel resections. Consensus guidelines by experts recommend bisphosphonate therapy for patients with bone metastases, reserving surgical treatment for patients with mechanical issues and/or potential spinal cord compression. Radiation can be employed for isolated painful metastases. PRRT may be an emerging therapy for treatment of bone metastases.

Medical Management of Gastroenteropancreatic Neuroendocrine Tumors   293

Chandrikha Chandrasekharan

The increased incidence and prevalence of neuroendocrine tumors (NETs) over the past few decades has been accompanied by an improvement in overall survival. There are differences in the management of small bowel NETs versus pNETs. The management of all patients with NETs must be individualized based on patient characteristics as well tumor-related factors. This article reviews the role of somatostatin analogues, historical results with chemotherapy in gastroenteropancreatic NETs (GEPNETs), and more recent evidence for the use of cytotoxic chemotherapy in GEPNETs. The article also discusses molecular targeted therapies approved for use in GEPNETs and some ongoing clinical trials.

Overview and Current Status of Peptide Receptor Radionuclide Therapy   317

David L. Bushnell and Kellie L. Bodeker

Peptide receptor radionuclide therapy (PRRT) is an effective form of treatment of patients with metastatic neuroendocrine tumors, delivering modest objective tumor response rates but notable survival and symptomatic benefits. The first PRRT approved by the US Food and Drug Administration was lutetium 177–DOTATATE and is for use in adults with somatostatin receptor–positive gastroenteropancreatic neuroendocrine tumors. The treatment paradigm typically leads to significant improvement in symptomology coupled with an extended period of progression-free survival. Side effects are limited, with a small fraction of individuals experiencing clinically significant long-term renal or hematologic toxicity.

SURGICAL ONCOLOGY CLINICS OF NORTH AMERICA

FORTHCOMING ISSUES

July 2020
Melanoma
Kieth Delman and Michael Lowe, *Editors*

October 2020
Emerging Therapies in Thoracic
Malignancies
Usman Ahmad and Sudish Murthy, *Editors*

July 2021
Palliative Care in Surgical Oncology
Bridget N. Fahy, *Editor*

RECENT ISSUES

July 2019
Immunotherapy for Solid Malignancies
Alfred E. Chang, *Editor*

April 2019
Minimally Invasive Oncologic Surgery, Part II
Claudius Conrad and James W. Fleshman,
Editors

January 2019
Minimally Invasive Oncologic Surgery, Part I
Claudius Conrad and James W. Fleshman,
Editors

SERIES OF RELATED INTEREST

Surgical Clinics of North America
http://www.surgical.theclinics.com
Thoracic Surgery Clinics
http://www.thoracic.theclinics.com
Advances in Surgery
http://www.advancessurgery.com

THE CLINICS ARE AVAILABLE ONLINE!
Access your subscription at:
www.theclinics.com

Erratum

In the January 2019 issue, in the article "Virtual and Augmented Reality in Oncologic Liver Surgery," (pages 31-44) one author's name was misspelled. It should be Muhammad Shahbaz, and the correct list of authors should read: Giuseppe Quero, MD, Alfonso Lapergola, MD, Luc Soler, PhD, Muhammad Shahbaz, MD, Alexandre Hostettler, PhD, Toby Collins, Msc, Jacques Marescaux, MD, FACS, (Hon) FRCS, (Hon) FJSES, Didier Mutter, MD, PhD, FACSc, Michele Diana, MD, PhD, and Patrick Pessaux, MD, PhD. Dr. Shahbaz's affiliations are: 1. Department of General Surgery, Qilu Hospital, Shandong University, China; 2. The Institute of Laparoscopic-Endoscopic Minimally Invasive Surgery of Shandong University, Shandong, China; 3. IHU-Strasbourg, Institute of Image-Guided Surgery, 1 Place de l'Hôpital, Strasbourg 67091, France. IRCAD, Research Institute Against Cancer of the Digestive System, 1 Place de l'Hôpital, Strasbourg 67091, France.

https://doi.org/10.1016/j.soc.2020.02.011

Foreword

Management of Gastrointestinal and Pancreatic Neuroendocrine Tumors

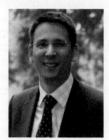

Timothy M. Pawlik, MD, MPH, MTS, PhD, FACS, FRACS (Hon.)
Consulting Editor

This issue of the *Surgical Oncology Clinics of North America* is devoted to covering the important topic of Management of Gastrointestinal (GI) and Pancreatic Neuroendocrine Tumors. Over the last several decades, there has been a noted increase in the incidence of neuroendocrine tumors. Concomitant to this epidemiological shift, significant advances have been achieved in the understanding of neuroendocrine diseases as well as in the surgical and systemic treatments of this disease. Neuroendocrine tumors can present, however, with a broad spectrum of clinical manifestations as well as have varied long-term prognoses. In turn, management of neuroendocrine tumors mandates a well-informed multidisciplinary approach that incorporates, among others, endocrinology, gastroenterology, medical oncology, and surgery. As such, it is critical for surgeons to have a firm grasp on the emerging knowledge regarding the diagnostic and treatment options for patients with neuroendocrine tumors. In light of this need, I am delighted to have Dr James Howe be the guest editor of this important issue of *Surgical Oncology Clinics of North America*. Dr Howe is Professor of Surgery at the University of Iowa, where he is the Division Director of Surgical Oncology. In addition, Dr Howe is codirector of the Neuroendocrine Cancer Clinic of Holden Comprehensive Cancer Center and coleader of the GI neuroendocrine multioncology group. Dr Howe was elected 2019 Chair of the North American Neuroendocrine Tumor Society and is currently the President-Elect of the Society of Surgical Oncology. Dr Howe has conducted substantial research toward the understanding of neuroendocrine tumors with over 100 manuscripts in peer-reviewed journals. Given Dr Howe's stature as an international leader in the management of neuroendocrine tumors, I can think of no one more suited to be the guest editor of this important issue of the *Surgical Oncology Clinics of North America*.

The issue covers a number of important topics, including the workup, as well as the medical and surgical management of patients with both GI and pancreatic

Surg Oncol Clin N Am 29 (2020) xiii–xiv
https://doi.org/10.1016/j.soc.2020.02.001
1055-3207/20/© 2020 Published by Elsevier Inc.

neuroendocrine tumors. In particular, a wide array of expert authors elucidates the surgical management of gastric, duodenal, small bowel, as well as pancreatic tumors. Other clinically relevant topics, such as the workup and use of functional imaging to diagnosis and stage patients with neuroendocrine tumors, are also covered. Furthermore, the medical management and the role of peptide radioreceptor therapy are delineated. I want to thank Dr Howe for enlisting the help of an amazing group of authors who are leaders in the field of neuroendocrine tumors. As you will witness yourself, Dr Howe and the authors do an expert job in highlighting the important and relevant aspects of caring for patients with GI and pancreatic neuroendocrine tumors. The knowledge contained in this issue of *Surgical Oncology Clinics of North America* will well serve surgical oncologists and other health care providers who care for patients with GI and pancreatic neuroendocrine tumors. I would like to thank Dr Howe and all the contributing authors for an excellent issue of the *Surgical Oncology Clinics of North America* and for tackling this important topic.

Timothy M. Pawlik, MD, MPH, MTS, PhD, FACS, FRACS (Hon.)
Department of Surgery
Oncology and Health Services Management and Policy
The Ohio State University
Wexner Medical Center
395 West 12th Avenue, Suite 670
Columbus, OH 43210, USA

E-mail address:
tim.pawlik@osumc.edu

Preface

Neuroendocrine Tumors

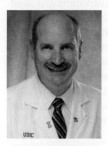

James R. Howe, MD
Editor

Neuroendocrine tumors (NETs) have long been an enigma for practicing physicians. The first accounts of patients with these tumors were published in the late 1800s, and the recognition that these were distinct pathologic entities from other gastrointestinal (GI) tumors was reported by Oberndorfer in 1907, who described them as *karzinoide*, or carcinoma-like. These rare tumors are commonly associated with unusual symptoms and are often misdiagnosed, which has led to the widespread adoption of the zebra as their symbol. Initially, NETs were considered to be benign, but Oberndorfer himself eventually conceded in 1929 that they metastasize. Despite this, NETs were still not consistently included in national cancer databases until toward the end of the century, with the realization that the majority have malignant potential and that they are frequently metastatic. The incidence of these tumors has increased 7-fold over the past several decades not just because of increasing inclusion in databases but also likely due to the ubiquitous use of computed tomographic scans for evaluation of abdominal symptoms. Their increased recognition and relatively indolent course have led NETs to become the second most prevalent GI malignancy. Although many patients present with metastatic disease, their survival can still be long, and therefore, proper recognition is paramount.

As physicians encounter NETs with increasing frequency, it is important to understand the diverse sites that they may originate from, and the broad spectrum of their clinical manifestations. These fascinating entities may produce carcinoid syndrome, with its flushing, diarrhea, and wheezing resulting from tumors originating in the small bowel, to hypoglycemia, ulcers, Cushing syndrome, and even hypercalcemic crisis in NETs from the pancreas. It is also not uncommon for patients to have very small primary tumors accompanied by large nodal and liver metastases. Through the important contributions of clinicians and researchers, much progress has been made in diagnosing these tumors, from the recognition of characteristic signs on physical exam, to advances in biochemical testing, anatomic and functional imaging, as well as

Surg Oncol Clin N Am 29 (2020) xv–xvi
https://doi.org/10.1016/j.soc.2020.01.001
1055-3207/20/© 2020 Published by Elsevier Inc.

surgonc.theclinics.com

identification of the pathologic features that differentiate them from other tumors and dictate their prognosis.

The clinical management of these patients is truly multidisciplinary and requires the skills of many different specialties. Radiologists, gastroenterologists, and pathologists help to make the diagnosis so that the surgeon can remove locoregional tumors and perform cytoreduction of metastatic disease. Endocrinologists diagnose and manage symptoms, and medical oncologists, interventional radiologists, and nuclear medicine physicians treat metastatic disease. Breakthroughs by basic scientists improve our understanding of the biologic basis of these tumors, leading to new treatments for NET patients. In this issue of *Surgical Oncology Clinics of North America*, we acknowledge the importance of all of these specialists and herein have assembled a diverse group of experts to present what the practicing clinician needs to know about the diagnosis and treatment of NETs from gastroenteropancreatic sites. I personally thank all of the authors who have contributed their time and expertise to this project, and the editors and production crew who have given us the opportunity.

James R. Howe, MD
Division of Surgical Oncology and
Endocrine Surgery
Department of Surgery
University of Iowa
Carver College of Medicine
200 Hawkins Drive
Iowa City, IA 52242, USA

E-mail address:
james-howe@uiowa.edu

Evolution of Neuroendocrine Tumor Therapy

Thomas M. O'Dorisio, MD[a],*, Alan G. Harris, MD, PhD[b],
M Sue O'Dorisio, MD, PhD[c]

KEYWORDS

- Neuroendocrine tumor • Therapy • Gastroenteropancreatic • PRRT • Octreotide
- GI Hormones

KEY POINTS

- Although most theranostic compounds are peptide agonists targeting G-protein-coupled receptors, several antagonist molecules are in preclinical and early clinical use.
- One example is a peptide ligand, 68Ga-DOTA-bombesin (neoBOMB) targeting the gastrin releasing peptide (GRP) receptor known to be expressed in prostate cancer cells.
- This GRPR antagonist has shown promising results in animal models and its first PET imaging in humans has been recently reported.
- Similarly, an antagonist at the somatostatin receptor has been introduced as a theranostic pair in neuroendocrine tumors.
- PRRT represents a single high affinity peptide specifically binding to a single membrane receptor. Either an agonist like octreotide, or an antagonist, can be used to bind to the specific somatostatin subtype receptor. As well, the same modified octreotide can be used for both diagnostic and therapeutic purposes (THERANOSTICS).

On April 2, 1986, a symposium comprised of multidisciplinary preclinical and clinical scientists and physicians was convened and the proceedings published.[1] It addressed neuroendocrine disorders of the gastroenteropancreatic (GEP) systems and introduced preclinical and clinical applications of the somatostatin peptide analogue SMS 201-995 (octreotide [Sandostatin]). Three years later, in 1989, octreotide was the first Food and Drug Administration (FDA)-approved drug for the symptomatic control of carcinoid syndrome and the watery diarrhea syndrome of the pancreatic neuroendocrine tumor (NET), VIPoma.[2] Now 30 years later, octreotide,

[a] Division of Endocrinology, University of Iowa Hospitals and Clinics, Room E401-5 GH, 200 Hawkins Drive, Iowa City, Iowa 52242, USA; [b] Department of Medicine, Division of Endocrinology and Metabolism, New York University Langone School of Medicine, New York, New York, 10016, USA; [c] Division of Pediatric Oncology, University of Iowa Hospitals and Clinics, Room 1300-28 BT, 200 Hawkins Drive, Iowa City, Iowa 52242, USA
* Corresponding author.
E-mail address: thomas-odorisio@uiowa.edu

Surg Oncol Clin N Am 29 (2020) 145–163
https://doi.org/10.1016/j.soc.2019.11.002
1055-3207/20/© 2019 Elsevier Inc. All rights reserved.

surgonc.theclinics.com

and the recently FDA-approved agent lanreotide, continue as first-line therapies for all symptomatic NETs. Furthermore, the isotopic radiolabeling of octreotide specifically targets somatostatin receptors overexpressed on NETs and has heralded yet another FDA-approved diagnostic-therapeutic strategy termed theranostics, which allows an octreotide derivative to act as a radiodiagnostic molecular imaging agent and a radio-therapeutic product for the treatment of malignant neuroendocrine tumors.[3,4]

To better understand the context of these developments, and the pivotal role native somatostatin and its long-acting analogues play in normal peptide regulation and neuropeptide excess associated with NETs, we delineate and define distinct eras in the history and discovery of gastrointestinal (GI) endocrinology. The major periods of gut endocrinology include: the physiology ("juice") era, the clinical era, the peptide chemistry era, and the peptide diagnostic and therapeutic era.[5]

Building on the historical milestones recently addressed in reviews by O'Dorisio[5] and Oberg,[6] we address and expand on the two reviews where appropriate. Regarding ^{177}Lu-DOTA(tyr)-octreotate and ^{90}Y-DOTA-(tyr)-octreotide therapy in child-hood and adult NETs, we highlight the collaboration between academia and industry in basic science and the clinical research that advanced LUTATHERA (Lu-177-dota-tate) to FDA approval as standard of care therapy for low-grade NETs.[4] Examples of new radioisotopes and therapy compounds currently in development for diagnosis and therapy for high-grade NETs are also discussed.

Endocrinology began in 1902 with the physiology era, with the discovery of the "blood-borne chemical messenger" secretin by Bayliss and Starling.[7] They demonstrated that HCl placed into canine duodenum resulted in the secretion of alkaline pancreatic juice. They called this substance "secretin" and later coined the term "hormone" derived from the Greek military word *Opuaw*, which means "I arouse/excite to activity."[5]

In 1905, Edkins,[8] a prominent physiologist, described a potent gastric acid secreta-gogue subsequently termed "gastrin." It was not until 1961 that Gregory and Tracy[9] identified the multigastrin forms confirming its biologic properties described by Edkins. Physiologists Ivy and Eldberg[10] described their observation on hormone-mediated gallbladder contraction. They noted that the extract from dog proximal small intestine when injected intravenously into another dog was associated with gall-bladder contraction. A second pair of physiologists, Harper and Raper,[11] found that dog small intestine extract was associated with gallbladder contraction and pancre-atic juice release and termed it "pancreozymin." For a time, the abbreviation CCK/PZ was used. It was ultimately determined that pancreozymin was indeed cholecys-tokinin (CCK). This highlights the insensitivity of the bioassay techniques at the time, and the tremendous impact that radioimmunoassay (RIA) was to have on the neuro-endocrine field.

A few years before the discovery of CCK, Banting and Best[12] were able to stabilize sheep insulin and achieve glucose homeostasis in pancreatectomized dogs. Shortly after insulin stabilization, a patient with insulin-dependent diabetes mellitus was suc-cessfully treated with the extracted sheep insulin. This and other key insulin mile-stones were reviewed by the endocrinologist Forsham[13] in 1982. In the United States, large-scale insulin production was achieved thanks to the strong collaboration between academia and industry (Eli Lilly) and NOVO-Nordisk in Europe. Diabetes mel-litus represented a peptide-deficient state of the enteropancreatic axis as opposed to the excess peptide hormone production by functional NETs.

During the era of physiologic discovery, morphologists, anatomists, and patholo-gists were working to identify the GEP cells responsible for the secretion of these newly identified peptide hormone substances. **Table 1** lists the key investigators who helped define the neuroendocrine cells of the GEP axis.[5,6]

Table 1
Investigators who helped describe and identify the amine/peptide-secreting cells of the GEP system

Investigator (s)	Year	Observation	References #
P. Langerhans	1870s	Cell clusters on acinar cells	Langerhans and Moorison,[14] 1869
E. Laguesse	1890s	Islets of Langerhans	Langerhans and Moorison,[14] 1869
R. P. Heidenhain	1870	EC EC-like: histamine secretion	Heidenhain,[15] 1870
A. Nikolas	1891	EC cells, GI tract	Nikolas,[16] 1891
N. Kulchitsky	1897	EC cells/crypts of Lieberkühn	Kulchitsky,[17] 1897
M. Ciaccio	1906	EC cells in human GI tract	Ciaccio,[18] 1906
A. Gosset and P. Masson	1914	Diffuse endocrine system	Gosset and Masson,[19] 1914
F. Feyter	1938	Helle zellen, clear cells; neuroendocrine	Feyter,[20] 1938
F. Feyter	1953	Coined paracrine and neurocrine	Feyter,[21] 1953

Abbreviation: EC, enterochromaffin.
Data from O'Dorisio TM. Gut endocrinology: clinical and therapeutic impact. Am J Med. 1986;81(6B):1-7 and Öberg K. The Genesis of the Neuroendocrine Tumors Concept: From Oberndorfer to 2018. Endocrinol Metab Clin North Am. 2018;47(3):711-731.

By 1950 it was clear that, within the GEP system, there were many unexplained control systems and a larger number of different neuroendocrine cells and their secreting products and actions that were yet to be recognized. A prominent gastrophysiologist, Grossman,[22] worked diligently to assign hormone and neurocrine action to the previously described substances, such as CCK and secretin. Until that time, the extracted peptide material was crude and only partially purified. This affected bioassay interpretation and assignment of the actual neuropeptides responsible for the observed actions. One example was the identification of incretin, a substance residing in the small intestine, released by a glucose load and affecting additional insulin secretion in a hormonal fashion. Moore[23] is credited with the first physiologic observation of a small intestinal extract that lowered blood sugars in the presence of an increased glucose load into the duodenum. It is now accepted that incretin is caused, in part, by the two GI peptides glucose-dependent insulinotropic peptide (GIP) and glucagon-like peptide-1.[24]

The peptide chemistry era was ushered in with two remarkable discoveries in the 1950s and 1960s. The first was the development of column chromatography, which used cross-linked dextran gel for gel filtration of substances based on particle size and cross-linking and molecular weight.[25] The resin columns used different size beads, which excluded extracts of different molecular weights and purification. The purification of gastrin from Zollinger-Ellison tumors by Gregory and Tracy in 1961 was an excellent example of the purification by column chromatography.[9] Furthermore, Jorpes and Mutt from the Karolinska Institute in Stockholm, Sweden, purified several GI peptides extracted from porcine intestine using large-diameter columns.[26,27] It has been estimated that the combined efforts of Gregory, Jorpes, and Mutt led to the purification of more than 14 GI neuropeptides that included GIP, vasoactive intestinal peptide (VIP), pancreastatin, and neuropeptide Y, and peptide tyrosine tyrosine (PYY).

The second critical discovery was the development of RIA by Yalow and Berson in 1959.[28,29] With highly purified GI peptides being rapidly produced, RIA used highly pure peptide standards in competitive protein binding curves with a short wavelength isotope, iodine 125- Kev 30, offering for the first time high peptide sensitivity and specificity measurements. Shortly after the initial description of RIA, McGuigan[30] published the gastrin RIA. With the development of high-titer peptide antibodies for RIA, antibodies directed against peptide-secreting neuroendocrine cells using the immunohistochemical (IHC) methodology was simultaneously developed. Two active investigators in neuroendocrine clinical research in the mid-1970s were the endocrinologist S.R. Bloom and pathologist J.M. Polak. Together they identified by RIA and IHC many GI neuroendocrine secreting cells,[31–33] and made a great contribution to GI neuroendocrinology by the mid-1970s. The United States had also developed RIAs for the newly identified neuropeptides. The Mayo Clinic developed commercial neuropeptide RIAs under the supervision of V.L.W. Go. Also, The Ohio State University/University Reference Laboratory performed CLIA-certified GI neuropeptide RIAs under the supervision of S. Cataland and T.M. O'Dorisio. The most durable commercial neuropeptide RIA laboratory in the United States is the Inter Science Institute, which will soon celebrate 50 years of performing peptide RIAs.[34]

In 1977, R. Yalow received the Nobel prize in physiology and medicine "for the development of RIA of peptide hormones." S. Berson had passed away and was not eligible posthumously. Dr Yalow shared the Nobel Prize that year with R. Guillemen and A. Schally "for their discoveries concerning the peptide hormone production of the brain." Dr Guillemin and his colleagues had discovered somatostatin.[35] Arimura and colleagues[36] established an acetone extraction RIA to measure plasma somatostatin plasma in 1978. The impact that RIA had on GI peptide discovery is depicted in **Fig. 1**.

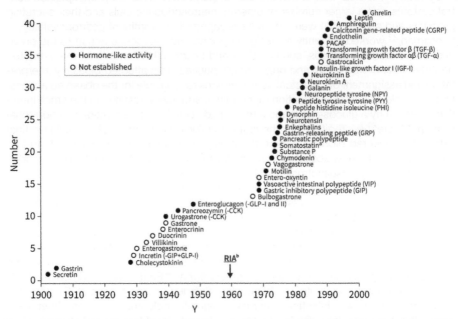

Fig. 1. Peptides identified in the mammalian gastroenteropancreatic system. [a] Somatostatin has all regulatory actions: endocrine, paracrine, neuroendocrine, autocrine. [b] RIA (radioimmunoassay) first described in 1959.[28,29] (*Adapted from* Rehfeld JF. Beginnings: a reflection on the history of gastrointestinal endocrinology. Regul Pept. 2012 Aug 10;177 Suppl:S1–5. doi: 10.1016/j.regpep.2012.05.087.)

With the discovery of new peptides/hormones during this period between 1960 and 2000, it would be only a matter of time before the development and utility of some of these peptides became clinically relevant (the peptide therapy era). The clinical era, albeit, at a much slower pace, progressed in parallel with the discovery of GI hormones beginning in 1902. The pathologist S. Oberndorfer is credited with the description of small bowel tumors, which he termed "karzinoide," meaning carcinoma-like. His publication in 1907[37] and description was the first to distinguish the slower growing tumors from true carcinomas. It was not until 1928 that he revised the initial description of benign tumors to more accurately reflect their malignant and metastatic potential.[38] In his section on carcinoid tumors, Oberg[6] cites a case report by Ransom[39] from 1890 of a woman with probable malignant carcinoid tumors who flushed after eating. Oberg[6] suggested this could be the first description of carcinoid syndrome. Lembeck,[40] in 1953, confirmed that serotonin was present in an ileal carcinoid tumor, specifically within the enterochromaffin cells. The problem of being able to determine carcinoid tumors as functional serotonin-secreting tumors in the past has been caused by the difficulty in measuring the plasma serotonin, which has a short half-life of 35 seconds. This has been overcome with the addition of ascorbic acid to a whole-blood sample.

It has now been shown that ileal carcinoid tumors are the second-most frequent leading tumor of the GI tract. Moreover, they have a higher incidence than esophageal and gastric carcinomas combined.[41] An insulin-secreting pancreatic NET was first described by Wilder and colleagues[42] in 1927. It was a case that used a bioassay whereby they could demonstrate that the liver metastasis contained bioactive insulin. Whipple and Frantz[43] published a large series of islet cell tumors associated with hypoglycemia. They also described what came to be known as Whipple triad: documented low blood sugar associated with symptoms of hypoglycemia, improved with glucose replacement.

In 1955, Zollinger and Ellison[44] described two patients with abdominal pain, diarrhea (because of excess gastric acid secretion), and atypical bleeding ulcerations of the small bowel associated with NETs of the pancreas. Shortly after the initial description, the syndrome was named ulcerogenic syndrome and/or Zollinger-Ellison syndrome. One of the first two patients initially reported was a 17-year-old woman at the time of diagnosis. A few years following her subtotal gastrectomy, it was noted she was a member of a multiple endocrine neoplasia (MEN) syndrome type 1 (MEN-1) kindred, and one of the authors (T.M.O.) helped care for this patient for almost 20 years. Her weight had remained quite stable even in the presence of liver metastasis and subtotal gastrectomy. It was determined by RIA that her tumor secreted gastrin and somatostatin, and that the somatostatin acted, in part, as an antagonist to gastrin secretion on her liver tumors via a peptide-peptide interaction. She was never begun on octreotide, but her liver lesions remained stable until the time of her death at age 65. A similar case of a gastrinoma secreting somatostatin was discussed by O'Dorisio and colleagues in 1987.[45]

Gregory and coworkers[46] identified gastrin from patients with Zollinger-Ellison syndrome, including one patient from the original Zollinger-Ellison publication. Using classic bioassay, they injected gastrinoma tumor extract intravenously into two dogs and showed profound gastric acid output. Their work validated Edkins[8] physiologic observation in 1905 using canine stomach mucosa extracts.

In 1958, internist J.V. Verner and pathologist A.B. Morrison described two patients with fulminant secretory diarrhea, hypokalemia, achlorhydria (most often hypochlorhydria), and pancreatic NETs. The patient also had metabolic acidosis caused by bicarbonate loss in the diarrhea.[47] Although initially termed "watery diarrhea, hypokalemia, achlorhydria," it came to be called watery diarrhea syndrome. Because the neuromodulator VIP shares amino acid homology with secretin and GIP, both neuropeptides were thought to be the modulating peptide excess in the watery diarrhea syndrome. It was not until the purification of VIP by S. Said and V. Mutt and the development of the VIP RIA that the actual pathohumoral state of VIP and watery diarrhea syndrome was established.[48,49]

Although glucagonoma syndrome was first described in 1942, McGavran and coworkers[50] reported a case of a patient with glucagonoma syndrome with elevated plasma glucagon levels, diabetes mellitus (type II), severe dermopathy, and a pancreatic NET in 1966. The immunoreactive-like glucagon RIA was performed by R.H. Unger and proved to be one of the best glucagon polyclonal antibodies (Unger 30K) for glucagon RIA in the United States. The association of the often-lethal thromboembolism in the glucagonoma syndrome was reported by Mallinson and coworkers in 1974.[51]

Somatostatinoma began to be described in the late 1970s. They are rare and are more often peripancreatic than pancreatic in location. These are considered asymptomatic but are associated with gallbladder disease (because of antagonism of CCK), diabetes mellitus (type II), and subclinical fat malabsorption (because of antagonism of pancreatic enzyme release).[52]

Although only 20% of pancreatic NETs are functional, these tumors of the GEP system predominantly secrete their excess peptides/amines in an endocrine manner. They may also secrete peptides or amines alien to their cell of origin in a paraendocrine (paracrine) fashion.[45,53] Because of the ability to measure plasma neuropeptides by specific and sensitive RIA, and recognizing their physiologic and pathophysiologic actions, we can ascribe peptide/amine function to GEP NETs based on their syndrome/symptoms. Although it is currently accepted that GEP NETs derive from neuroendocrine cells/tissue, the amine precursor uptake decarboxylase hypothesis of Pearse[54,55] remains appealing. His concept considered that the diffuse endocrine system is of neural crest origin. It was supported by the finding that neuron-specific enolase is present in all parts of the neuroendocrine cell system.[56] Unfortunately, we have come to appreciate the inadequate specificity of neuron-specific enolase antibodies, which may have impacted on Pearse's conclusion that the origin of neuroendocrine cells are derived from neural crest tissue. Later work by Andrew and colleagues[57] was an endodermal origin of neuroendocrine cells, and not necessarily neural crest origin. The amine precursor uptake decarboxylase concept, however, remains a convenient and practical framework to describe and study NETs.

Most enteropancreatic NETs are considered sporadic. However, inherited syndromes associated with pancreatic and thyroid NETs exist, and their genetics have been determined. These include MEN1 and MEN2 syndromes, von Hippel-Lindau disease, neurofibromatosis-1, and tuberous sclerosis. Although the inherited NET-associated syndromes are rare, we have clinically observed MEN1 and MEN2 more often in our NET clinics than von Hippel-Lindau disease or tuberous sclerosis. This may be caused, in part, by the functional nature of the pancreatic NETs in MEN1, and the diagnosis and management of pheochromocytoma in MEN2 syndromes. Norton and coworkers[58] published a review of the genetics and clinical management of MEN1 and MEN2 in 2015. **Table 2** represents the major NETs of the GEP system and their MEN associations.

Clinically affected MEN1 patients most often present initially with hypercalcemia and elevated parathyroid hormone or a history of parathyroid surgery and evidence of four gland parathyroid hyperplasia. The most common pituitary tumor, when

Table 2
Major neuroendocrine tumors of the GEP system and their associations with multiple endocrine neoplasias

Peptide/Amine	Syndrome/Symptom	Apudoma/NET	MEN1 or MEN2[a]
Gastrin	Zollinger-Ellison diarrhea, atypical GI ulcers	Gastrinoma	1
Insulinoma	Hypoglycemia, symptomatic	Insulinoma	1
VIP	Watery diarrhea syndrome	VIPoma	1 (rare)
Glucagon	Dermatosis, diabetes, thromboembolism	Glucagonoma	1 (rare)
Somatostatin	Diabetes, fat malabsorption, cholelithiasis	Somatostatinoma	1 (rare) 2 (very rare)
Pancreatic polypeptide	Asymptomatic	PP-oma	1
Calcitonin	Asymptomatic/diarrhea, flushing	Medullary thyroid carcinoma	2
Norepinephrine/ epinephrine	Hypertension, tachycardia, pallor	Pheochromocytoma	2
Serotonin, substance P, neurotensin	Flushing, diarrhea, cool perspiration	Carcinoid	1 (lung carcinoid) 2 (ileal carcinoid)

[a] MEN1, autosomal-dominant; gene resides on chromosome 11q13; 610 aa nuclear protein "MENIN" Tumor Suppressor. MEN2, autosomal-dominant, gene on chromosome 10q; a receptor tyrosine kinase protooncogene[6,58].
Modified from O'Dorisio TM, Vinik AI. Pancreatic polypeptide in mixed hormone-producing tumors of the gastrointestinal tract. In Cohen S, Soloway RD (Eds) Contemporary issues in gastroenterology. Edinburgh: Churchill-Livingston 1984;5:117-128; with permission.

present, is a prolactinoma, but can also be a growth hormone– or corticotropin-secreting tumor. The pancreatic NET, when it occurs, is most commonly an insulinoma or gastrinoma, but rare glucagonomas or VIPoma can also be seen in other members of MEN1 kindreds. The pancreatic NETs are most often multiple adenomas, one or two of which may grow while the other adenomas remain stable. Correcting the hypercalcemia when present before working up a functional PNET is recommended. Whereas carcinoid tumor can co-occur in MEN1 and MEN2 syndromes, the pulmonary carcinoid tumor seems more prevalent in MEN1 patients, in our experience.

Regarding MEN2 syndrome, the most frequent component of MEN2 almost always involves medullary thyroid carcinoma (MTC) from the neuroendocrine C-cells (parafollicular cells) of the thyroid gland. MTC is always present in MEN2 and constitutes the primary diagnosis. Parathyroid hyperplasia can also be present in MEN2A but is not as clinically frequent as seen in MEN1 patients. The third gland involved in MEN2 is the adrenal medulla, which gives rise to pheochromocytomas. Patients may present first with symptoms of pheochromocytoma and thereafter an MTC is discovered. Both MTC and pheochromocytoma are often bilateral. MEN2B is much less common (5%) than MEN2A, which accounts for 95% of MEN2 patients. MEN2B is clinically more aggressive, also consists of pheochromocytomas, but does not have parathyroid hyperplasia; it is also associated with a marfanoid body habitus and ganglioneuromas of the GI tract.[58] Carcinoembryonic antigen with serial measurements of calcitonin is helpful in detecting early aggressivity and metastasis of MEN2-associated MTC.

The final portion of this review addresses selected aspects of the various peptide therapies that currently exist in the United States. The following schema represents a partial approach to the various therapeutic modalities (**Fig. 2**).

As noted, the arrows are two-way, and designed to represent that electing one therapy does not eliminate its option at a different phase of treatment. It is important to demonstrate that any of the therapeutic options can be repeated. Most of the listed options are discussed by other authors in this issue. This review briefly addresses surgery/debulking and somatostatin and lanreotide therapy, and discusses the most recent FDA-approved peptide receptor radionuclide therapy (PRRT).

SURGERY/CYTOREDUCTION

It is historically and presently accepted that the first best therapy in the management of NET is surgery, whenever possible. Less well-established is the overall survival (OS) improvement when the primary tumor is removed versus being unable to remove the primary tumor. This is caused, in part, by the reality that all surgical studies of this nature are retrospective and the assignment of patients to no surgery is inherently unethical. That said, there are publications that strongly suggest benefits in progression-free survival (PFS) and OS when the primary tumor and hepatic metastasis debulking is possible.[59–62] At the University of Iowa, our endocrine surgeon (editor of the present monograph) is aggressive in removing primary PNETS and SBNETs, with liver tumor debulking (and liver sparing) when safe surgery and low patient risk are possible[62]

OCTREOTIDE/LANREOTIDE

Octreotide and lanreotide remain as first-line management and therapy for functional and nonfunctional NETs. They are remarkable for their durability over decades and

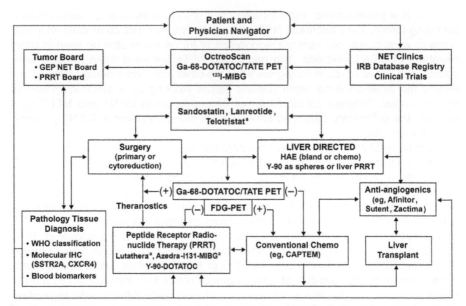

Fig. 2. Carcinoid and neuroendocrine tumors: cancer management and treatment options of care. [a] Most recently FDA approved. FDG, fluorodeoxyglucose; WHO, World Health Organization. (*Courtesy of* Iowa NET Team, Iowa City, IA.)

merit discussion. Octreotide (Sandostatin) and, somewhat later, lanreotide (Somatuline) were both developed as analogues (more properly, congeners) of the active ringed portion of native somatostatin-14.[63–65] Their other natural form is somatostatin-28, representing an extension of somatostatin-14 away from its active eight amino acid ring.[66] As noted from **Fig. 1**, somatostatin has been shown to have all four regulatory functions: (1) endocrine, (2) paracrine, (3) neurocrine, and (4) autocrine.[66] Shortly after its initial discovery and publication in 1973 by Brazeau and colleagues,[35] Sandoz (now Novartis) focused their medicinal chemists to synthesize a longer acting fragment of the eight amino acid ring of the native somatostatin to be used clinically. Almost 9 years later, octreotide (SMS 201-995, Sandostatin) was synthesized by Bauer and colleagues.[63] Shown next in **Fig. 3** is the amino acid structure of Sandostatin-native somatostatin-14 and the eight amino acid synthetic structures of octreotide and lanreotide both containing the D-isomers of the naturally occurring amino acids and the bioactive ringed portion. D-isomers prevent enzyme degradation, as compared with the naturally occurring L-form amino acids in somatostatin-14. Also documented in **Fig. 3** showing the 1 to 14 somatostatin and octreotide and lanreotide is the purported amino acid, lysine, within the ringed portion considered to be the primary peptide binding site of somatostatin, octreotide, and lanreotide to the somatostatin receptor subtype 2 (sstr2A), the most prevalent receptor of the five somatostatin receptor subtypes on neuroendocrine cells and their NETs (see **Fig. 3**).[66]

It is important to appreciate that for 10 years following the discovery of native somatostatin, there was a large number of publications reporting somatostatin's mechanisms of action and regulatory role in mammalian physiology[67–69] and its regulatory role in NETs. Based on the information available on native somatostatin, the widespread clinical use of octreotide and (somewhat later) the use of lanreotide, was a reasonable and rational extension. Both analogues had a much longer plasma

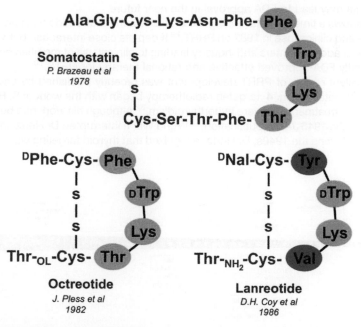

Fig. 3. Somatostatin and its congeners.

half-life than the naturally occurring somatostatin, and a much more potent and durable action on NETs.[70–73] During the late 1980s, while octreotide and lanreotide were being used on a compassionate use basis to treat NETs and growth-hormone-secreting pituitary tumors causing acromegaly, there were efforts to characterize the various receptors on NETs. Reubi and coworkers[74] mapped somatostatin receptor subtypes using autoradiographic techniques that included the use of ^{125}Iodine isotope labeled to the tyrosine substituted for phenylalanine in octreotide at position 3. Patel and Srikant[75] demonstrated peptide analogue subtype selectivity using five clonal human somatostatin subtype receptors (hsstr1-5). During the same year, Bruns and colleagues[76] discussed the molecular pharmacology of somatostatin-receptor subtypes. This was made possible for sstr2A by highly specific IHC with a commercially available polyclonal antibody, UMB-1 (Biotrend, Epitomics, Inc, Cambridge, MA, USA). Characterization of the UMB-1 antibody was published in 2012 by Korner and coworkers.[77] As noted in our therapeutic schema, all patients coming to our NET clinics for the first time will have their tumor tissue stained (when available) for sstr2A. Qian and colleagues[78] published a study examining the presence of somatostatin subtype receptors 1 to 5 and OS and PFS in patients with metastatic NETs. They concluded that patients with NETs that express sstr2A (but not sstr1, sstr3, sstr4, or sstr5) have a longer OS. They determined that tumors with sstr2A IHC that are treated with somatostatin analogues have a longer PFS.[78]

PEPTIDE RECEPTOR RADIONUCLIDE THERAPY AND THERANOSTICS

The remarkably persistent standard of care use of somatostatin analogues, especially octreotide, would almost naturally lead to PRRT of GEP NETs. We discuss the history of theranostics, from the FDA-approved diagnostic ^{68}Ga-DOTATATE PET scan (NETSPOT) and its therapeutic partner, ^{177}Lu-DOTATATE PRRT, and allude to novel tumor targets that may lead to FDA approval in the near future.

Fig. 4 shows a timeline establishing the similar role that octreotide has had since its synthesis and clinical use in 1982 on PRRT.[79] It depicts close interaction between discovery by academic centers and industry leading to clinical use of modified octreotide as a recently FDA-approved effective and rational therapy for NETS.[80]

An excellent review of PRRT development was recently published by Levine and Krenning.[81] Noted in **Fig. 4**, targeted radiotherapy began with the work of S. Hertz using ^{131}Iodine treatment of severe hyperthyroidism.[82] Although his work had been done well before the 1946 *JAMA* publication,[82] World War II interrupted Dr Hertz' investigative efforts. During the 1940s, Dr Hertz recognized that thyroid targeting with ^{131}Iodine

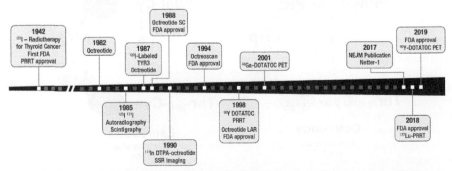

Fig. 4. A timeline of octreotide culminating in development of PRRT and theranostics.

made it possible to successfully treat patients with thyroid cancer. The Society of Nuclear Medicine and Molecular Imaging established a yearly Sol Hertz Award in 2016, recognizing "individuals who have made outstanding contributions to radionuclide therapy."

The first use of the term "peptide receptor" concept probably derives from the work by the Erasmus University group, headed by Krenning[83] and Maecke and colleagues.[84] There are early publications by Krenning and colleagues[83] that not only address the peptide receptor acronym, but also demonstrate proof of concept using ^{111}In-octreotide as an imaging and therapeutic agent given to a single patient. Mueller-Brand with Maecke and their colleagues reported on the "powerful new tool," DOTA-TOC (a chelator attached to [tyr3]-octreotide), for sstr2A in metastatic NET subjects. This was the first use of β emitting energy, [90]Yttrium, coupled with the DOTA chelator.[85]

Krenning and his group at Erasmus pursued diagnostic imaging with [123]Iodine-labeled Tyr3-octreotide achieving successful scintigraphic imaging.[86] By 1990, they had successfully developed [111]Indium-labeled DTPA (chelator) attached to pentetreotide (OctreoScan) and reported their 1000-patient experience in 1993.[87] The Octreoscan was ultimately used for diagnostic entry criteria in the registered NETTER-1 trial for PRRT[4] coupled with therapy using ^{177}Lu-DOTATATE. Since 2001, the improved diagnostic scan for detection of somatostatin receptor positivity was developed using the ^{68}Ga-DOTA-somatostatin analogue, thereby increasing the sensitivity and specificity by using PET instead of single-photon emission computed tomography (SPECT). In 2007, Baum and colleagues published their work on the highly sensitive and specific ^{68}Ga-DOTA-(tyr3)-octreotide (TOC) and DOTA-(tyr3)-octreotide, substituted threonine for threoninolol-octreotide [TATE]) PET imaging.[88] It was, however, the use of the diagnostic OctreoScan with ^{177}Lu-DOTATATE that led to the first FDA-approved, European Medicines Agency–approved radiopharmaceutical for PRRT.[80]

Noted in **Fig. 5**, the term "theranostics" was coined by Rosch and Baum in 2011.[89] The theranostics concept is the use of the identical linker molecule (peptide in this case) with the chelator "cage" for ^{68}Ga for diagnosis, and the ^{177}Lu/^{90}Y for therapy. A good description of PRRT and of theranostics is depicted in **Fig. 5**.[84]

On the top right-hand panel is the DOTA-chelator with its "cage" containing the therapeutic radiometal, 90Y. The top middle panel is the DOTA chelator attached to (tyr3)-octreotide (TOC) and considered to be the vector binding to the tumor's sstr2A. The top left panel is the tumor membrane with the sstr2A dangling externally above the membrane. For a single receptor (sstr2A) binding to a single ligand (tyr3)-octreotide, four properties are necessary[84]: (1) high sstr2A expression on the NET, (2) the native peptide (somatostatin) sequence being known, (3) high affinity/specificity/avidity for the target (sstr2A), and (4) the analogues (vector, ligand) are synthetically feasible (50 amino acid residues or less).

The next major breakthrough in theranostics is likely to be the introduction of new radioisotopes and new targeting agents in addition to DOTATOC and DOTATATE. [177]Lutetium and [90]Yttrium are primarily β emitters with path lengths greater than the average diameter of a single cell, thus generating "cross-fire" effects of cytotoxicity to adjacent cells and normal tissues. α Particle energy emitters, such as [225]Ac (astatine) and [212]Pb (lead) coupled to a high-affinity somatostatin analogue, are likely to deliver a higher energy dose to a single cell with little or no cross-fire when targeted to tumors expressing high levels of sstr2A. Recent *in vitro* experiments in cell lines expressing sstr2 have shown a six-fold increase in radiation dose/cell from [213]Bi-DOTATOC compared with ^{177}Lu-DOTATATE.[90] Importantly, these results substantiate

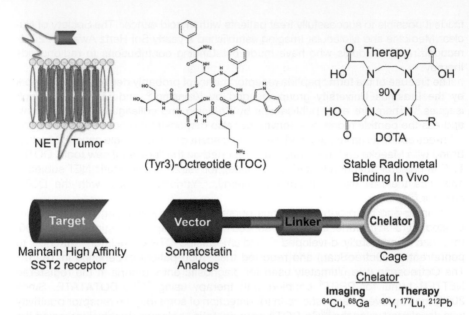

Fig. 5. Targeted molecular imaging and therapy (PRRT) and theranostics concept. Theranostics is the use of diagnostic radionuclides (^{64}Cu, ^{68}Ga, ^{203}Pb) and therapeutic radionuclides (^{90}Y, ^{177}Lu, ^{212}Pb) labeled to the same somatostatin congener (TOC or TATE).[89] (*Courtesy of H. Maecke, University Hospital, Basel, CH.*)

emerging evidence that α emitters may be more effective for PRRT because of preferred dose deposition within the cell nucleus (**Table 3**).[91]

The contribution of internalization to targeting efficiency was then investigated within the geometry of cells by modifying the uptake of α or β emitting radionucleotides from complete membrane bound (0% internalized) to fully internalized (100%). The uptake values arising with 100% internalization were approximately 1.5-fold higher for the entire cell, and 2- to 3-fold higher for the nucleus when compared with binding to the cell membrane. α Emitters deposit significantly higher doses for the tumor metastasis of various sizes relative to β emitters representing 60 to 140 times higher doses for ^{212}Pb and ^{213}Bi, and 190 to 620 times higher doses for ^{225}Ac when compared with the β emitter, ^{177}Lu (Azure). Importantly, these results substantiate emerging evidence that α emitters may be more effective for PRRT because of preferred dose deposition within the cell nucleus.

Most NETs are low grade 1 and 2 with Ki-67 less than 20%. Grade 3 NETS and neuroendocrine carcinomas (NECs) have less response to either ^{177}Lu- or ^{90}Y-

Table 3		
Radionuclides currently in use for theranostics		
Radioisotope (Emission)	**Average Path Length (mm)**	**Mean Particle Energy (MeV)**
^{225}Ac (α)	<0.1	5.59
^{212}Pb (α)	<0.1	6.0–8.8[a]
^{177}Lu (β)	1.7	0.134
^{90}Yt (β)	0.05–12	0.933

[a] ^{212}Pb decays to ^{212}Bi (36%) and ^{212}Po (64%) with respective α energies.

DOTATOC or DOTATATE. These high-grade tumors have a Ki-67 of 55% to 90% and often lack the sstr2A expression, leading investigators to try to identify theranostics targets for grade 3 NETS and NECs. CXCR4 is a chemokine receptor that like sstr2A is a G-protein-coupled receptor expressed on the cell surface and internalized on binding of a high-affinity ligand.[92] We and others have identified CXCR4 expression on NEC, multiple myeloma, and leukemia.[93–97] The ligand for CXCR4 is a small peptide SDF-1, also known as CXCLI2. Pentixafor is a CXCR4 antagonist that can be complexed to the DOTA chelator. ^{68}Ga-Pentixifor and ^{177}Lu-Pentixifor are, thus, a theranostic pair. [177]Lu can be used for SPECT imaging and diagnosis: however, ^{68}Ga-Pentixifor is improved as a PET imaging agent with a sensitivity of 3 to 5 mm as compared with 10 to 15 mm sensitivity for SPECT. ^{177}Lu-Pentixather has shown promise as a radiotherapeutic drug in early studies for patients with multiple myeloma and leukemia,[93] but CXCR4 is expressed on hematopoietic progenitors and stromal cells, leading to concern for bone marrow toxicity. A recent preclinical study has demonstrated that bone marrow from mice treated with ^{177}Lu-Pentixather is able to serve as a graft in lethally irradiated animals, providing support for the use of ^{177}Lu-Pentixather in aggressive malignancies with dosimetry of bone marrow dose to prevent toxicity.[98] Patients with multiple myeloma or leukemia treated with ^{177}Lu-Pentixather routinely receive autologous hematopoietic stem cell rescue.

177Lu-PSMA-617 has primarily been tested in Germany under compassionate use circumstances and relapsed metastatic castrate-resistant prostate cancer and has only recently been introduced into US clinical trials. A retrospective analysis of 145 patients treated in 12 European centers demonstrated greater than 50% decrease in prostate-specific antigen levels in most patients.[99] Hematologic toxicity was low even in these heavily pretreated patients; dry mouth related to high uptake of the ^{177}Lu-PMSA-617 in salivary glands was the primary toxicity along with fatigue and nausea.[100] These preliminary results support the conduct of controlled phase 2 trials that are currently ongoing in Europe and the United States.

Although most theranostic compounds are peptide agonists targeting G-protein-coupled receptors, several antagonist molecules are in preclinical and early clinical use. One example is a peptide ligand, 68Ga-DOTA-bombesin (neoBOMB), targeting the gastrin-releasing peptide receptor known to be expressed in prostate cancer cells.[101] This gastrin-releasing peptide receptor antagonist has shown promising results in animal models and its first PET imaging in humans has been recently reported. Similarly, an antagonist at the somatostatin receptor has been introduced as a theranostic pair in NETs. [68]Ga/^{177}Lu-DOTA-JR-11 seems to bind to many more sites/cells than either DOTATOC or DOTATATE in low-grade NETs. It is in early phase trials with little information on safety or efficacy available at this time.

ACKNOWLEDGMENTS

A special acknowledgment for Ms Sue Kieffer for her careful editorial input and bibliography research and accuracy. As well, the Authors acknowledge the expertise of Graphic Artist, Ms. Teresa Ruggle, for the high quality of the Chapter's Figures.

DISCLOSURES

This Manuscript was supported, in part, by a NCI SPORE Award # NCI P50 CA 174521, P.I. M Sue O'Dorisio. T.M. O'Dorisio is a Co-Investigator and Director of the SPORE CORE Clinical Trials.

REFERENCES

1. Neuroendocrine disorders of the gastroenteropancreatic system. Clinical applications of the somatostatin analogue SMS 201-995 (Octreotide, Sandostatin). April 2-4, 1986, San Diego, California. Am J Med 1986;81(6B):1–101. O'Dorisio TM, eds.
2. Approved drug products with therapeutic equivalence evaluations, 39th edition US Department of Health and Human Services Food and Drug Administration. 2019:vol. 3;326. Available at: https://www.fda.gov/media/71474/download.
3. Bushnell DL Jr, O'Dorisio TM, O'Dorisio MS, et al. 90Y-edotreotide for metastatic carcinoid refractory to octreotide. J Clin Oncol 2010;28(10):1652–9.
4. Strosberg J, El-Haddad G, Wolin E, et al. Phase 3 trial of 177Lu-Dotatate for midgut neuroendocrine tumors. N Engl J Med 2017;376(2):125–35.
5. O'Dorisio TM. Gut endocrinology: clinical and therapeutic impact. Am J Med 1986;81(6B):1–7.
6. Öberg K. The genesis of the neuroendocrine tumors concept: from Oberndorfer to 2018. Endocrinol Metab Clin North Am 2018;47(3):711–31.
7. Bayliss WM, Starling EH. Preliminary communication on the causality of the so called "preferential reflex secretion" of the pancreas. Lancet 1902;1:813–4.
8. Edkins JS. On the chemical mechanism of gastric secretion. Lancet 1905;11:156–7.
9. Gregory RA, Tracy HJ. The preparation and properties of gastrin. J Physiol 1961;156:523–43.
10. Ivy AC, Eldberg E. A hormone mechanism for gallbladder contraction and evaluation. Am J Physiol 1928;86:599–613.
11. Harper AA, Raper HS. Pancreozymin, a stimulant of the secretion of pancreatic enzymes in extracts of the small intestine. J Physiol 1943;102(1):115–25.
12. Banting FG, Best CH. Pancreatic extracts. 1922. J Lab Clin Med 1990;115(2):254–72. PMID:2405086.
13. Forsham PH. Milestones in the 60-year history of insulin (1922-1982). Diabetes Care 1982;5(Suppl 2):1–3.
14. Langerhans P, Moorison H. Contributions to the microscopic anatomy of the pancreas. Baltimore (MD): John Hopkins Press; 1937.
15. Heidenhain, R. Untersuchungen fiber den Bau der Labdriisen Arch. Mikr. Anat. 6:(1870) 368-372.
16. Nikolas A. Recherches sur l'epithelium de l'intestin grele. Intern Monatssch Anat Physiol 1891;8:1–23.
17. Kulchitsky N. Zur Frage uber den Bau des Darmkanals. Arch Mikr Anat 1897;49:7–35.
18. Ciaccio M. Sur une nouvelle espece cellulaire dans les glandes de Lieberkuhn. C R Seances Soc Biol Fil 1906;60:76–7.
19. Gosset A, Masson P. Tumeurs endocrines de l'appendice. Presse Med 1914;25:237–9.
20. Feyter F. Ueber diffuse endokrine epitheaiale organe. Zentralbl Innere Med 1938;545:31–41.
21. Feyter F. Ueber die peripherin endkrinem (Parakrinim) drusen des menschen. Vienna (Austria): W, Maudrich Verlag; 1953.
22. Grossman MI. General concepts. In: Bloom SR, Polak JM, editors. Gut hormones. Edinburgh (Scotland): Churchill-Livingstone; 1981. p. 17–22.
23. Moore B. On the treatment of diabetus mellitus by acid extract of duodenal mucous membrane. Biochem J 1906;1(1):28–38.

24. Rehfeld JF. The origin and understanding of the incretin concept. Front Endocrinol (Lausanne) 2018;9:387.
25. Porath J, Flodin P. A new method for the detection of amino-acids, peptides, proteins and other buffering substances on paper. Nature 1951;168(4266): 202–3.
26. Jorpes JE, Mutt V. The preparation of secretin. Biochem J 1952;52(2):328–30.
27. Jorpes E, Mutt V, Toczko K, et al. Further purification of cholecystokinin and pancreozymin. Acta Chem Scand 1964;18:2408–12.
28. Yalow RS, Berson SA. Assay of plasma insulin in human subjects by immunological methods. Nature 1959;184(Suppl 21):1648–9.
29. Yalow RS, Berson SA. Immunoassay of endogenous plasma insulin in man. J Clin Invest 1960;39:1157–75.
30. McGuigan JE. Antibodies to the carboxyl-terminal tetrapeptide of gastrin. Gastroenterology 1967;53(5):697–705.
31. Bloom SR, Bryant MG, Polak JM. Proceedings: distribution of gut hormones. Gut 1975;16:821.
32. Solica E, Polak JM, Larsson L-I, et al. Update on Lohsane classification of endocrine cells. In: Bloom SR, Polak JM, editors. Gut hormone. 2nd edition. Edinburgh (Scotland): Churchill Livingstone; 1981. p. 96–100.
33. Bloom SR, Polak JM. Glucagonomas, VIPomas and somatostatinomas. Clin Endocrinol Metab 1980;9(2):285–97.
34. Vinik AI, O'Dorisio TM, Woltering E, et al. Neuroendocrine tumors: a comprehensive guide to diagnosis and management. 5th edition. Inglewood, CA: Inter-Science Institute; 2012.
35. Brazeau P, Vale W, Burgus R, et al. Hypothalamic polypeptide that inhibits the secretion of immunoreactive pituitary growth hormone. Science 1973; 179(4068):77–9.
36. Arimura A, Coy DH, Chihara M, et al. Somatostatin. In: Bloom SR, Polak JM, editors. Gut hormone. Edinburgh (Scotland): Churchill Livingstone; 1976. p. 437–41.
37. Oberndorfer S. Karzenoide tumoren des dünndarms. Frankf Z Pathol 1907;1: 426–32.
38. Oberndorfer S. Karzinoide handuch der speziellen. handbuch der speziellen pathologischen anatomie und histologie. Berlin: Springer; 1928. p. 814–47.
39. Ransom W. A case of primary carcinoma of the ileum. Lancet 1890;2:1020–3.
40. Lembeck F. 5-Hydroxytryptamine in carcinoid tumor. Nature 1953;172:910–1.
41. Dasari A, Shen C, Halperin D, et al. Trends in the incidence, prevalence, and survival outcomes in patients with neuroendocrine tumors in the United States. JAMA Oncol 2017;3(10):1335–42.
42. Wilder RM, Allan FN, Power WH, et al. Carcinoma of the islands of the pancreas: hyperinsulinism and hypoglycemia. JAMA 1927;89:348–55.
43. Whipple AO, Frantz VK. Adenoma of islet cells with hyperinsulinism: a review. Ann Surg 1935;101(6):1299–335.
44. Zollinger RM, Ellison EH. Primary peptic ulcerations of the jejunum associated with islet cell tumors of the pancreas. Ann Surg 1955;142(4):709–23.
45. O'Dorisio TM, Mekhjian HS, Ellison EC, et al. Role of peptide radioimmunoassay in understanding peptide-peptide interactions and clinical expression of gastroenteropancreatic endocrine tumors. Am J Med 1987;82(Suppl 5B):60–7.

46. Gregory RA, Grossman MI, Tracy HJ, et al. Nature of the gastric secretagogue in Zollinger-Ellison tumours. Lancet 1967;2(7515):543–4.

47. Verner JV, Morrison AB. Islet cell tumor and a syndrome of refractory watery diarrhea and hypokalemia. Am J Med 1958;25(3):374–80.

48. Said SI, Faloona GR. Elevated plasma and tissue levels of vasoactive intestinal polypeptide in the watery-diarrhea syndrome due to pancreatic, bronchogenic and other tumors. N Engl J Med 1975;293(4):155–60.

49. Gaginella TS, O'Dorisio TM. Vasoactive intestinal polypeptide neuromodulation of intestinal secretion. In: Binder HJ, editor. Mechanism of intestinal secretion. New York: Alan R Liss; 1979. p. 231–47.

50. McGavran MH, Unger RH, Recant L, et al. A glucagon-secreting alpha-cell carcinoma of the pancreas. N Engl J Med 1966;274(25):1408–13.

51. Mallinson CN, Cox B, Bloom SR. Proceedings: plasma levels of amino acids and glucagon in patients with pancreatic glucagonomas. Gut 1974; 15(4):340.

52. Ganda OP, Weir GC, Soeldner JS, et al. "Somatostatinoma": a somatostatin-containing tumor of the endocrine pancreas. N Engl J Med 1977;296(17): 963–7.

53. Vinik I, Strodel WE, O'Dorisio TM. Endocrine tumors of the gastroenteropancreatic (GEP) axis. In: Santern RJ, Manni A, editors. Endocrine related tumors. Boston: Martinus Nijhoff; 1984. p. 305–45.

54. Pearse AG. Common cytochemical properties of cells producing polypeptide hormones, with particular reference to calcitonin and the thyroid C cells. Vet Rec 1966;79(21):587–90.

55. Pearse AG. The APUD concept and hormone production. Clin Endocrinol Metab 1980;9(2):211–22.

56. Schmechel D, Marangos PJ, Brightman M. Neurone-specific enolase is a molecular marker for peripheral and central neuroendocrine cells. Nature 1978; 276(5690):834–6.

57. Andrew A, Kramer B, Rawdon BB. The origin of gut and pancreatic neuroendocrine (APUD) cells: the last word? J Pathol 1998;186:117–8.

58. Norton JA, Krampitz G, Jensen RT. Multiple endocrine neoplasia: genetics and clinical management. Surg Oncol Clin N Am 2015;24(4):795–832.

59. Givi B, Pommier SJ, Thompson AK, et al. Operative resection of primary carcinoid neoplasms in patients with liver metastases yields significantly better survival. Surgery 2006;140(6):891–7.

60. Hill JS, McPhee JT, McDade TP, et al. Pancreatic neuroendocrine tumors: the impact of surgical resection on survival. Cancer 2009;115(4):741–51.

61. Woltering EA, Voros BA, Beyer DT, et al. Aggressive surgical approach to the management of neuroendocrine tumors: a report of 1,000 surgical cytoreductions by a single institution. J Am Coll Surg 2017;224(4):434–47.

62. Scott AT, Breheny PJ, Keck KJ, et al. Effective cytoreduction can be achieved in patients with numerous neuroendocrine tumor liver metastases (NETLMs). Surgery 2019;165:166–77.

63. Bauer W, Briner U, Doepfner W, et al. SMS 201-995: a very potent and selective octapeptide analogue of somatostatin with prolonged action. Life Sci 1982; 31(11):1133–40.

64. Liebow C, Reilly C, Serrano M, et al. Somatostatin analogues inhibit growth of pancreatic cancer by stimulating tyrosine phosphatase. Proc Natl Acad Sci U S A 1989;86(6):2003–7.

65. Rossowski WJ, Coy DH. Specific inhibition of rat pancreatic insulin or glucagon release by receptor-selective somatostatin analogs. Biochem Biophys Res Commun 1994;205(1):341–6.
66. O'Dorisio TM, Redfern S. Somatostatin and somatostatin-like peptides: clinical research and clinical applications. In: Mazzaferro EL, editor. Advances in endocrinology and metabolism, Vol. 1. St Louis (MO): Mobley; 1980. p. 175–230.
67. Reichlin S. Somatostatin. N Engl J Med 1983;309(24):1495–501.
68. Reichlin S. Somatostatin (second of two parts). N Engl J Med 1983;309(25): 1556–63.
69. Yamada RT, Chide T. Somatostatin. In: Malkhlouf GM, Schults SG, editors. Handbook of physiology: section 6: the gastrointestinal system volume ii: neural and endocrine biology. Bethesda (MD): Oxford University Press; 1989. p. 431–53.
70. Lamberts SW, van der Lely AJ, de Herder WW, et al. Octreotide. N Engl J Med 1996;334(4):246–54.
71. Rinke A, Müller HH, Schade-Brittinger C, et al. Placebo-controlled, double-blind, prospective, randomized study on the effect of octreotide LAR in the control of tumor growth in patients with metastatic neuroendocrine midgut tumors: a report from the PROMID Study Group. J Clin Oncol 2009;27(28): 4656–63.
72. Caplin ME, Pavel M, Ćwikła JB, et al. Lanreotide in metastatic enteropancreatic neuroendocrine tumors. N Engl J Med 2014;371(3):224–33.
73. Harris AG, O'Dorisio TM, Woltering EA, et al. Consensus Statement: Octreotide Dose Titration in Secretory Diarrhea. Diarrhea Management Consensus Development Panel. Dig Dis Sci 1995;40(7):1464–73.
74. Reubi JC, Maurer R, von Werder K, et al. Somatostatin receptors in human endocrine tumors. Cancer Res 1987;47(2):551–8.
75. Patel YC, Srikant CB. Subtype selectivity of peptide analogs for all five cloned human somatostatin receptors (hsstr 1-5). Endocrinology 1994;135(6): 2814–7.
76. Bruns C, Weckbecker G, Raulf F, et al. Molecular pharmacology of somatostatin-receptor subtypes. Ann N Y Acad Sci 1994;733:138–46.
77. Körner M, Waser B, Schonbrunn A, et al. Somatostatin receptor subtype 2A immunohistochemistry using a new monoclonal antibody selects tumors suitable for in vivo somatostatin receptor targeting. Am J Surg Pathol 2012;36(2): 242–52.
78. Qian ZR, Li T, Ter-Minassian M, et al. Association between somatostatin receptor expression and clinical outcomes in neuroendocrine tumors. Pancreas 2016; 45(10):1386–93.
79. Harris AG. The clinical development of the somatostatin analogue octreotide. Rotterdam (Netherlands): PhD Thesis, Erasmus University, Department of Internal Medicine; 2003.
80. Hennrich U, Kopka K. Lutathera®: The First FDA- and EMA-approved radiopharmaceutical for peptide receptor radionuclide therapy. Pharmaceuticals (Basel) 2019;12(3) [pii:E114].
81. Levine R, Krenning EP. Clinical history of the theranostic radionuclide approach to neuroendocrine tumors and other types of cancer: historical review based on an interview of Eric P. Krenning by Rachel Levine. J Nucl Med 2017;58(Suppl 2): 3S–9S.

82. Hertz S, Roberts A. Radioactive iodine in the study of thyroid physiology; the use of radioactive iodine therapy in hyperthyroidism. J Am Med Assoc 1946; 131:81–6.

83. Krenning EP, Kooij PP, Bakker WH, et al. Radiotherapy with a radiolabeled somatostatin analogue, [111In-DTPA-D-Phe1]-octreotide. A case history. Ann N Y Acad Sci 1994;733:496–506.

84. Heppeler A, Froidevaux S, Eberle AN, et al. Receptor targeting for tumor localisation and therapy with radiopeptides. Curr Med Chem 2000;7(9): 971–94.

85. Otte A, Jermann E, Behe M, et al. DOTATOC: a powerful new tool for receptor-mediated radionuclide therapy. Eur J Nucl Med 1997;24(7):792–5.

86. Lamberts SW, Bakker WH, Reubi JC, et al. Somatostatin-receptor imaging in the localization of endocrine tumors. N Engl J Med 1990;323(18):1246–9.

87. Krenning EP, Kwekkeboom DJ, Bakker WH, et al. Somatostatin receptor scintigraphy with [111In-DTPA-D-Phe1]- and [123I-Tyr3]-octreotide: the Rotterdam experience with more than 1000 patients. Eur J Nucl Med 1993;20(8): 716–31.

88. Antunes P, Ginj M, Zhang H, et al. Are radiogallium-labelled DOTA-conjugated somatostatin analogues superior to those labelled with other radiometals? Eur J Nucl Med Mol Imaging 2007;34(7):982–93.

89. Rösch F, Baum RP. Generator-based PET radiopharmaceuticals for molecular imaging of tumours: on the way to THERANOSTICS. Dalton Trans 2011; 40(23):6104–11.

90. Chan HS, de Blois E, Morgenstern A, et al. In vitro comparison of 213Bi- and 177Lu-radiation for peptide receptor radionuclide therapy. PLoS One 2017; 12(7):e0181473.

91. Azure MT, Archer RD, Sastry KS, et al. Biological effect of lead 212 localized in the nucleus of mammalian cells: role of recoil energy in the radiotoxicity of internal alpha particle emitters. Radiat Res 1994;140(2):273–83.

92. Scarlett KA, White EZ, Coke CJ, et al. Agonist-induced CXCR4 and CB2 heterodimerization inhibits Galpha13/RhoA-mediated migration. Mol Cancer Res 2018;12:1541–7786.

93. Philipp-Abbrederis K, Herrmann K, Knop S, et al. In vivo molecular imaging of chemokine receptor CXCR4 expression in patients with advanced multiple myeloma. EMBO Mol Med 2015;7(4):477–87.

94. Asfour I, Afify H, Elkourashy S, et al. CXCR4 (CD184) expression on stem cell harvest and CD34(+) cells post-transplant. Hematol Oncol Stem Cell Ther 2017;10(2):63–9.

95. Lapa C, Herrmann K, Schirbel A, et al. CXCR4-directed endoradiotherapy induces high response rates in extramedullary relapsed multiple myeloma. Theranostics 2017;7(6):1589–97.

96. Muhlethaler-Mottet A, Liberman J, Ascencao K, et al. The CXCR4/CXCR7/CXCL12 axis is involved in a secondary but complex control of neuroblastoma metastatic cell homing. PLoS One 2015;10(5):e0125616.

97. Werner RA, Weich A, Higuchi T, et al. Imaging of chemokine receptor 4 expression in neuroendocrine tumors: a triple tracer comparative approach. Theranostics 2017;7(6):1489–98.

98. Habringer S, Lapa C, Herhaus P, et al. Dual targeting of acute leukemia and supporting niche by CXCR4-directed theranostics. Theranostics 2018;8(2): 369–83.

99. Rahbar K, Ahmadzadehfar H, Kratochwil C, et al. German multicenter study investigating 177Lu-PSMA-617 radioligand therapy in advanced prostate cancer patients. J Nucl Med 2017;58(1):85–90.
100. Heck MM, Retz M, Tauber R, et al. PSMA-targeted radioligand therapy in prostate cancer. Urologe A 2017;56(1):32–9 [in German].
101. Nock BA, Kaloudi A, Lymperis E, et al. Theranostic perspectives in prostate cancer with the gastrin-releasing peptide receptor antagonist Neo Bomb1: preclinical and first clinical results. J Nucl Med 2017;58(1):75–80.

Workup of Gastroenteropancreatic Neuroendocrine Tumors

Joseph S. Dillon, MB, BCh, BAO

KEYWORDS

- Gastroenteropancreatic neuroendocrine tumors • Clinical presentation
- Tumor markers • Imaging • Biopsy

KEY POINTS

- Gastroenteropancreatic neuroendocrine tumors may present incidentally, or with features related to the size and site of the primary tumor or metastases, or with symptoms related to the secretions of these tumors.
- All biochemical tumor markers have potential for false-positive and false-negative results.
- Cross-sectional imaging (performed with specific protocols) and functional imaging have complementary roles in the diagnosis and management of Gastroenteropancreatic neuroendocrine tumors.
- Biopsy assessment must fulfill updated (World Health Organization 2017) criteria to optimally guide therapy choices.

INTRODUCTION

The workup of patients with neuroendocrine tumors of the gastrointestinal tract or pancreas (GEPNETs) generally involves initial recognition of the clinical features associated with the tumors, followed by appropriate use of cross-sectional and functional imaging, analysis of appropriate tumor markers, and tissue biopsy. Some patients present incidentally, and workup then involves imaging, biochemical testing and biopsy. This article reviews these aspects of GEPNET management.

CLINICAL PRESENTATION

The presentation of GEPNETs may be incidental or based on symptoms. Symptoms may relate to mass effects, size and site of the primary tumor or metastatic disease, or to hormonal secretions of these tumors. Both hormonal and mass symptoms may differ based on the site of origin of the primary tumor.

Division of Endocrinology, University of Iowa, 200 Hawkins Drive, Iowa City, IA 52242, USA
E-mail address: joseph-dillon@uiowa.edu

Surg Oncol Clin N Am 29 (2020) 165–183
https://doi.org/10.1016/j.soc.2019.10.002
1055-3207/20/© 2019 Elsevier Inc. All rights reserved.

INCIDENTAL PRESENTATION OF NEUROENDOCRINE TUMORS

Screening colonoscopy may commonly reveal incidental findings of small rectal neuroendocrine tumors (NETs)[1] or, very rarely, reveal terminal ileal NETs.[2] Appendicular NETs may be found incidentally in appendicitis specimens (where the small NET lesions at the appendiceal tip may not have played a role in the development of appendicitis[3]). Up to 40% of pancreatic NETs may be noted incidentally.[4] Gastric and duodenal lesions may also be noted incidentally on endoscopy for nonspecific symptoms. Consistent with the increased rate of incidental diagnosis of NETs, the increased incidence of NETs is partially related to sooner diagnosis of early stage lesions.[5,6] The relatively slow growth of these tumors may enhance the likelihood of being diagnosed at some time during another presentation or routine endoscopy.

SYMPTOMATIC PRESENTATION OF NEUROENDOCRINE TUMORS
Presentation Related to Size and Site of Primary or Metastatic Tumors

The specific presentations of NETs are partially dependent on their sites of origin, as follows.

Gastric neuroendocrine tumors
Gastric NETs consist of 3 etiologically distinct groups[7]: type 1 associated with chronic atrophic gastritis, low gastric acid, and high gastrin; type 2 associated with functional gastrinoma, high gastric acid, and gastrin; and type 3 with generally normal gastric acid and gastrin. Of these, type 3 may be associated with mass effect of the primary tumor and lymph nodal or hepatic metastatic disease. Type 1 lesions are generally small and multiple, and these patients present with nonspecific dyspeptic symptoms of chronic atrophic gastritis, frequently in the setting of a personal or family history of other autoimmune disorders, for example, thyroid disease.[8] Type 2 lesions also tend to be small and multiple, with a low propensity for metastatic spread, and present with peptic ulceration or duodenal mass effect of the associated gastrinoma. However, type 3 lesions generally present as larger (>2 cm), higher grade, single lesions with a high metastatic risk. Their presentation may be like gastric adenocarcinoma with abdominal pain, weight loss, and iron deficiency.[9,10] Type 3 gastric NETs may occasionally present with atypical flushing (patchy, cherry red, pruritic, prolonged, with chemosis) associated with histamine release.

Duodenal neuroendocrine tumors
These are generally small unifocal lesions that may metastasize to local nodes. They may be associated with intestinal obstructive features, anemia, jaundice (if close to the ampulla of Vater), or hormonal features of Zollinger-Ellison syndrome (if gastrinoma).[11] Duodenal NETs may also present with features of type 1 neurofibromatosis.[12]

Pancreatic neuroendocrine tumors
These are referred to as either functional PNETs or nonfunctional PNETs. The nonfunctional PNETs (approximately 80% of all PNETs) consist of those that are not associated with the production of any hormonal output, or the production of hormonal output lower than a threshold needed to produce symptoms, or the secretion of substances with no known associated symptoms (eg, chromogranin A [CGA], pancreatic polypeptide). Nonfunctional tumors tend to be bigger than functional tumors on diagnosis.[13] They may present with abdominal pain (from primary or related to bulky nodal or hepatic metastases), early satiety, variceal gastrointestinal (GI) bleeding, or jaundice.[14]

Jejunoileal neuroendocrine tumors
These tumors may present with abdominal pain[15,16] related to the primary tumor, met-astatic nodal, peritoneal or hepatic lesions, or desmoplastic reaction. Pain may relate to acute or recurrent subacute small bowel obstruction. GI bleeding and anemia may occur from ulceration of the primary tumor or varices from venous obstruction owing to mass effect, venous infiltration, or perivascular fibrosis of mesenteric vessels. There may be associated nausea, vomiting, weight loss, and early satiety.

Colorectal neuroendocrine tumors
Seventy percent of rectal NETs are noted incidentally during screening colonoscopies and are localized in more than 80% of cases at diagnosis.[17] Less frequent presenta-tions are with altered bowel habit (13%), rectal bleeding (6%), abdominal or rectal pain (5%). Colonic NETs tend to present later, frequently with bulky metastatic nodal or liver disease, and symptoms of abdominal pain, GI blood loss, or obstruction.[18]

Neuroendocrine tumors of the gastrointestinal tract or pancreas metastases
In tertiary referral centers, up to 77% of pancreatic and 91% of intestinal NETs present with distant metastases.[19] With all GEPNETs, the predominant sites of metastatic dis-ease are liver, local and distant lymph nodes, peritoneum, and mesentery, followed by bone, with lung and brain more rarely involved.[20] Metastatic disease can be symptom-atic by bulky nodal, mesenteric, or liver lesions causing abdominal pain, early satiety, nausea, and weight loss. Nodal or mesenteric lesions, with disease encasing the mesenteric vasculature, may cause intestinal ischemia and postprandial abdominal pain. Hydronephrosis may occur because of retroperitoneal or mesenteric nodal dis-ease, or related desmoplastic reaction, resulting in flank pain, sepsis, and decreased renal function. Either the bulk of liver disease, or adenopathy in the porta hepatis, or adenopathy or mesenteric lesions around the superior mesenteric vein, can be asso-ciated with portal vein or mesenteric vein thrombosis, resulting in hypersplenism, vari-ces, and/or ascites.

Desmoplastic reaction
Jejunoileal NETs are particularly associated with desmoplastic reactions.[21] Evidence of intra-abdominal fibrosis may be noted on cross-sectional imaging in up to 50% of those presenting with small bowel NET.[22] The fibrosis frequently leads to the develop-ment of bowel ischemia, small bowel obstruction, or hydronephrosis.[23] It can be diffi-cult to determine if some of these symptoms are related to bulk of disease or desmoplastic reaction. The etiology of the fibrotic desmoplastic reaction in GEPNETs is still unclear. Although multiple lines of evidence suggest that serotonin causes fibrotic reactions in the right sided heart valves and abdomen, other NET-secreted tachykinins and transforming growth factor-β may also play a role.[24]

Presentation Related to Hormonal Secretion of Primary or Metastatic Tumors

Gastrointestinal neuroendocrine tumors
The presentation of GI-NETs related to their hormonal output depends on the specific hormone(s) that are produced by the tumors and their metastases. The hormones pro-duced vary by site of the primary GI-NET (**Table 1**). For example, gastric NETs can produce histamine from enterochromaffin-like cells and midgut NETs (jejunum to cecum) produce serotonin from enterochromaffin cells, whereas serotonin is not pro-duced by colorectal NETs, which are derived from peptide YY- and enteroglucagon-expressing L cells.

The classical carcinoid syndrome describes a symptom complex that may include flushing (90%), diarrhea (70%), abdominal cramping (40%), valvular heart disease

Table 1		
Hormonal secretions by tissue		
Tissue	Hormones	Symptoms/Syndrome
Gastric	Histamine, CGA	Atypical flush, wheeze, angioedema
Duodenal	CGA, Somatostatin, Gastrin	Cholelithiasis, steatorrhea, diabetes, ZE syndrome (gastrinoma)
Jejunoileal, appendiceal, cecal	Serotonin, CGA, pancreastatin	Carcinoid syndrome
Colorectal	Pancreatic polypeptide	No hormonal symptoms
Pancreatic	See **Table 2**	See **Table 2**

Abbreviation: ZE, Zollinger-Ellison; CGA, Chromogranin A.

(30%), telangiectasia (25%), wheezing (15%), or pellagra (5%).[25] Although many tumor-secreted chemicals may play a role in the symptoms of carcinoid syndrome, serotonin is thought to play a dominant role in the diarrhea and profibrotic effects (cardiac valvular disease and desmoplastic reaction). Histamine, prostaglandins, and substance P may play dominant roles in the carcinoid flushing reaction.[26] Flushing associated with small intestinal NETs is predominantly facial, lasting less than 1 minute, and has a cyanotic hue, whereas that from gastric NETs may be bright red, prolonged, more widely spread, and associated with chemosis and wheeze or other histaminergic features[26] (see **Table 1**).

In a recent analysis of the Surveillance, Epidemiology, and End Results database, features of carcinoid syndrome were recorded most often in patients with small bowel and cecal NETs (32%), appendiceal (17%), colorectal (11%), and lung (8%)[27] disease (patients with PNETs were not analyzed). Carcinoid syndrome data for colorectal tumors may have been overestimated in this study owing to misclassification of cecal tumors, since descending colon and rectal tumors are generally derived from neoplastic L-cells, which do not secrete serotonin, whereas cecal (and small bowel) tumors are derived from serotonin-secreting enterochromaffin cells.

The prevalence of carcinoid syndrome increases with the presence of liver metastatic disease.[27] This is thought to relate to the metabolic degradation of serotonin and other carcinoid syndrome hormonal mediators delivered to the liver via the portal vein, whereas the serotonin generated in liver metastases is delivered into the hepatic veins, entering the systemic circulation without further liver metabolism. Carcinoid syndrome may occasionally occur in individuals without evident liver metastatic disease. This may be due to unrecognized liver metastatic disease[27,28] or to tumor with systemic rather than portal venous drainage (some bulky retroperitoneal or pelvic nodes, peritoneal implants, primary ovarian, or lung NETs).

Pancreatic neuroendocrine tumors

Functional PNETs (approximately 20%[29]) present with characteristic symptoms related to the predominant hormone secreted. The occurrence of carcinoid syndrome in patients with PNETs is unusual (<1%) and relates to the small proportion of patients with PNETs expressing serotonin (8%).[30] Ultra-rare PNETs secreting renin, luteinizing hormone, insulin-like growth factor-2, cholecystokinin, glucagon-like peptide-1 have also been described, some associated with clinical syndromes.[31] Specific hormones secreted by functional PNETs and the characteristic clinical presentation of each are noted in **Table 2**. Nonfunctional PNETs may be associated with elevated serum concentrations of CGA, pancreatic polypeptide, or pancreastatin (see **Table 2**).

Presentation of genetically driven neuroendocrine tumors of the gastrointestinal tract or pancreas

The majority of GEPNETs are sporadic but about 10% to 20% of patients with PNETs harbor genomic mutations, some of which produce well-characterized syndromes. These are generally autosomal dominant in inheritance pattern, although a family history maybe lacking owing to de novo gene mutation, variable penetrance of features, incomplete family history, and other factors. Pancreatic NETs are rarely the first manifestation of any of these syndromes and so other features should be evident on history. The possibility of an associated genetic syndrome should be considered in all patients with PNETs and further genetic testing pursued if there are features suggestive of genetic mutations, because the management of the NET may differ in the context of genetic disorders.[35] **Table 3** lists the specific PNET-associated genetic disorders that need to be considered.

Duodenal NETs may also be associated with multiple endocrine neoplasia, type 1 or neurofibromatosis, type 1. Familial occurrence of small bowel GI-NETs has rarely been described.[36] A genomic mutation in inositol polyphosphate multikinase has been proven in 1 family, whose NETs presented in a manner typical of sporadic GI-NETs

Table 2
Hormonal secretions in functional PNETs

Hormone	Features	% of F-PNET	% Malignant	Additional Notes
Insulin	Recurrent hypoglycemia	40	10	
Glucagon	Diarrhea, glossitis, necrolytic migratory erythema, weight loss, hyperglycemia, blood clots	~5	80	
VIP	Diarrhea, hypokalemia, achlorhydria	<5	80	Also in colon, liver, adrenal tumors
ACTH	Cushingoid facies, weight gain, diabetes, hypertension	<1	>80	Coexisting ZE syndrome 35%, insulinoma 5%
GHRH	Acromegalic features, diabetes	<1	—	Also in lung NETs, 75% have MEN1
PTHRP	Hypercalcemia	<1	—	Also in multiple other cancers
Gastrin	Pain, diarrhea (ZE syndrome)	20	>90	Also in duodenum NETs, 25% have MEN1
Somatostatin	Diabetes, cholelithiasis, steatorrhea, weight loss	<5	75	Also in duodenum, jejunum, 50% have NF1
Serotonin	Flushing, diarrhea (carcinoid syndrome)	<1	>95	8% with elevated urine 5HIAA without syndrome

Abbreviations: 5HIAA, 5-hydroxyindoleacetic acid; ACTH, adrenocorticotrophic hormone; F-PNET, functional pancreatic neuroendocrine tumor; GHRH, growth hormone releasing hormone; MEN1, multiple endocrine neoplasia type 1; NF1, neurofibromatosis type 1; PTHRP, parathyroid hormone-related peptide; VIP, vasoactive intestinal polypeptide; ZE, Zollinger-Ellison.
Data from Refs.[14,30,32–34]

Table 3
PNET-associated genetic disorders

Syndrome	Gene/ Inheritance	Incidence of PNETs	Associated Features	Differences from Incidental
Multiple endocrine neoplasia type 1	MEN1/AD	~60%	Hyperparathyroidism 95%; pituitary adenoma 40%; duodenal NET, adrenal adenoma, lung and thymus NET, lipoma, angiofibroma	Multifocal microadenomas
Von Hippel-Lindau	VHL/AD	~15%	Cranial and retinal hemangioblastoma 70%; renal cell carcinoma 90%; pheochromo cytoma 15%; endolymphatic cell tumor 10%.	
Neurofibromatosis type 1	NF1/AD	<10%	Neurofibroma, optic glioma, café-au-lait spot, Lisch nodule	Somatostatinomas
Tuberous sclerosis	TSC1/AD	Rare	Multiorgan hamartoma, epilepsy, angiofibroma, mental retardation	
Glucagon cell hyperplasia and neoplasia	GCGR/AR	Rare	—	Nesidioblastosis with α cell hyperplasia; high plasma glucagon without diarrhea, rash or diabetes[39]

Abbreviations: AD, autosomal dominant; AR, autosomal recessive; GCGR, glucagon receptor gene; MEN1, multiple endocrine neoplasia type 1; NF1, neurofibromatosis type 1; TSC1, tuberous sclerosis complex subunit 1; VHL, Von Hippel-Lindau.

but with more tumor multifocality.[37] Recently, genomic mutations in MUTYH (encoding a DNA repair enzyme and also associated with familial adenomatosis polyposis) and CHEK2 and BRCA2 (encoding tumor suppressor genes and also associated with breast, ovarian and prostate cancers) were described in some patients with PNETs[38] (see **Table 3**).

THE ROLE OF IMAGING IN WORKUP OF PATIENTS WITH NEUROENDOCRINE TUMORS OF THE GASTROINTESTINAL TRACT OR PANCREAS

For patients with NETs, both cross-sectional (computed tomography [CT] scans, MRI, and ultrasound [US] examination) and functional (⁶⁸gallium-DOTATATE PET scans, Octreoscan, PET with fludeoxyglucose F 18 [¹⁸FDG-PET]) imaging are used to determine that the patient has neuroendocrine cancer, localize the primary tumor, stage the disease, achieve adequate diagnostic biopsy, determine amenability for surgery or other intervention, and follow response to therapy.

Cross-sectional and functional imaging are used in a complementary manner to take advantages of the relative strengths of each modality. The relative role and reported accuracy of different modalities vary significantly based on availability of newer technologies in CT scans and MRI over time, recent availability of ^{68}Ga-DOTATATE PET imaging, and variable local expertise with these modalities and with endoscopic US (EUS) examination.

Functional Imaging

The role of functional imaging is further described elsewhere in this issue. [68]Gallium-DOTATATE PET and Octreoscan functional imaging for GEPNETs are based on the unique feature of high-level somatostatin receptor expression in 85% to 100% of well-differentiated GEPNETs.[40] With the 2016 approval of ^{68}Ga-DOTATATE preparations for use in PET imaging, the ^{68}Ga-DOTATATE PET/CT scan (or MRI) has replaced the Octreoscan as the functional imaging agent of choice for well-differentiated NETs, owing to far higher sensitivity,[41] particularly for lesions less than 2 cm,[42] coupled with ease of use (less radiation exposure and 1- to 2-hour total duration rather than 2 days with Octreoscan). Newer somatostatin receptor-based PET imaging agents are being developed, for example, ^{64}Cu-DOTATATE, which promise to broaden the availability of this imaging technology further. Given its expense, professional societies have developed "appropriate use criteria" for ^{68}Ga-DOTATATE PET imaging. Appropriate indications include localization of the primary tumor, initial staging after histologic diagnosis, preoperative staging, evaluation of masses not amenable to biopsy, evaluation of patients with biochemical evidence, and symptoms of NET without evidence of tumor on conventional imaging or prior biopsy, and others.[43]

Functional Imaging in Patients with Unknown Primary Neuroendocrine Tumors

Approximately 12% of patients with NETs have unknown primary lesions, despite standard cross-sectional imaging and biopsy.[5] Functional imaging with ^{68}Ga-labelled somatostatin analogs and PET/CT scans can improve primary tumor identification for a further 38% to 59% of patients.[44] It is important to be aware of the potential for false-positive localization of ^{68}Ga-DOTATATE in the uncinate process of the pancreas and in areas of inflammation.[45] Intrapancreatic accessory spleen can also be misdiagnosed as a small PNET on both CT and ^{68}Ga-DOTATATE PET scans and may require further nuclear imaging to resolve.[46]

Identifying the primary tumor is important because multiple retrospective studies suggest that resection of the primary NET, along with debulking of lymph nodes and hepatic metastases, may have a survival benefit for patients with NET.[47] Identifying the primary tumor is also important because NETs from different sites vary in their prognosis[5] and their response to therapies.[48] Furthermore, many clinical trials recruit only patients with NETs of specific tissue origin.

PET with Fludeoxyglucose F 18 Imaging for High-Grade and Poorly Differentiated Neuroendocrine Tumors

Expression levels for somatostatin receptors, and thus positivity on ^{68}Ga-DOTATATE imaging, declines with grade 3 and poorly differentiated lesions.[49] However, grade 3 and poorly differentiated GEPNET lesions may be positive on [18]FDG-PET scans in up to 100% of cases. Thus, [18]FDG-PET scanning is helpful in the staging of patents with high-grade tumors and identification of those at risk for more rapid progression.[50]

Neuroendocrine Tumors of the Gastrointestinal Tract or Pancreas Features on Cross-Sectional Imaging

Jejunoileal NETs are generally small (mean, 2 cm; range, 0.4–6.6 cm[51]) and primary tumors are frequently not detected by cross-sectional imaging. Cross-sectional CT scans or MRI may suggest a small bowel localization of a primary tumor by demonstrating the consequences of desmoplastic reaction and mesenteric fibrosis, or by enlargement of lymph nodes (calcified in ≤70%[52]) in characteristic nodal fields along the superior mesenteric artery[53] or by the demonstration of other specific sites of metastatic disease.[54] Oral contrast (eg, water for upper intestinal lesions or dilute barium in sorbitol for distal small bowel lesions, with use of an anticholinergic to inhibit peristalsis) may enhance finding the primary intestinal lesion(s) by producing bowel distension and limiting motion artifact.[55] Other options for identifying small bowel primary lesions include capsule endoscopy, CT enteroclysis, and double balloon enteroscopy,[56] although the role of these investigations is unclear in comparison with careful intraoperative palpation of the complete small bowel.[51] The role of CT scans or MRI in gastric, duodenal, rectal, or colonic NETs is to adequately stage the disease, detecting local and regional adenopathy and distant metastases, and to assess the degree of local invasion and vascular compromise. Direct or EUS-aided visualization by endoscopy is preferred to cross-sectional imaging in diagnosis of primary NETs in these sites.

GEPNETs and their metastases generally enhance (appear hyperintense) during the arterial phase of intravenous contrast infusion on CT scans and MRI, with low intensity on T1 and intermediate to high intensity on T2-weighted noncontrast images on MRI. Hepatic metastases may be isointense on portal venous phase CT imaging, or may present as low attenuation lesions in this phase. Hence, the use of "triple phase" CT imaging, incorporating precontrast, arterial phase, and portal venous phase imaging, can be crucial to diagnosing these lesions.[57] Magnetic resonance, especially using hepatic arterial phase images, fat-suppressed fast spin echo T2-weighted images, diffusion-weighted images, and hepatocyte-specific contrast media (eg, gadoxetic acid), demonstrates significantly more hepatic metastatic lesions than CT imaging,[58] although even these protocols miss abundant micrometastases.[59] Magnetic resonance cholangiopancreatography imaging sequences can define specific obstruction and infiltration around the biliary and pancreatic ducts, although the better spatial resolution of CT scans can also provide clear preoperative information on pancreatic and bile ducts patency and vascular encasement.

Endoscopic Ultrasound Examination

Although transabdominal US examination has a relatively limited diagnostic imaging role besides facilitating accurate tissue biopsy, EUS examination has an important role in the imaging and biopsy of pancreatic NETs and in the imaging of gastroduodenal and rectal lesions and local nodal screening. EUS examination in rectal and gastric lesions can define the depth of invasion and clarify the appropriate treatment strategy (endoscopic submucosal resection vs surgical resection). It offers the highest available imaging sensitivity for pancreatic NETs, although the delineation and biopsy of pancreatic tail lesions may be less accurate. However, EUS is highly operator dependent and technically challenging.

Finally, patients with serotonin secreting NETs or elevated N-terminal pro-B-type natriuretic peptides should have transthoracic echocardiography to evaluate for carcinoid valve disease.[60] Specific details of available imaging modalities for GEPNETs are noted in **Tables 4** and **5**.

Table 4
Imaging modalities available for GEPNETs

Modality	Advantages	Disadvantages	Indications	Sensitivity (%)	Specificity (%)
CT abdomen and pelvis (triple phase)	Cost, wide availability, fast imaging, good spatial resolution, good liver views (triphasic)	Misses smaller or isodense liver lesions, or small nodes and bone lesions	Initial diagnosis/ staging, biopsy, preoperative planning	82	86
MRI with or without contrast; hepatocyte-specific contrast (eg, gadoxetate)	Best for liver, pancreas, bone, brain; better differentiation of normal vs tumor; no radiation (preferred for MEN1 screening)	Longer scan times – movement artifact in bowel/abdominal nodes, claustrophobia; less spatial resolution; cost (MRI > CT)	Initial diagnosis/ staging, preoperative planning	79 (PNETs) 75 (liver metastases)	100 (PNETs) 98 (liver metastases)
68Ga-DOTATATE PET	Visualizes small primary GI-NETs, lesions in bone, small nodes and peritoneum, missed on CT or MRI	Cost (PET >> MRI > CT); availability; SSTR2 negative lesions	Grade 1, 2, WD grade 3; specific indications[43]	92 (All NETs) 52 (primary unknown)	88 (all NETs)
18FDG-PET	Visualizes higher grade 2/grade 3, and PDNET	Cost, generally negative or poor uptake in WDNET	Grade 3, PDNET	52% (grade 1, grade 2 GEPNETs) 100% (PDNET)[61]	—

(continued on next page)

Table 4
(continued)

Modality	Advantages	Disadvantages	Indications	Sensitivity (%)	Specificity (%)
EGD, colonoscopy, and EUS examination	Direct visualization and biopsy of gastric, duodenal, colorectal, some terminal ileal NETs, visualization of strictures, bleeding sites, wall thickness, adjacent nodes; high definition pancreas evaluation and biopsy	Operator dependent, EUS expertise limited, difficulty with NET detection in tail of pancreas	Imaging and guided biopsy in stomach, duodenum, pancreas, colorectal (incidental findings in terminal ileum)	EUS examination 86 (PNETs)	EUS examination 92 (PNETs)
Transabdominal US examination	Availability	Operator dependent, poor imaging quality	Guided biopsy	88 (liver metastases) 39 (PNET detection rate)	95 (liver metastases)

Abbreviations: EGD, esophagogastroduodenoscopy; PD, poorly differentiated; SSTR2, somatostatin receptor 2; WD, well-differentiated.
Data from Sundin A, Arnold R, Baudin E, et al. ENETS Consensus Guidelines for the Standards of Care in Neuroendocrine Tumors: Radiological, Nuclear Medicine & Hybrid Imaging. Neuroendocrinology. 2017;105(3):212-244.

Table 5 Indicated imaging by disease site	
NET Location	Recommended Imaging
Gastric types 1, 2, 3	Recommend EGD in types 1–3; consider EUS (for infiltration, nodal assessment); CT scan or MRI staging with type 3; consider ^{68}Ga-DOTATATE PET for types 2 and 3
Duodenal	Recommend EGD; consider EUS (for infiltration, nodal assessment); recommend CT scan or MRI abdomen for staging; consider ^{68}Ga-DOTATATE PET
Jejunoileal, appendix, cecum	Recommend CT scan or MRI abdomen/pelvis; consider specific enterography or enteroscopy protocols for jejunoileal or colonoscopy for cecal; recommend ^{68}Ga-DOTATATE PET for staging; consider echocardiogram
Distal colorectal	Recommend CT scan or MRI abdomen/pelvis; recommend colonoscopy; consider EUS examination for rectal lesions; recommend ^{68}Ga-DOTATATE PET
Pancreatic	Recommend CT scan or MRI for staging; consider EGD/EUS for staging/biopsy; recommend ^{68}Ga-DOTATATE PET for staging
Poorly differentiated neuroendocrine carcinoma	Recommend CT scan of the chest/abdomen/pelvis; consider ^{18}FDG-PET, ^{68}Ga-DOTATATE PET, nuclear bone scan

Abbreviation: EGD, esophagogastroduodenoscopy.
Data from Kunz PL, Reidy-Lagunes D, Anthony LB, et al. Consensus guidelines for the management and treatment of neuroendocrine tumors. Pancreas. 2013;42(4):557-577.

THE ROLE OF BIOCHEMICAL MARKERS IN WORKUP OF PATIENTS WITH NEUROENDOCRINE TUMORS OF THE GASTROINTESTINAL TRACT OR PANCREAS

Because GEPNETs arise from secretory cells of the GI tract and pancreas, it is not surprising that multiple (>20) proteins, peptides, and amines have been documented as secretory products of these tumors.[62] Measurement of these chemicals in blood or urine has been used extensively as an aid to diagnosis and monitoring of patients with GEPNETs. Some of the chemicals secreted result in evident symptoms (eg, serotonin-induced diarrhea, or insulin-induced hypoglycemia), whereas others are not associated with evident symptomatic effects (eg, CGA). A minority of GEP patients with NET have "functional tumors," with 19% of newly diagnosed patients with GI-NETs presenting with carcinoid syndrome[27] and 27% of patients with PNETs presenting with hormonal syndromes.[15] There are commercially available assays for a subset of these secreted products. Some biochemical markers have also been suggested to have prognostic implications, for example, neurokinin A[63] or pancreastatin,[64] although such claims have not yet been sanctioned by consensus panels.[65]

The appropriate role of biochemical markers in diagnostic testing remains somewhat controversial because of poor sensitivity for early disease, and multiple influences on specificity. The hepatic clearance of serotonin can be up to 80%[66] and thus blood serotonin or its excreted breakdown product, urine 5-hydroxyindoleacetic acid, may not be abnormal until GEPNETs are associated with (serotonin-secreting) hepatic metastases. Additionally, the commonly used CGA is elevated by proton pump inhibitors, chronic atrophic gastritis, and renal dysfunction, among many other conditions.[67] CGA decreases with a half-life of 5 days on withdrawal of proton pump inhibitors.[68] All current biochemical markers have issues affecting their sensitivity or specificity, including medications, diet, fasting state, technique of phlebotomy, handling of the sample, and a lack of standardization between laboratories.[69] Results of these tests must to be considered in the context of these confounding factors.

Additionally, it is clear that there are cases of functional NETs where the secreted substance(s) causing the syndrome are not assayed in standard, regularly performed, assays. One-quarter of patients diagnosed with carcinoid syndrome diarrhea have normal 24-hour urinary 5-hydroxyindoleacetic acid.[70] Serotonin accounts for only 50% of the prodiarrheal activity in small intestinal NETs[71] and plays little role in flushing. Tachykinins, a family of peptides secreted by small intestinal NETs, can cause both flushing and diarrhea, but are not routinely assayed.[72]

Professional society recommendations for use of tumor markers in GEPNETs are noted in **Table 6**. In general, laboratory evaluation of functional pancreatic tumors is guided by the specific syndrome exhibited (eg, insulin and glucose testing for hypoglycemia with suspected insulinoma), and CGA and pancreatic polypeptide are considered in nonfunctional tumors. In jejunoileal, appendicular and cecal NETs (all derived from transformed enterochromaffin cells), CGA and some assay of serotonin concentration are suggested (serum or blood serotonin, plasma or 24-hour urine 5-hydroxyindoleacetic acid[79]), with consideration of testing pancreastatin if there are factors present that influence the level of CGA (proton pump inhibitor use, decreased renal function, etc). Although professional societies have not endorsed other biochemical testing, studies support consideration of pancreastatin and neurokinin A as prognostic markers in jejunoileal NETs.[80,81]

To improve the clinical usefulness of tumor markers, there has been significant interest in the use of multianalyte marker testing related to miRNA profiling, isolation of circulating tumor cells, and analysis of circulating gene transcripts overexpressed in NETs. The only commercially available multianalyte test is the NETest. This test involves quantitative reverse-transcription and polymerase chain reaction amplification of 51 genes whose expression is enhanced in NETs. Early data suggest high sensitivity (>95%) and specificity (>95%) in the detection of all GEPNETs.[82] There are no evident confounders for the NETest of the type that interfere with biochemical markers. The NETest has not yet been recommended by professional organizations (see **Table 6**).

THE ROLE OF BIOPSY IN WORKUP OF PATIENTS WITH NEUROENDOCRINE TUMORS OF THE GASTROINTESTINAL TRACT OR PANCREAS

An adequate biopsy and pathologic examination by an expert pathologist are crucial in the workup of patients with GEPNETs. Biopsies may be percutaneous (US examination, CT scan, or MRI guided), endoscopic, or by EUS examination. Minimum requirements for pathologic reports have been published[83,84] and reports should conform to the most recent World Health Organization classification.[85] In general, core biopsies are preferred to cytology,[86] to allow for a full diagnostic assessment. However, cytology is frequently sufficient for preoperative diagnosis of PNETs and discrimination of poorly differentiated grade 3 from well-differentiated grade 1 or 2 morphology.[31,83] The diagnostic accuracy of pancreatic fine needle aspiration cytology is 97% and the concordance rate for grade assessment, between Ki67 on fine needle aspiration versus postoperative histology, is 83%.[87]

The pathologic assessment includes conventional histology of hematoxylin and eosin–stained slides to establish that the morphology is consistent with the diagnosis of NET and to review the differentiation state, an important component of grading. These studies may also reveal evidence of mixed neuroendocrine carcinoma, where

Table 6
Recommendations for use of biomarkers in diagnosis and management of NETs

Society/ Organization	NET Type				
	Colo-Rectal	Jejunoileal, Appendiceal, Cecal	Gastroduodenal	Pancreatic	High-Grade GEPNEC
NANETS[73-75]	CGA (Rec), U5HIAA (Cons)	CGA, U5HIAA (Rec)	Gastrin (Rec), U5HIAA, CGA (Cons)	CGA (Rec), U5HIAA, gastrin, glucagon, insulin proinsulin, VIP, PP, PTHRP, GHRH, ACTH, (others as clinically indicated)	No Rec
ENETS[10,16,18,31,76,77]	CGA (Rec)	Appendix: CGA (Rec), U5HIAA (Cons) J-I: CGA, U5HIAA (Rec)	Gastric type 1, 2: Gastrin, CGA (Rec) Gastric type 3: CGA (Rec) Duodenal: CGA (Rec) Others as indicated clinically or genetically	NF-PNET: CGA (Rec) F-PNET: based on specific symptoms	CGA, NSE (Cons)
NCCN[78]	CGA, urine or plasma 5HIAA[a]			CGA, PP (others as clinically indicated)[a]	

Abbreviations: ACTH, adrenocorticotrophic hormone; Cons, consider; ENETS, European Neuroendocrine Tumor Society; F-PNET, functional PNET; GEPNEC, gastro-enteropancreatic neuroendocrine carcinoma; GHRH, growth hormone-releasing hormone; J-I, jejunoileal; NANETS, North American Neuroendocrine Tumor Society; NCCN, National Comprehensive Cancer Network; NF-PNET, nonfunctional PNET; NSE, neuron-specific enolase; PP, pancreatic polypeptide; PTHRP, parathyroid hormone-related peptide; Rec, recommend; U5HIAA, 24-hour urine 5-hydroxyindoleacetic acid; VIP, vasoactive intestinal polypeptide.
[a] All NCCN recommendations are category 3 ("Based upon any level of evidence, there is major NCCN disagreement that the intervention is appropriate").

more than 30% of cells are of nonendocrine origin. For gastric carcinoids, biopsy of fundic mucosa and assessment for chronic atrophic gastritis is appropriate.

The tumor grade (which influences therapy options, because chemotherapy is preferred over other options for metastatic high-grade lesions) is established from immunohistochemical studies using the MIB-1 antibody to label Ki67, a cellular proliferation-related protein, to determine the Ki67 proliferation index, and (optionally) counting the number of mitotic cells per 10 high-power fields or 2 mm^2 on hematoxylin and eosin–stained slides. Tumor grade may increase between primary and metastatic lesions,[88] and thus biopsy of a metastatic lesion may be preferred to initially guide therapy options.

A panel of immunohistochemical studies establish the tumor as a NET. These must include CGA and synaptophysin to confirm that the biopsied lesion is a NET. Other markers may also be considered, for example, cytokeratin to differentiate GEPNETs from pheochromocytoma or paraganglioma NETs.[73,83]

The site of origin of the tumor (if biopsy is from a metastatic lesion) is an important influence on the surgical approach. Specific immunohistochemical markers (eg, CDX2 (prominent in small bowel), and PAX6 or ISL1 [prominent in pancreas]) may help to differentiate the cell of origin for metastases from an unknown primary. Further immunohistochemistry can be performed to confirm the specific hormones secreted by the tumor.[19] These studies are generally not necessary because functional tumors are defined by the associated clinical syndrome and blood biochemistry.[89] However, these studies may be of use in some patients, for example, with multiple endocrine neoplasia type 1, where most gastrinomas arise from the duodenum and any accompanying PNETs are either nonfunctional or are secreting hormones other than gastrin.[89]

SUMMARY

Understanding the unique clinical, laboratory, imaging, and pathology features of GEPNETs is important in the preoperative evaluation of these rare tumors.

DISCLOSURE

This work was supported by National Cancer Institute SPORE Grant P50 CA174521-01.

REFERENCES

1. Yoon SN, Yu CS, Shin US, et al. Clinicopathological characteristics of rectal carcinoids. Int J Colorectal Dis 2010;25(9):1087–92.

2. Ten Cate EM, Wong LA, Groff WL, et al. Post-surgical surveillance of locally advanced ileal carcinoids found by routine ileal intubation during screening colonoscopy: a case series. J Med Case Rep 2014;8:444.

3. Njere I, Smith LL, Thurairasa D, et al. Systematic review and meta-analysis of appendiceal carcinoid tumors in children. Pediatr Blood Cancer 2018;65(8):e27069.

4. Gallotti A, Johnston RP, Bonaffini PA, et al. Incidental neuroendocrine tumors of the pancreas: MDCT findings and features of malignancy. AJR Am J Roentgenol 2013;200(2):355–62.

5. Dasari A, Shen C, Halperin D, et al. Trends in the incidence, prevalence, and survival outcomes in patients with neuroendocrine tumors in the United States. JAMA Oncol 2017;3(10):1335–42.

6. Sackstein PE, O'Neil DS, Neugut AI, et al. Epidemiologic trends in neuroendocrine tumors: an examination of incidence rates and survival of specific patient subgroups over the past 20 years. Semin Oncol 2018;45(4):249–58.

7. Delle Fave G, O'Toole D, Sundin A, et al. ENETS consensus guidelines update for gastroduodenal neuroendocrine neoplasms. Neuroendocrinology 2016;103(2): 119–24.

8. Castoro C, Le Moli R, Arpi ML, et al. Association of autoimmune thyroid diseases, chronic atrophic gastritis and gastric carcinoid: experience from a single institution. J Endocrinol Invest 2016;39(7):779–84.

9. Rindi G, Bordi C, Rappel S, et al. Gastric carcinoids and neuroendocrine carcinomas: pathogenesis, pathology, and behavior. World J Surg 1996;20(2):168–72.

10. Delle Fave G, Kwekkeboom DJ, Van Cutsem E, et al. ENETS Consensus Guidelines for the management of patients with gastroduodenal neoplasms. Neuroendocrinology 2012;95(2):74–87.

11. Rossi RE, Rausa E, Cavalcoli F, et al. Duodenal neuroendocrine neoplasms: a still poorly recognized clinical entity. Scand J Gastroenterol 2018;53(7):835–42.

12. Witzigmann H, Loracher C, Geissler F, et al. Neuroendocrine tumours of the duodenum. Clinical aspects, pathomorphology and therapy. Langenbecks Arch Surg 2002;386(7):525–33.

13. Zhu LM, Tang L, Qiao XW, et al. Differences and similarities in the clinicopathological features of pancreatic neuroendocrine tumors in china and the united states: a multicenter study. Medicine 2016;95(7):e2836.

14. Guilmette JM, Nose V. Neoplasms of the neuroendocrine pancreas: an update in the classification, definition, and molecular genetic advances. Adv Anat Pathol 2019;26(1):13–30.

15. Dahdaleh FS, Calva-Cerqueira D, Carr JC, et al. Comparison of clinicopathologic factors in 122 patients with resected pancreatic and ileal neuroendocrine tumors from a single institution. Ann Surg Oncol 2012;19(3):966–72.

16. Pape UF, Perren A, Niederle B, et al. ENETS Consensus Guidelines for the management of patients with neuroendocrine neoplasms from the jejuno-ileum and the appendix including goblet cell carcinomas. Neuroendocrinology 2012; 95(2):135–56.

17. Weinstock B, Ward SC, Harpaz N, et al. Clinical and prognostic features of rectal neuroendocrine tumors. Neuroendocrinology 2013;98(3):180–7.

18. Caplin M, Sundin A, Nillson O, et al. ENETS Consensus Guidelines for the management of patients with digestive neuroendocrine neoplasms: colorectal neuroendocrine neoplasms. Neuroendocrinology 2012;95(2):88–97.

19. Pavel M, Baudin E, Couvelard A, et al. ENETS Consensus Guidelines for the management of patients with liver and other distant metastases from neuroendocrine neoplasms of foregut, midgut, hindgut, and unknown primary. Neuroendocrinology 2012;95(2):157–76.

20. Riihimaki M, Hemminki A, Sundquist K, et al. The epidemiology of metastases in neuroendocrine tumors. Int J Cancer 2016;139(12):2679–86.

21. Daskalakis K, Karakatsanis A, Stalberg P, et al. Clinical signs of fibrosis in small intestinal neuroendocrine tumours. Br J Surg 2017;104(1):69–75.

22. Druce MR, Bharwani N, Akker SA, et al. Intra-abdominal fibrosis in a recent cohort of patients with neuroendocrine ('carcinoid') tumours of the small bowel. QJM 2010;103(3):177–85.

23. Modlin IM, Shapiro MD, Kidd M. Carcinoid tumors and fibrosis: an association with no explanation. Am J Gastroenterol 2004;99(12):2466–78.

24. Druce M, Rockall A, Grossman AB. Fibrosis and carcinoid syndrome: from causation to future therapy. Nat Rev Endocrinol 2009;5(5):276–83.
25. Caplin ME, Buscombe JR, Hilson AJ, et al. Carcinoid tumour. Lancet 1998; 352(9130):799–805.
26. Hannah-Shmouni F, Stratakis CA, Koch CA. Flushing in (neuro)endocrinology. Rev Endocr Metab Disord 2016;17(3):373–80.
27. Halperin DM, Shen C, Dasari A, et al. Frequency of carcinoid syndrome at neuroendocrine tumour diagnosis: a population-based study. Lancet Oncol 2017; 18(4):525–34.
28. Elias D, Lefevre JH, Duvillard P, et al. Hepatic metastases from neuroendocrine tumors with a "thin slice" pathological examination: they are many more than you think. Ann Surg 2010;251(2):307–10.
29. Fischer L, Kleeff J, Esposito I, et al. Clinical outcome and long-term survival in 118 consecutive patients with neuroendocrine tumours of the pancreas. Br J Surg 2008;95(5):627–35.
30. Zandee WT, van Adrichem RC, Kamp K, et al. Incidence and prognostic value of serotonin secretion in pancreatic neuroendocrine tumours. Clin Endocrinol 2017; 87(2):165–70.
31. Falconi M, Eriksson B, Kaltsas G, et al. ENETS Consensus Guidelines Update for the Management of Patients with Functional Pancreatic Neuroendocrine Tumors and Non-Functional Pancreatic Neuroendocrine Tumors. Neuroendocrinology 2016;103(2):153–71.
32. Borson-Chazot F, Garby L, Raverot G, et al. Acromegaly induced by ectopic secretion of GHRH: a review 30 years after GHRH discovery. Ann Endocrinol (Paris) 2012;73(6):497–502.
33. Maragliano R, Vanoli A, Albarello L, et al. ACTH-secreting pancreatic neoplasms associated with Cushing syndrome: clinicopathologic study of 11 cases and review of the literature. Am J Surg Pathol 2015;39(3):374–82.
34. Luna IE, Monrad N, Binderup T, et al. Somatostatin-immunoreactive pancreaticoduodenal neuroendocrine neoplasms: twenty-three cases evaluated according to the WHO 2010 classification. Neuroendocrinology 2016;103(5):567–77.
35. Falconi M, Bartsch DK, Eriksson B, et al. ENETS Consensus Guidelines for the management of patients with digestive neuroendocrine neoplasms of the digestive system: well-differentiated pancreatic non-functioning tumors. Neuroendocrinology 2012;95(2):120–34.
36. Jarhult J, Landerholm K, Falkmer S, et al. First report on metastasizing small bowel carcinoids in first-degree relatives in three generations. Neuroendocrinology 2010;91(4):318–23.
37. Sei Y, Zhao X, Forbes J, et al. A Hereditary Form of Small Intestinal Carcinoid Associated With a Germline Mutation in Inositol Polyphosphate Multikinase. Gastroenterology 2015;149(1):67–78.
38. Scarpa A, Chang DK, Nones K, et al. Whole-genome landscape of pancreatic neuroendocrine tumours. Nature 2017;543(7643):65–71.
39. Yu R, Nissen NN, Dhall D, et al. Nesidioblastosis and hyperplasia of alpha cells, microglucagonoma, and nonfunctioning islet cell tumor of the pancreas: review of the literature. Pancreas 2008;36(4):428–31.
40. Reubi JC. Somatostatin and other Peptide receptors as tools for tumor diagnosis and treatment. Neuroendocrinology 2004;80(Suppl 1):51–6.
41. Van Binnebeek S, Vanbilloen B, Baete K, et al. Comparison of diagnostic accuracy of (111)In-pentetreotide SPECT and (68)Ga-DOTATOC PET/CT: a

lesion-by-lesion analysis in patients with metastatic neuroendocrine tumours. Eur Radiol 2016;26(3):900–9.

42. Hope TA, Calais J, Zhang L, et al. (111)In-pentetreotide scintigraphy vs. (68)Ga-DOTATATE PET: impact on Krenning scores and effect of tumor burden. J Nucl Med 2019;60(9):1266–9.

43. Hope TA, Bergsland EK, Bozkurt MF, et al. Appropriate use criteria for somatostatin receptor PET imaging in neuroendocrine tumors. J Nucl Med 2018;59(1):66–74.

44. Menda Y, O'Dorisio TM, Howe JR, et al. Localization of unknown primary site with (68)Ga-DOTATOC PET/CT in patients with metastatic neuroendocrine tumor. J Nucl Med 2017;58(7):1054–7.

45. Hofman MS, Lau WF, Hicks RJ. Somatostatin receptor imaging with 68Ga DOTATATE PET/CT: clinical utility, normal patterns, pearls, and pitfalls in interpretation. Radiographics 2015;35(2):500–16.

46. Collarino A, del Ciello A, Perotti G, et al. Intrapancreatic accessory spleen detected by 68Ga DOTANOC PET/CT and 99mTc-colloid SPECT/CT scintigraphy. Clin Nucl Med 2015;40(5):415–8.

47. Howe JR, Cardona K, Fraker DL, et al. The surgical management of small bowel neuroendocrine tumors: consensus guidelines of the North American Neuroendocrine Tumor Society. Pancreas 2017;46(6):715–31.

48. Chatzellis E, Angelousi A, Daskalakis K, et al. Activity and safety of standard and prolonged capecitabine/temozolomide administration in patients with advanced neuroendocrine neoplasms. Neuroendocrinology 2019;109(4):333–45 [Epub ahead of print].

49. Hankus J, Tomaszewska R. Neuroendocrine neoplasms and somatostatin receptor subtypes expression. Nucl Med Rev Cent East Eur 2016;19(2):111–7.

50. Howe JR. The supporting role of (18)FDG-PET in patients with neuroendocrine tumors. Ann Surg Oncol 2015;22(7):2107–9.

51. Keck KJ, Maxwell JE, Utria AF, et al. The distal predilection of small bowel neuroendocrine tumors. Ann Surg Oncol 2018;25(11):3207–13.

52. Pantongrag-Brown L, Buetow PC, Carr NJ, et al. Calcification and fibrosis in mesenteric carcinoid tumor: CT findings and pathologic correlation. AJR Am J Roentgenol 1995;164(2):387–91.

53. Lardiere-Deguelte S, de Mestier L, Appere F, et al. Toward a preoperative classification of lymph node metastases in patients with small intestinal neuroendocrine tumors in the era of intestinal-sparing surgery. Neuroendocrinology 2016;103(5):552–9.

54. Bhosale P, Shah A, Wei W, et al. Carcinoid tumours: predicting the location of the primary neoplasm based on the sites of metastases. Eur Radiol 2013;23(2):400–7.

55. Anzidei M, Napoli A, Zini C, et al. Malignant tumours of the small intestine: a review of histopathology, multidetector CT and MRI aspects. Br J Radiol 2011;84(1004):677–90.

56. Gangi A, Siegel E, Barmparas G, et al. Multifocality in small bowel neuroendocrine tumors. J Gastrointest Surg 2018;22(2):303–9.

57. Sundin A, Arnold R, Baudin E, et al. ENETS consensus guidelines for the standards of care in neuroendocrine tumors: radiological, nuclear medicine & hybrid imaging. Neuroendocrinology 2017;105(3):212–44.

58. Ronot M, Clift AK, Baum RP, et al. Morphological and functional imaging for detecting and assessing the resectability of neuroendocrine liver metastases. Neuroendocrinology 2018;106(1):74–88.

59. Gibson WE, Gonzalez RS, Cates JMM, et al. Hepatic micrometastases are associated with poor prognosis in patients with liver metastases from neuroendocrine tumors of the digestive tract. Hum Pathol 2018;79:109–15.
60. Davar J, Connolly HM, Caplin ME, et al. Diagnosing and managing carcinoid heart disease in patients with neuroendocrine tumors: an expert statement. J Am Coll Cardiol 2017;69(10):1288–304.
61. Zhang P, Yu J, Li J, et al. Clinical and prognostic value of PET/CT imaging with combination of (68)Ga-DOTATATE and (18)F-FDG in gastroenteropancreatic neuroendocrine neoplasms. Contrast Media Mol Imaging 2018;2018:2340389.
62. Vinik AI, Silva MP, Woltering EA, et al. Biochemical testing for neuroendocrine tumors. Pancreas 2009;38(8):876–89.
63. Woltering EA, Voros BA, Thiagarajan R, et al. Plasma neurokinin a levels predict survival in well-differentiated neuroendocrine tumors of the small bowel. Pancreas 2018;47(7):843–8.
64. Woltering EA, Voros BA, Beyer DT, et al. Plasma pancreastatin predicts the outcome of surgical cytoreduction in neuroendocrine tumors of the small bowel. Pancreas 2019;48(3):356–62.
65. Oberg K, Couvelard A, Delle Fave G, et al. ENETS consensus guidelines for standard of care in neuroendocrine tumours: biochemical markers. Neuroendocrinology 2017;105(3):201–11.
66. Kema IP, de Vries EG, Muskiet FA. Clinical chemistry of serotonin and metabolites. J Chromatogr B Biomed Sci Appl 2000;747(1–2):33–48.
67. Modlin IM, Gustafsson BI, Moss SF, et al. Chromogranin A–biological function and clinical utility in neuro endocrine tumor disease. Ann Surg Oncol 2010; 17(9):2427–43.
68. Mosli HH, Dennis A, Kocha W, et al. Effect of short-term proton pump inhibitor treatment and its discontinuation on chromogranin A in healthy subjects. J Clin Endocrinol Metab 2012;97(9):E1731–5.
69. Aluri V, Dillon JS. Biochemical testing in neuroendocrine tumors. Endocrinol Metab Clin North Am 2017;46(3):669–77.
70. Kulke MH, Horsch D, Caplin ME, et al. Telotristat ethyl, a tryptophan hydroxylase inhibitor for the treatment of carcinoid syndrome. J Clin Oncol 2017;35(1):14–23.
71. Lembeck F. 5-Hydroxytryptamine in a carcinoid tumour. Nature 1953; 172(November 14):910–1.
72. Cunningham JL, Janson ET, Agarwal S, et al. Tachykinins in endocrine tumors and the carcinoid syndrome. Eur J Endocrinol 2008;159(3):275–82.
73. Kunz PL, Reidy-Lagunes D, Anthony LB, et al. Consensus guidelines for the management and treatment of neuroendocrine tumors. Pancreas 2013;42(4):557–77.
74. Anthony LB, Strosberg JR, Klimstra DS, et al. The NANETS consensus guidelines for the diagnosis and management of gastrointestinal neuroendocrine tumors (nets): well-differentiated nets of the distal colon and rectum. Pancreas 2010; 39(6):767–74.
75. Strosberg JR, Coppola D, Klimstra DS, et al. The NANETS consensus guidelines for the diagnosis and management of poorly differentiated (high-grade) extrapulmonary neuroendocrine carcinomas. Pancreas 2010;39(6):799–800.
76. Pape UF, Niederle B, Costa F, et al. ENETS consensus guidelines for neuroendocrine neoplasms of the appendix (excluding goblet cell carcinomas). Neuroendocrinology 2016;103(2):144–52.
77. Garcia-Carbonero R, Sorbye H, Baudin E, et al. ENETS consensus guidelines for high-grade gastroenteropancreatic neuroendocrine tumors and neuroendocrine carcinomas. Neuroendocrinology 2016;103(2):186–94.

78. National Comprehensive Cancer Network. Neuroendocrine and adrenal tumors (Version 1.2019). Available at: https://www.nccn.org/professionals/physician_ gls/pdf/neuroendocrine.pdf. Accessed August 4, 2019.
79. Carling RS, Degg TJ, Allen KR, et al. Evaluation of whole blood serotonin and plasma and urine 5-hydroxyindole acetic acid in diagnosis of carcinoid disease. Ann Clin Biochem 2002;39(Pt 6):577–82.
80. Sherman SK, Maxwell JE, O'Dorisio MS, et al. Pancreastatin predicts survival in neuroendocrine tumors. Ann Surg Oncol 2014;21(9):2971–80.
81. Ardill JE, McCance DR, Stronge WV, et al. Raised circulating Neurokinin A predicts prognosis in metastatic small bowel neuroendocrine tumours. Lowering Neurokinin A indicates improved prognosis. Ann Clin Biochem 2016;53(Pt 2): 259–64.
82. Modlin IM, Bodei L, Kidd M. Neuroendocrine tumor biomarkers: from monoanalytes to transcripts and algorithms. Best Pract Res Clin Endocrinol Metab 2016; 30(1):59–77.
83. Perren A, Couvelard A, Scoazec JY, et al. ENETS consensus guidelines for the standards of care in neuroendocrine tumors: pathology: diagnosis and prognostic stratification. Neuroendocrinology 2017;105(3):196–200.
84. Kulke MH, Anthony LB, Bushnell DL, et al. NANETS treatment guidelines: welldifferentiated neuroendocrine tumors of the stomach and pancreas. Pancreas 2010;39(6):735–52.
85. Lloyd RV, Klöppel G, Rosai J. WHO classification of tumours of endocrine organs, vol. 10. Lyon (France): IARC; 2017.
86. Singh S, Asa SL, Dey C, et al. Diagnosis and management of gastrointestinal neuroendocrine tumors: an evidence-based Canadian consensus. Cancer Treat Rev 2016;47:32–45.
87. Hijioka S, Hara K, Mizuno N, et al. Diagnostic performance and factors influencing the accuracy of EUS-FNA of pancreatic neuroendocrine neoplasms. J Gastroenterol 2016;51(9):923–30.
88. Keck KJ, Choi A, Maxwell JE, et al. Increased grade in neuroendocrine tumor metastases negatively impacts survival. Ann Surg Oncol 2017;24(8):2206–12.
89. Jensen RT, Cadiot G, Brandi ML, et al. ENETS Consensus Guidelines for the management of patients with digestive neuroendocrine neoplasms: functional pancreatic endocrine tumor syndromes. Neuroendocrinology 2012; 95(2):98–119.

Pathologic Considerations in Gastroenteropancreatic Neuroendocrine Tumors

Andrew M. Bellizzi, MD

KEYWORDS

- Neuroendocrine • Differentiation • Grade • Ki-67 • WHO classification
- Immunohistochemistry • Site of origin

KEY POINTS

- Neuroendocrine neoplasms include well-differentiated neuroendocrine tumor, pheochromocytoma/paraganglioma, and poorly differentiated neuroendocrine carcinoma, which are characterized by general neuroendocrine marker expression and the production of peptide hormones and/or biogenic amines.
- "Differentiation" refers to the morphologic appearance of a neoplasm and is dichotomized into well- and poorly differentiated categories and "grade" takes mitotic count and Ki-67 proliferation index into account with well-differentiated neuroendocrine tumor stratified into low- (G1), intermediate- (G2), and high-grade (G3) groups and poorly differentiated neuroendocrine carcinoma considered G3, by definition.
- The 2019 WHO Classification of Digestive System Tumours ("WHO GI Blue Book") contains the current gold standard classification of gastroenteropancreatic neuroendocrine neoplasms; it includes the category "neuroendocrine tumor G3," which was absent from the 2010 WHO classification.
- Immunohistochemistry is useful for determining the site of origin of metastatic well-differentiated neuroendocrine tumor of occult origin, most of which arise from the jejunoileum (CDX2+) or pancreas (islet 1+), and for distinguishing morphologically ambiguous well-differentiated neuroendocrine tumor G3 (p53 wild-type pattern, Rb intact) from large cell neuroendocrine carcinoma (p53 mutant pattern and/or Rb lost).

INTRODUCTION

This review serves as a primer on contemporary neuroendocrine neoplasm classification, with an emphasis on gastroenteropancreatic well-differentiated neuroendocrine tumors. Topics discussed include general features of neuroendocrine neoplasms; general neuroendocrine marker immunohistochemistry; the distinction of well-differentiated neuroendocrine tumor from pheochromocytoma/paraganglioma and other diagnostic mimics poorly differentiated neuroendocrine carcinoma from

Department of Pathology, University of Iowa Hospitals and Clinics, 200 Hawkins Drive, Iowa City, IA 52242, USA
E-mail address: andrew-bellizzi@uiowa.edu

Surg Oncol Clin N Am 29 (2020) 185–208
https://doi.org/10.1016/j.soc.2019.11.003
1055-3207/20/© 2019 Elsevier Inc. All rights reserved.

surgonc.theclinics.com

diagnostic mimics; the concepts of differentiation and grade and the application of Ki-67 immunohistochemistry to determine the latter; the various World Health Organization (WHO) classifications of neuroendocrine neoplasms, including the 2019 WHO classification of gastroenteropancreatic tumors; organ-specific considerations for gastroenteropancreatic well-differentiated neuroendocrine tumors; immunohistochemistry to determine site of origin in metastatic well-differentiated neuroendocrine tumor of occult origin; immunohistochemistry in the distinction of well-differentiated neuroendocrine tumor G3 from large cell neuroendocrine carcinoma; and finally, required and recommended reporting elements for biopsies and resections of gastroenteropancreatic neuroendocrine epithelial neoplasms.

GENERAL FEATURES OF NEUROENDOCRINE NEOPLASMS

Neuroendocrine neoplasms include well-differentiated neuroendocrine tumors, poorly differentiated neuroendocrine carcinomas, pheochromocytoma, and paraganglioma (**Fig. 1**). These tumor types express general neuroendocrine markers and produce peptide hormones and/or biogenic amines. Well-differentiated neuroendocrine tumors and poorly differentiated neuroendocrine carcinomas (including small cell neuroendocrine carcinoma and large cell neuroendocrine carcinoma) are distinguished from pheochromocytoma/paraganglioma by their epithelial nature, as demonstrated by expression of the intermediate filament keratin. Neuroendocrine neoplasms, especially well-differentiated examples, characteristically express one or more somatostatin receptor subtypes, which is the physiologic basis of somatostatin receptor

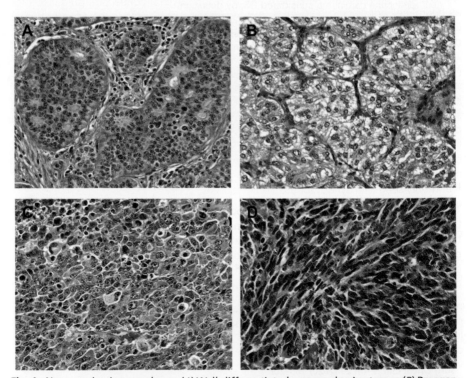

Fig. 1. Neuroendocrine neoplasms. (*A*) Well-differentiated neuroendocrine tumor. (*B*) Paraganglioma. (*C*) Large cell neuroendocrine carcinoma. (*D*) Small cell neuroendocrine carcinoma.

imaging (ie, OctreoScan or NETSPOT) and somatostatin receptor-based peptide receptor radionuclide therapy (eg, Lutathera).

Morphologically, well-differentiated neuroendocrine neoplasms, including well-differentiated neuroendocrine tumor and pheochromocytoma/paraganglioma, typically demonstrate "organoid" architecture. Although the latter typically grow in a nested pattern (also known as "zellballen" in these tumor types), the former may assume one or more architectural patterns, including nested, trabecular, and pseudoglandular, either singly or in combination. Small cell neuroendocrine carcinoma typically demonstrates diffuse architecture, while large cell neuroendocrine carcinoma may be organoid or diffuse. Both well- and poorly differentiated neuroendocrine neoplasms tend to demonstrate finely granular chromatin (also known as "salt and pepper" chromatin).

GENERAL NEUROENDOCRINE MARKER IMMUNOHISTOCHEMISTRY

Immunohistochemistry for general neuroendocrine markers is essentially mandatory to confirm the neuroendocrine nature of a tumor. Traditional neuroendocrine markers include synaptophysin (component of synaptic-like vesicles) and chromogranin A (component of dense core and chromaffin granules). Synaptophysin is generally more sensitive (approaching 100% in well-differentiated tumors), while chromogranin A is more specific. Well-differentiated neuroendocrine neoplasms typically demonstrate diffuse, strong staining for one or both of these markers. Although jejunoileal and appendiceal enterochromaffin (EC)-cell neuroendocrine tumors are nearly always chromogranin A-positive, only 80% to 90% of pancreatic tumors are positive and rectal and appendiceal L-cell tumors are often weak-to-negative. CD56 (also known as neural cell adhesion molecule) is often used as a general neuroendocrine marker (it is especially popular among pulmonary pathologists), but its use is discouraged due to lack of specificity.

Poorly differentiated neuroendocrine carcinomas are less likely to be synaptophysin ($\sim$60%) and chromogranin A ($\leq$50%)-positive and are less likely yet to be strongly expressing. I will not even consider synaptophysin and/or chromogranin A positivity in support of a diagnosis of poorly differentiated neuroendocrine carcinoma if it is seen in less than 30% of tumor cells (and even then I am wary; the stronger and more diffuse the expression, the better) (**Fig. 2**A, B). The reason for my trepidation—10% to 20% of nonneuroendocrine carcinomas from virtually every anatomic site demonstrate some degree of general neuroendocrine marker expression (a phenomenon I refer to as "occult" neuroendocrine differentiation) (**Fig. 2**C, D).[1–3] It is more commonly seen with synaptophysin than chromogranin A (although it can be seen with either or both markers), generally in scattered cells (although occasionally diffuse), and is 3 to 4 times more likely in adenocarcinoma than squamous cell carcinoma. Pathologists are generally unaware of this phenomenon and may render an interpretation of "poorly differentiated carcinoma with neuroendocrine differentiation" (or "features"), which is a description rather than a diagnosis and creates confusion among treating clinicians.

Additional immunohistochemical support for a diagnosis of poorly differentiated neuroendocrine carcinoma in this setting would include dot-like/perinuclear keratin positivity, thyroid transcription factor 1 (TTF-1) positivity (80%–90% of small cell lung cancers; 40% of extrapulmonary visceral poorly differentiated neuroendocrine carcinomas), and Rb loss (90% of small cell lung cancers; 50% of extrapulmonary visceral neuroendocrine carcinomas).[4,5]

Insulinoma-associated protein 1 (INSM1) is rapidly emerging as a general neuroendocrine marker. This zinc-finger transcription factor was initially discovered by

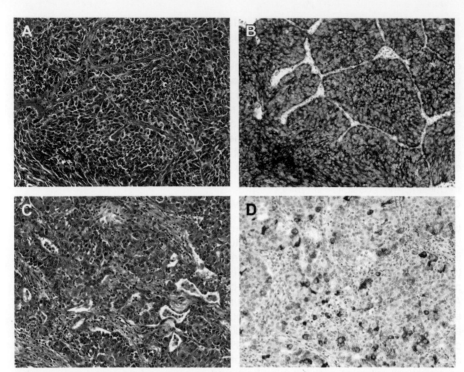

Fig. 2. Poorly differentiated neuroendocrine carcinoma versus nonneuroendocrine carcinoma with "occult" neuroendocrine differentiation. (*A*) This small cell lung cancer demonstrates (*B*) diffuse, strong synaptophysin expression. Poorly differentiated neuroendocrine carcinomas are often general neuroendocrine marker weak-to-negative, in which case dot-like keratin positivity, TTF-1 expression, and Rb loss may serve as surrogate markers for the presence of neuroendocrine differentiation. (*C*) This poorly differentiated lung adenocarcinoma was initially diagnosed as "poorly differentiated carcinoma with neuroendocrine features" based on (*D*) this synaptophysin immunostain. Ten to twenty percent of nonneuroendocrine carcinomas express general neuroendocrine markers, usually in weak, patchy fashion (as in this case), but occasionally quite strongly. This finding has no clear bearing on prognosis or therapy.

genomic subtraction of a glucagonoma cDNA library from an insulinoma library.[6] It was introduced to the diagnostic pathology community by Rosenbaum and colleagues[7] in 2015, who demonstrated INSM1 positivity in 88% of 129 neuroendocrine neoplasms from diverse anatomic sites and only 1 of 24 nonneuroendocrine tumors. As well-differentiated neuroendocrine neoplasms are nearly always positive for the traditional general neuroendocrine markers, its role in these is unclear (possibly useful as a "specificity" marker in a synaptophysin+/chromogranin A− tumor). Although data are still accumulating, INSM1 seems to be very useful to confirm the neuroendocrine nature of a poorly differentiated neuroendocrine carcinoma. For example, Rooper and colleagues[8] reported INSM1 positivity in 95% of 39 small cell lung cancers with an average H-score of 154 (note: H-score is the product of intensity*percent cells staining and ranges from 0 to 300), while synaptophysin and chromogranin A were positive in only 62% (average H-score 60) and 49% (average H-score 85), respectively.

IMMUNOHISTOCHEMISTRY TO DISTINGUISH EPITHELIAL FROM NONEPITHELIAL NEUROENDOCRINE NEOPLASMS

In a suspected well-differentiated neuroendocrine tumor, broad-spectrum keratin immunohistochemistry (eg, keratin AE1/AE3, OSCAR, CAM5.2) is highly recommended to confirm the epithelial nature of the tumor. In tumors presenting as metastases of unknown primary, pathologists often perform CK7 and CK20 to help assign site of origin. These keratins are usually not expressed by neuroendocrine epithelial neoplasms, which preferentially express keratins 8 and 18. Rarely, broad-spectrum keratins are negative, in which case alternative broad-spectrum epithelial markers may be used, including antibodies to EpCAM (ie, MOC-31, Ber-EP4) and EMA.

In a broad-spectrum epithelial marker-negative well-differentiated neuroendocrine neoplasm, the possibility of pheochromocytoma/paraganglioma should be strongly considered. Although it is "pathology dogma" that the "positive" marker of pheochromocytoma/paraganglioma is S-100, which highlights nonneoplastic sustentacular cells, that marker is neither adequately sensitive nor specific, as pheochromocytomas/paragangliomas may lack sustentacular cells and well-differentiated neuroendocrine tumors, especially appendiceal and bronchopulmonary examples, often possess them.[9] The best positive pheochromocytoma/paraganglioma marker is GATA-3 (which is most familiar to pathologists as a breast and urothelial carcinoma marker) (**Fig.** 3A, B).[10,11] Pheochromocytomas and sympathetic paragangliomas also express tyrosine hydroxylase. Succinate dehydrogenase subunit B (SDHB) immunohistochemistry is highly recommended in pheochromocytoma/paraganglioma to screen for SDH deficiency due to inactivation of any SDH subunit, with SDHB loss (seen in 30% of thoracoabdominal and $\geq$15% of head and neck paragangliomas and 5% of pheochromocytomas) suggesting the possibility of a hereditary tumor (ie, hereditary paraganglioma-pheochromocytoma syndrome, Carney-Stratakis syndrome) and associated with adverse prognosis (**Fig.** 3C).[12] Although islet 1 is often used as a marker of pancreatic origin in a well-differentiated neuroendocrine tumor (see later discussion), it is also a sympathoadrenal lineage marker and is, thus, often positive in pheochromocytoma/paraganglioma—a significant diagnostic pitfall (that can be avoided by performing a broad-spectrum keratin in suspected well-differentiated neuroendocrine tumors).[13]

As discussed above, some well-differentiated neuroendocrine tumors are characteristically synaptophysin+/chromogranin A−. This general neuroendocrine marker immunophenotype is also characteristic of adrenal cortical carcinoma, solid pseudopapillary neoplasm, and glomus tumor, which, unfortunately, are also histologic mimics of well-differentiated neuroendocrine tumor. These should always be considered in a "synaptophysin+ only" tumor, especially in the retroperitoneum and pancreas (the former 2), stomach (glomus tumor), and at potentially metastatic sites. The former 2 may be broad-spectrum keratin positive, although typically weakly so. Positive diagnostic markers include melan A and SF1 (adrenal cortical carcinoma), nuclear β-catenin (solid pseudopapillary neoplasm), and smooth muscle actin (glomus tumor).

In a poorly differentiated neuroendocrine carcinoma, broad-spectrum keratin positivity may be useful to support the neuroendocrine nature of the tumor (if dot-like) and to distinguish it from diagnostic mimics, including small round blue cell sarcomas (panel determined by clinical presentation, often including CD99 for Ewing sarcoma and desmin for rhabdomyosarcoma) and hematolymphoid tumors (typically CD45+).

DIFFERENTIATION

Neuroendocrine neoplasms should be dichotomized into well-differentiated and poorly differentiated examples. This assignment of "differentiation" is based solely

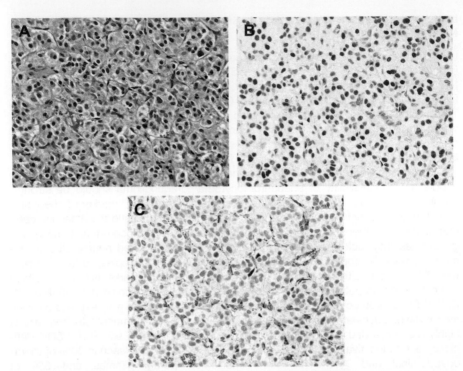

Fig. 3. Paraganglioma/pheochromocytoma versus well-differentiated neuroendocrine tumor. While well-differentiated neuroendocrine tumors should be broad-spectrum keratin-positive, this (*A*) paraganglioma expressed (*B*) GATA-3, supporting the diagnosis. (*C*) Loss of SDHB expression (with intact signal in endothelium and sustentacular cells) raises the possibility of a hereditary tumor and is prognostically adverse.

on the hematoxylin-eosin (H&E) appearance of the tumor, usually readily performed at low-to-medium power. Well-differentiated neoplasms typically demonstrate organoid architecture and possess low nucleus:cytoplasm (N:C) ratios; necrosis is typically absent and tends to be "punctate," if present. Most neuroendocrine tumors and pheochromocytomas/paragangliomas are easily recognized as well differentiated. Small cell neuroendocrine carcinoma is an exemplar of poor differentiation. It typically demonstrates diffuse architecture, is characterized by incredibly high N:C ratios, and may show extensive (geographic) necrosis. Large cell neuroendocrine carcinomas may be recognized as poorly differentiated based on nuclear features (large nuclei, irregular nuclear countours, coarse chromatin) and may demonstrate extensive necrosis.

The WHO classification of gastroenteropancreatic neuroendocrine tumors does NOT include a "moderately differentiated" category, although some other classifications do and a pathologist may be eager to diagnose a well-differentiated neuroendocrine tumor as moderately differentiated when it is more "atypical" then their conception of how a neuroendocrine tumor should look. If a pathology report notes the presence of a "moderately differentiated neuroendocrine tumor," ask your pathologist to reclassify the lesion according to the relevant contemporary WHO classification (see later discussion).

All that being said, there are certainly rare cases in which differentiation is not readily assigned. In fact, well-differentiated neuroendocrine tumor and poorly differentiated neuroendocrine carcinoma exist along a morphologic continuum (with the vast majority of neoplasms segregating at the extremes of the differentiation spectrum). Higher-grade well-differentiated tumors (especially G3 examples, see later discussion) can be impossible to distinguish from large cell neuroendocrine carcinoma, especially in small biopsy samples. Rather than shoehorning them into a moderately differentiated category, which implies diagnostic certainty, it is better to diagnose these cases as "neuroendocrine epithelial neoplasm, differentiation uncertain." In these rare, morphologically ambiguous cases, immunohistochemistry may be helpful in assigning these to the "well-differentiated" or "poorly differentiated" categories (see later discussion).

GRADE

In pathology, the terms differentiation and grade are generally used interchangeably. In gastroenteropancreatic neuroendocrine epithelial neoplasms, grade has a specific meaning, distinct from differentiation. Grade reflects the degree of proliferation in a tumor and is assigned based on an assessment of the mitotic rate and Ki-67 proliferation index. Well-differentiated neuroendocrine tumors may be G1 (low grade), G2 (intermediate grade), or G3 (high grade), while poorly differentiated neuroendocrine carcinomas are G3, by definition.

The mitotic rate is evaluated in 50 high-power microscopic fields (HPFs), with the result expressed as the number of mitotic figures per $2mm^2$ (equivalent to 10 HPF on microscopes with a field number of 20); as mitotic activity may be heterogeneously distributed in a tumor, some attempt should be made to identify the most mitotically active areas (ie, "hotspots"). The Ki-67 proliferation index should be assessed in at least 500 tumor cells, again with attention given to hotspots (which are much easier to identify on Ki-67-immunostained than H&E-stained slides) (**Fig. 4**). When the grades based on the mitotic rate and Ki-67 proliferation index are discrepant, the higher grade is assigned. In most of these instances, the grade based on the Ki-67 proliferation index is higher. Approximately one-third of well-differentiated neuroendocrine tumors that are G1 based on mitotic rate are G2 based on the Ki-67 proliferation index, with a similar frequency of tumors that are G2 based on mitotic rate found to be G3 based on the Ki-67 proliferation index.[14–16] Therefore, Ki-67 immunohistochemistry is considered mandatory in well-differentiated neuroendocrine tumors. "Eyeball estimates" of Ki-67 proliferation indices are notoriously inaccurate, especially around grade thresholds (ie, 3% and 20%), and formal counting is generally recommended (**Fig. 5**).[17] This usually takes the form of manual counting of a camera-captured image. Digital image analysis may also be used, if it has been successfully validated against the gold standard of a manual count.

Mitotic counting and Ki-67 immunohistochemistry are not required in poorly differentiated neuroendocrine carcinomas, as they are definitionally G3. I always perform Ki-67 immunohistochemistry in a suspected poorly differentiated neuroendocrine carcinoma, though, for 2 reasons: (1) crushed well-differentiated neuroendocrine tumors may be mistaken for small cell neuroendocrine carcinoma (a grave diagnostic error averted by recognition of a low Ki-67 proliferation index) and (2) the Ki-67 proliferation index may predict response to chemotherapy, with higher proliferation indices (ie, ≥55%) associated with greater likelihood of response to platinum-based chemotherapy and lower proliferation indices (ie, <60%) associated with greater likelihood of response to temozolomide.[18,19]

Although Ki-67 immunohistochemistry is essentially mandatory for grading, in patients with tumor at multiple sites there is little guidance on which sample to test. We were intrigued by a report from the Cedars-Sinai group several years ago of a cohort of 57 ileal well-differentiated neuroendocrine tumor patients in whom a Ki-67 proliferation index greater than 2% at either the primary or a metastatic site was the only

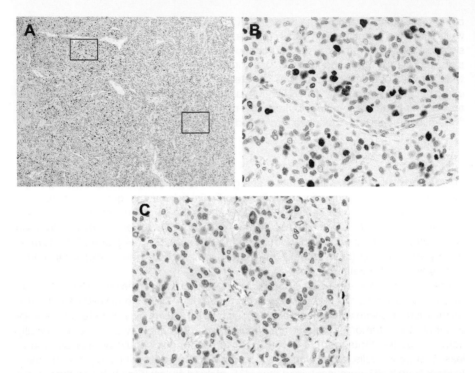

Fig. 4. Ki-67 proliferation index heterogeneity. (*A*) Low-power photomicrograph of Ki-67-immunostained well-differentiated neuroendocrine neoplasm highlights areas of (*B*) frequent (14% in this image) and (*C*) absent (0%) tumor cell staining. The Ki-67 proliferation index should be based on a count of at least 500 tumor nuclei in a "hotspot."

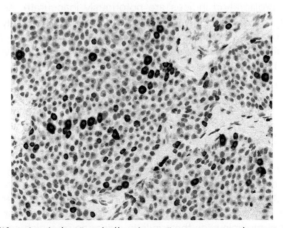

Fig. 5. Ki-67 proliferation index "eyeball estimate" versus manual count. This Ki-67 immunostain was originally reported as "approximately 30%" by the referring pathologist. A manual count of a camera-captured image found a proliferation index of 19.9% (175 Ki-67-immunostained tumor cells/878 tumor cells counted).

significant predictor of progression-free survival on multivariate analysis (in a model that initially included age, presence of stage IV disease, necrosis, atypia, and grade based on mitotic rate).[20] Other groups have noted a tendency for higher Ki-67 proliferation indices in liver metastases than in primary gastroenteropancreatic tumors and a relationship between tumor size and Ki-67 proliferation index.[21–23] Based on these data, we perform Ki-67 immunohistochemistry on initial diagnostic biopsies as well as those taken in the setting of recurrent or progressive disease. In resection specimens, we separately test primary, regional, and distant disease, if present. In the setting of multiple primary tumors (and/or multiple lymph node metastases/tumor deposits and/or multiple distant metastases) we test tissue blocks containing the largest focus of tumor. In a cohort of 103 gastroenteropancreatic tumor patients in whom Ki-67 was performed in both primary and metastatic tumor, we recently reported a higher grade in the metastasis in 24%, a higher grade in the primary in 10%, and the same grade in 66%.[24] The progression-free and overall survivals for patients with a G1 primary/G2 metastasis were superimposable on those for patients with a G2 primary. Therefore, I have taken to saying that, in terms of outcome, "any G2 trumps."

WORLD HEALTH ORGANIZATION CLASSIFICATION OF NEUROENDOCRINE NEOPLASMS

The WHO Classification of Tumors, published as a series of "Blue Books," represents the international gold standard for tumor classification. The 4th edition was composed of 12 organ-system-based volumes published between 2007 and 2018. The 5th edition of the *WHO Classification of Tumours of the Digestive System* (the first volume in the 5th series) was in press at the time I was writing this review.

Each Blue Book has "jurisdiction" over the classification of neuroendocrine neoplasms within its organ-system scope. Given the epidemiology of neuroendocrine neoplasms, the most "important" classifications are in the GI and Lung Blue Books. The *WHO Classification of Tumours of the Digestive System* has purview over all gastroenteropancreatic neoplasms, while the *WHO Classification of Tumours of the Lung, Pleura, Thymus and Heart* has purview over bronchopulmonary (and thymic) neoplasms. The *WHO Classification of Tumours of Endocrine Organs* has purview over pancreatic neuroendocrine neoplasms (as well as neuroendocrine neoplasms of the pituitary, thyroid, parathyroid, adrenal, and paraganglia) but NOT other gastrointestinal (GI) neoplasms. Relevant chapters (or sections of chapters) in other Blue Books are brief. Because of the sequencing of publication and substantial overlap in authorship, the Endocrine Blue Book classification of pancreatic neuroendocrine neoplasms may serve as a "preview" of the GI Blue Book classification.

The classification of neuroendocrine neoplasms of the digestive system in the 2019 *WHO Classification of Tumours of the Digestive System* will adopt the classification from the 2017 Endocrine Blue Book (**Table 1**). Although technically it only had purview over pancreatic tumors, as soon as it was published I began to apply it to all gastroenteropancreatic neuroendocrine neoplasms, as it addressed 3 shortcomings of the 2010 *WHO Classification of Tumours of the Digestive System* (4th edition): (1) the "G1/G2 Ki-67 hole", (2) well-differentiated neuroendocrine tumor G3, and (3) mixed tumors composed of various elements. In the 2010 classification, the Ki-67 proliferation index of a G1 tumor was defined as $\leq 2\%$, while that of a G2 tumor was defined as 3% to 20%. There was no accounting for proliferation indices greater than 2 and less than 3%. In the 2017 and 2019 classifications, the Ki-67 proliferation index of a G1 tumor is defined as less than 3%, closing the "hole." As soon as the 2010 classification was published, investigators noted rare tumors that were morphologically well differentiated but

Table 1
2019 WHO classification of gastroenteropancreatic neuroendocrine epithelial neoplasms

Classification/ Grade	Ki-67 Proliferation Index	Mitotic Count
(Well-differentiated) neuroendocrine tumor:		
G1	<3%	<2 per 2mm²
G2	3%–20%	2–20 per 2mm²
G3	>20%	>20 per 2mm²
(Poorly differentiated) neuroendocrine carcinoma:		
G3	>20%	>20 per 2mm²
Mixed neuroendocrine-nonneuroendocrine neoplasm		

From Klimstra DS, Kloppel G, LaRosa S, Rindi G. Classification of neuroendocrine neoplasms of the digestive system. In: WHO Classification of Tumours of the Digestive System. 5th ed. Lyon: IARC; 2019.

that had Ki-67 proliferation indices greater than 20% (**Fig. 6**). The 2017 and 2019 classifications created the category "neuroendocrine tumor G3."[25–27] In my practice, well-differentiated neuroendocrine tumor G3 constitutes up to 5% of all neuroendocrine tumors and, among digestive tumors, is more common among pancreatic tumors. Not surprisingly, these tumors typically pursue a clinical course in-between that of well-differentiated neuroendocrine tumor G2 and poorly differentiated neuroendocrine carcinoma and are less likely than poorly differentiated neuroendocrine carcinoma to respond to chemotherapy. The 2010 classification referred to neoplasms composed of combinations of nonneuroendocrine and neuroendocrine elements as "mixed adenoneuroendocrine carcinoma". The 2017 and 2019 classifications acknowledge that the nonneuroendocrine carcinoma component of these tumors may be squamous (eg, in

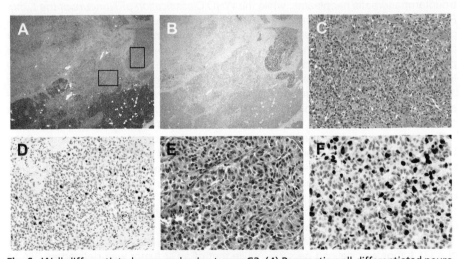

Fig. 6. Well-differentiated neuroendocrine tumor G3. (*A*) Pancreatic well-differentiated neuroendocrine tumor with (*B*) Ki-67 proliferation index heterogeneity readily noted at low power. (*C, D*) Whereas most of the tumor had a low-to-intermediate proliferation index (3.5% in *D*), there was a distinct clone with a high proliferation index (44%) (*E, F*). This tumor pursued an aggressive clinical course with the patient dying 9 months after distal pancreatectomy.

the esophagus or anus) and that, rarely, the neuroendocrine component is well-differentiated, designating these mixed tumors as "mixed neuroendocrine-nonneuroendocrine neoplasms". These rare tumors are distinguished from the nonneuroendocrine carcinomas with occult neuroendocrine differentiation discussed above in that the neuroendocrine and nonneuroendocrine components must be morphologically distinct, with the minor component representing at least 30% of the tumor.

The classification of neuroendocrine neoplasms of the lung from the 2015 *WHO Classification of Tumours of the Lung, Pleura, Thymus and Heart* is presented in **Table 2**.[28] This classification includes 2 well-differentiated neuroendocrine tumor types, typical and atypical carcinoid tumor, and 2 poorly differentiated neuroendocrine carcinoma types, small cell and large cell neuroendocrine carcinoma. Although the classification does not make use of the Ki-67 proliferation index, I routinely perform Ki-67 immunohistochemistry, which is especially useful in small biopsies containing too few high-power microscopic fields for reliable mitotic counting and in crushed specimens in which morphologic assessment is difficult; it also likely provides independent prognostic information.[29] Typical carcinoid tumor is roughly equivalent to gastroenteropancreatic well-differentiated neuroendocrine tumor G1, with Ki-67 proliferation indices typically less than 4%, while atypical carcinoid tumor is roughly equivalent to gastroenteropancreatic well-differentiated neuroendocrine tumor G2, with Ki-67 proliferation indices typically between 4% and 25%.[30] The lung classification does not include a well-differentiated G3 category, although I have seen rare examples.[31] The poorly differentiated neuroendocrine carcinoma types are analogous, although the mitotic threshold is lower in the lung (>10 per 2 mm^2) than in the GI tract (>20 per 2mm^2).

SITE-SPECIFIC CONSIDERATIONS

Although gastroenteropancreatic neuroendocrine neoplasms arise throughout the GI tract and are subject to a common classification, site of origin is at least as, if not more, relevant to biology than grade is. In this section, I will thumbnail essential site-specific considerations for these well-differentiated neuroendocrine tumors.

Esophagus

Well-differentiated neuroendocrine tumors of the esophagus are so rare that I have never seen one, and, if I did, I would write a case report.

Table 2
2015 WHO classification of bronchopulmonary neuroendocrine epithelial neoplasms

Classification	Mitotic Count	Necrosis	Other Features
Carcinoid tumor:			
Typical carcinoid	<2 per 2 mm^2	Absent	Tumor must be ≥0.5 cm
Atypical carcinoid	2–10 per 2 mm^2	Present	Diagnosis based on presence of either or both features
Poorly differentiated neuroendocrine carcinoma:			
Small cell carcinoma	>10 per 2 mm^2	Frequent	Characteristic histology
Large cell neuroendocrine carcinoma	>10 per 2 mm^2	Frequent	Organoid morphology and expression of at least 1 general neuroendocrine marker

Reprinted from Travis WD, Colby TV, Corrin B et al. (1999). Histological Typing of Lung and Pleural Tumours. WHO International Histological Classification of Tumours 3rd ed. Springer-Verlag: Berlin. With kind permission of Springer Science + Business Media.

Stomach

Gastric well-differentiated neuroendocrine tumors arise in 3 main settings.[32] That vast majority (60%–70%) arise in association with autoimmune atrophic gastritis (so-called type I tumors). These enterochromaffin-like (ECL) cell tumors arise in the gastric body driven by hypergastrinemia, tend to be multiple, are nearly always clinically benign, and are readily dealt with endoscopically. Type II tumors (10%) arise in the setting of combined multiple endocrine neoplasia type 1 (MEN1)/Zollinger-Ellison syndrome. Again, these are ECL-cell tumors driven by hypergastrinemia (in this case a gastrinoma) and tend to be multiple and indolent; they may even spontaneously regress with resection of the underlying gastrinoma. Type III tumors (25%) are sporadic, solitary, and aggressive, sometimes requiring gastrectomy. To assist in this typing, your pathologist should comment on the background oxyntic mucosa if it is present (atrophic in type I, possibly hypertrophic/hyperplastic in type II; ECL-cell hyperplasia in types I and II) and you should order a serum gastrin.

Duodenum

A recent large series of duodenal well-differentiated neuroendocrine tumors highlighted 4 different types: (1) nonfunctioning (60% of 176), (2) ampullary somatostatin-expressing (21%), (3) gastrinoma (11%), and (4) gangliocytic paraganglioma (7%).[33] Tumor type had no bearing on survival, although ampullary somatostatin-expressing tumors and gastrinomas were more likely to present with lymph node metastasis than nonfunctioning tumors. Most nonfunctioning tumors expressed one or more hormones immunohistochemically (gastrin >> somatostatin > serotonin >> other) and, as such, hormone immunohistochemistry need not be routinely used (ie, functionality is defined as presentation with a hypersecretion syndrome). Ampullary somatostatin-expressing tumors typically demonstrate pseudoglandular architecture and are, thus, apt to be mistaken for adenocarcinoma; although there is a disease association with NF1 (10% in this series), most tumors arise sporadically. Thirty-five percent of the gastrinomas in this series arose in association with MEN1. They have a propensity for regional lymph node metastasis, occasionally in the setting of a minute (and thus occult) primary. Gangliocytic paragangliomas consist of an admixture of neuroendocrine epithelial and neural elements (Schwann cells, axons, ganglion cells) and nearly always arise in the ampullary region.

Pancreas

Most pancreatic well-differentiated neuroendocrine tumors arise sporadically and are nonfunctioning. Tumors measuring less than 0.5 cm are classified as "microadenomas" and are presumed benign. Insulinomas account for up to 20% of resected tumors, while other functional tumors are rare. Pathologists should take care to distinguish pancreatic well-differentiated neuroendocrine tumors from morphologic mimics, including acinar cell carcinoma (trypsin+) and solid pseudopapillary neoplasm (nuclear β-catenin+). The presence of multiple pancreatic well-differentiated neuroendocrine tumors is typically seen with MEN1 and, less commonly, with von Hippel-Lindau syndrome. In the latter instance, tumors may demonstrate microvesicular cytoplasm, and patients often manifest concurrent pancreatic serous cystadenomas.

Jejunoileum

Jejunoileal well-differentiated neuroendocrine tumors are nearly always composed of serotonin-producing EC cells, are often multifocal (50%), and have a predilection for the distal small intestine.[34] Unlike the situation in the pancreas, multifocality does not imply a genetic basis. Although 5% of patients have an affected first-degree relative, a germline mutation is only exceptionally identified.[35] Small primary tumors are notorious for metastasis (eg, in the Armed Forces Institute of Pathology [AFIP] series of 159 tumors, 21% of tumors <1 cm involved regional lymph nodes and 29% of tumors measuring 1 to 2 cm demonstrated distant metastasis).[36] Serotonin and substance P production by the tumors causes mesenteric vascular elastosis and resulting ischemia, while patients with large volume hepatic metastasis may manifest carcinoid syndrome (5%).

Appendix

The vast majority of appendiceal well-differentiated neuroendocrine tumors are incidentally discovered, and appendectomy is generally sufficient. Most are EC-cell tumors (similar to jejunoileal primaries) with 10% to 20% representing L-cell (enteroglucagon-expressing) tumors. The latter demonstrate trabecular or tubular architecture, are nearly always miniscule (up to a few millimeters in size), and are categorically benign. The North American Neuroendocrine Tumor Society (NANETS) and the European Neuroendocrine Tumor Society (ENETS) recommend right hemicolectomy in appendiceal well-differentiated neuroendocrine tumor given one or more of the following: size greater than 2 cm, location at the base of the appendix, positive margin, mesoappendiceal (NANETS) or deep (>3 mm) mesoappendiceal invasion (ENETS), and gross nodal involvement (NANETS).[37,38] Although NANETS recommends right hemicolectomy given lymph-vascular space invasion or G2, ENETS is more circumspect, recommending a discussion about (rather than mandating) a right hemicolectomy. Finally, despite the name, goblet cell carcinoid tumor is an adenocarcinoma variant and should be managed accordingly.

Colorectum

Most colorectal neuroendocrine tumors are incidentally discovered and benign. They have a special predilection for the rectum, are typically composed of L-cells, and characteristically demonstrate trabecular architecture. In the AFIP series of colorectal tumors 81 arose in the rectum and 3 in the distal sigmoid colon.[39] Rare cecal tumors have more in common with jejunoileal EC-cell tumors. The ENETS recently published a colorectal management guideline.[40] Most tumors are effectively managed endoscopically. Surgery is indicated for tumors greater than 2 cm, tumors 1 to 2 cm invasive into the muscularis propria, rare tumors less than 1 cm invasive into the muscularis propria in which a local resection has failed, and in G3 patients considered candidates for resection (many of these latter patients will have distant metastases).

IMMUNOHISTOCHEMISTRY FOR SITE OF ORIGIN ASSIGNMENT IN METASTASIS OF OCCULT ORIGIN

Ten to 20% of well-differentiated neuroendocrine tumors present as metastases of occult origin, typically from the jejunoileum (especially) and pancreas, and less commonly from the lung or other sites.[4,41–43] Most jejunoileal primaries are difficult-to-impossible to reach with conventional endoscopy, are difficult-to-impossible to detect on cross-sectional imaging, and, as mentioned previously, have a tendency to metastasize even at small sizes. Determination of site of origin is prognostically and therapeutically significant. For example, the median survival in patients with distant metastases from tumors of jejunoileal, pancreatic, and lung origin is 65, 27, and 17 months, respectively; resection of the primary tumor may be considered even in the face of widespread metastatic disease and is associated with prolonged survival and, in midgut primaries, protects patients from significant bleeding and obstruction risks; capecitabine/temozolomide and mTOR and receptor tyrosine kinase inhibitors are much more likely to be used in foregut than midgut tumors.[41] Immunohistochemistry is useful to assign site of origin.

The University of Iowa immunohistochemical algorithm to assign site of origin in a well-differentiated neuroendocrine tumor is presented in **Fig. 7** (see also **Fig. 8**). I originally developed it in the setting of a comprehensive review on this topic published in 2013 but have updated it extensively since, as superior markers of lung and rectal and complementary markers of pancreatic and midgut neuroendocrine tumors have emerged.[4] Given the epidemiology of metastatic well-differentiated neuroendocrine tumors of occult origin, its "first round" emphasizes identifying tumors of jejunoileal and pancreatic origin. CDX2 is expressed by 90% of jejunoileal tumors, although it is also expressed by 15% of pancreatic tumors. Islet 1 is the most sensitive pancreas marker (70% of metastases in the aggregated published literature, although 85% in my anecdotal experience). To boost the sensitivity of the classifier to identify pancreatic tumors, I had originally intended to add polyclonal PAX8 (55% sensitive in the aggregated published literature). When I tested polyclonal PAX8 in my laboratory, pancreatic tumors were nonreactive and I substituted PAX6, which is the main PAX-family transcription factor expressed by normal islets and to which polyclonal PAX8 cross-reacts.[44] Islet 1 and PAX6 are never significantly expressed by midgut tumors, although both are usually expressed by rectal tumors (ie, the same transcriptional machinery regulates islet and L-cell development). SATB2, which is typically used in diagnostic pathology as a marker of adenocarcinoma of lower GI origin, has emerged as the preferred marker of lower GI well-differentiated neuroendocrine tumors; I recently found moderate-to-strong expression in 92% of 25 rectosigmoid, 55% of 33 appendical, and 0% of 331 other well-differentiated neuroendocrine neoplasms from diverse anatomic sites.[45] Islet

Iowa Well-Differentiated Neuroendocrine Tumor Classifier

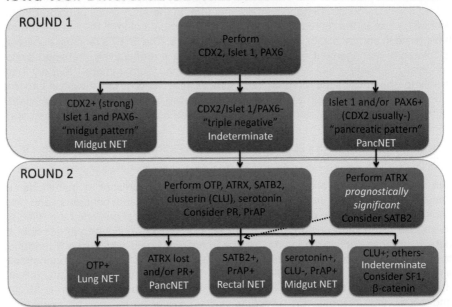

Fig. 7. University of Iowa immunohistochemical algorithm for well-differentiated neuroendocrine tumor site of origin.

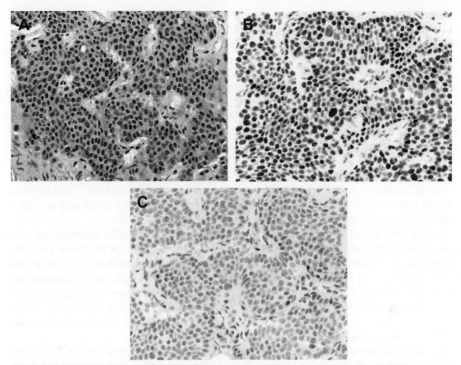

Fig. 8. Metastatic well-differentiated neuroendocrine tumor of unknown primary—site of origin immunohistochemistry. (A) This well-differentiated neuroendocrine tumor metastatic to liver expresses (B) CDX2 and not (C) islet 1 (depicted) or PAX6, supporting a midgut (ie, jejunoileal) origin. Subsequent Ga 68-DOTATATE scan demonstrated focal uptake in the distal ileum.

1 may also be expressed by pheochromocytoma/paraganglioma (broad-spectrum keratin−), medullary thyroid carcinoma and pituitary tumors (unlikely to present as metastasis of occult origin), and, rarely, by bronchopulmonary tumors.[46]

Along with SATB2, other "second round" markers include OTP, ATRX, clusterin, serotonin, progesterone receptor (PR), and prostatic acid phosphatase (PrAP). Although SATB2 may be used in islet 1/PAX6-positive tumors to interrogate a rectal origin, the other markers typically come into play with CDX2/PAX6/Islet 1 "triple-negative" tumors. Although TTF-1 is most commonly applied (although aggregated published sensitivity is only 31%), OTP is the clear first choice lung well-differentiated neuroendocrine tumor marker, at least twice as sensitive without sacrificing specificity.[47] I recently found OTP positivity in 82% of 77 typical and 50% of 12 atypical carcinoids and only 1 of 603 gastroenteropancreatic well-differentiated neuroendocrine tumors (a pancreatic tumor that also expressed islet 1 and PAX6).[48] Frequent ATRX inactivation (10%–20%) was noted in recent studies defining the molecular genetic landscape of pancreatic neuroendocrine tumors and not in jejunoileal or bronchopulmonary tumors.[49–51] In addition to using it as a pancreatic site of origin marker, I also apply it as a prognostic marker once a pancreatic origin is established (inactivation is associated with unfavorable prognosis overall, although more favorable prognosis in the subset of patients presenting with metastatic disease).[52,53] Of note, inactivation was seen in 13% of 103 pheochromocytomas/paragangliomas.[54] Clusterin is usually strongly expressed by well-differentiated neuroendocrine tumors of diverse anatomic sites with the exception of jejunoileal tumors, in which it is rarely, weakly expressed. I found clusterin positivity in

82% of 148 nonjejunoileal tumors (average H-score 183) and only 8% of 107 jejunoileal tumors (average H-score 31).[55] Since CDX2 is only 90% sensitive for tumors of jejunoileal origin, I recently added serotonin as an additional midgut marker. I found serotonin positivity in 75% of 256 metastatic jejunoileal, 3% of 63 metastatic pancreatic, and 0% of 44 bronchopulmonary well-differentiated neuroendocrine tumors.[56] Adding serotonin to CDX2 increased the sensitivity for detecting jejunoileal origin from 90% to 96%, and all serotonin-positive pancreatic tumors expressed islet 1 and/or PAX6. Although data are limited, the largest published study of PR reported expression in 58% of 96 pancreatic, 0% of 29 tubal gut, and 7% of 15 lung tumors.[57] PrAP, although typically used as a prostatic adenocarcinoma marker, is usually (>80%) expressed by rectal well-differentiated neuroendocrine tumors. When I formally evaluated it, I found expression in 88% of 17 rectal but also 37% of 41 metastatic midgut and only 8% of 13 metastatic pancreatic and 0% of 20 lung well-differentiated neuroendocrine tumors.[58] Before I had SATB2 and serotonin in my laboratory, I used PrAP as my primary rectal and as a secondary midgut marker.

A simplified site of origin algorithm is presented in **Fig. 9**. All the markers are performed simultaneously. It substitutes PR and polyclonal PAX8 for the more sensitive combination of islet 1 and PAX6 and TTF-1 for the more sensitive OTP. All of the markers used in the simplified algorithm are in widespread clinical use by pathologists for alternative diagnostic applications. As a note of caution, many pathology laboratories have shifted to performing monoclonal PAX8 immunohistochemistry (a fact your pathologist may be unaware of), which is negative in pancreatic well-differentiated neuroendocrine tumors.

In poorly differentiated neuroendocrine carcinomas, beyond the use of TTF-1 and CK20 to distinguish tumors of visceral from cutaneous origin, immunohistochemistry has almost no role in site of origin assignment. In the aggregated published literature, TTF-1 is expressed by 83% of small cell lung cancers, 36% of large cell neuroendocrine lung cancers, 36% of extrapulmonary visceral poorly differentiated neuroendocrine

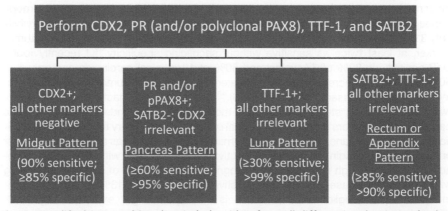

Well-Differentiated Neuroendocrine Tumor Classifier For the Real World:
Assumes Positivity for Broad-Spectrum Epithelial Marker and
Diffuse, Strong Positivity for Chromogranin A and/or Synaptophysin

Perform CDX2, PR (and/or polyclonal PAX8), TTF-1, and SATB2

CDX2+; all other markers negative	PR and/or pPAX8+; SATB2-; CDX2 irrelevant	TTF-1+; all other markers irrelevant	SATB2+; TTF-1-; all other markers irrelevant
Midgut Pattern	Pancreas Pattern	Lung Pattern	Rectum or Appendix Pattern
(90% sensitive; ≥85% specific)	(≥60% sensitive; >95% specific)	(≥30% sensitive; >99% specific)	(≥85% sensitive; >90% specific)

Fig. 9. Simplified immunohistochemical algorithm for well-differentiated neuroendocrine tumor site of origin.

carcinomas, and only 0.8% of Merkel cell carcinomas.[4] CK20 is expressed by 88% of Merkel cell carcinomas, 63% of poorly differentiated neuroendocrine carcinomas of the major salivary glands (usually parotid), 6% of other extrapulmonary visceral poorly differentiated neuroendocrine carcinomas, and 5% of small cell lung cancers. Beyond TTF-1 and CK20, any neurofilament and strong SATB2 expression are more common in Merkel cell than visceral poorly differentiated neuroendocrine carcinomas, while achaete-scute homolog 1 (ASCL1; also known as MASH1) positivity favors a visceral over a cutaneous origin.[45,59] Up to 80% of Merkel cell carcinomas are driven by a polyomavirus (ie, Merkel cell polyomavirus), and I was initially excited about immunohistochemistry to the virus's large T antigen (clone CM2B4) to increase the accuracy of the TTF-1/CK20 classifier.[60] It has subsequently been found that CK20-negative Merkel cell carcinomas are also apt to be CM2B4-negative.[61] The immunostain is useful, though, in distinguishing Merkel cell carcinoma (CM2B4+) from poorly differentiated neuroendocrine carcinoma of major salivary gland origin (CM2B4−).

Unlike the situation in well-differentiated neuroendocrine tumors, other than TTF-1, ASCL1, and SATB2, transcription factor immunohistochemistry is not useful to assign site of origin in poorly differentiated neuroendocrine carcinomas. In fact, these tumors have a tendency to express multiple transcription factors independent of site of origin, generally in weak, patchy fashion but occasionally more strongly. I have dubbed this phenomenon "marked transcription factor lineage infidelity."[62]

IMMUNOHISTOCHEMISTRY TO DISTINGUISH WELL-DIFFERENTIATED NEUROENDOCRINE TUMOR G3 FROM POORLY DIFFERENTIATED NEUROENDOCRINE CARCINOMA

As mentioned previously, up to 5% of well-differentiated neuroendocrine tumors are G3 (ie, possess Ki-67 proliferation indices >20% and/or mitotic counts >20 per 2mm^2) and these can be very difficult to distinguish from large cell neuroendocrine carcinoma, especially in small biopsies—typically from metastatic sites. **Fig. 10** presents the University of Iowa immunohistochemical algorithm for distinguishing morphologically ambiguous well-differentiated neuroendocrine tumor G3 from poorly differentiated neuroendocrine carcinoma. The molecular genetic hallmark of small cell lung cancer is biallelic inactivation of TP53 and RB1.[63] Although not as extensively studied, large cell neuroendocrine carcinoma of lung origin and extrapulmonary visceral neuroendocrine carcinomas often, although not always, share this molecular genetic fingerprint.[26,64,65] p53 and Rb immunohistochemistry are, thus, critical elements of this algorithm (**Fig. 11**). I recently found mutant-pattern p53 staining (missense or null patterns) in 71% of 31 small cell lung and 76% of extrapulmonary visceral, Rb loss in 85% of small cell lung and 52% of extrapulmonary visceral, and mutant-pattern p53 and/or Rb loss in 97% and 81% of small cell lung cancers and extrapulmonary visceral poorly differentiated neuroendocrine carcinomas, respectively.[5]

We supplement these with clusterin, SSTR2A, and CXCR4. As discussed previously, clusterin is usually strongly expressed by nonjejunoileal well-differentiated neuroendocrine tumors and is only occasionally, weakly expressed by poorly differentiated neuroendocrine carcinomas (19%, average H-score 36).[55] SSTR2A is ubiquitously (>99%) and very frequently (>85%) strongly expressed by well-differentiated neuroendocrine tumors of jejunoileal and pancreatic origin, respectively; we have observed less frequent expression by bronchopulmonary tumors (40%).[66] Poorly differentiated neuroendocrine carcinomas are less frequently positive (30%–40%), and even when positive they are typically less strongly expressing (H-scores in the 100–150 range).[67] Our group is investigating the chemokine receptor CXCR4 as a

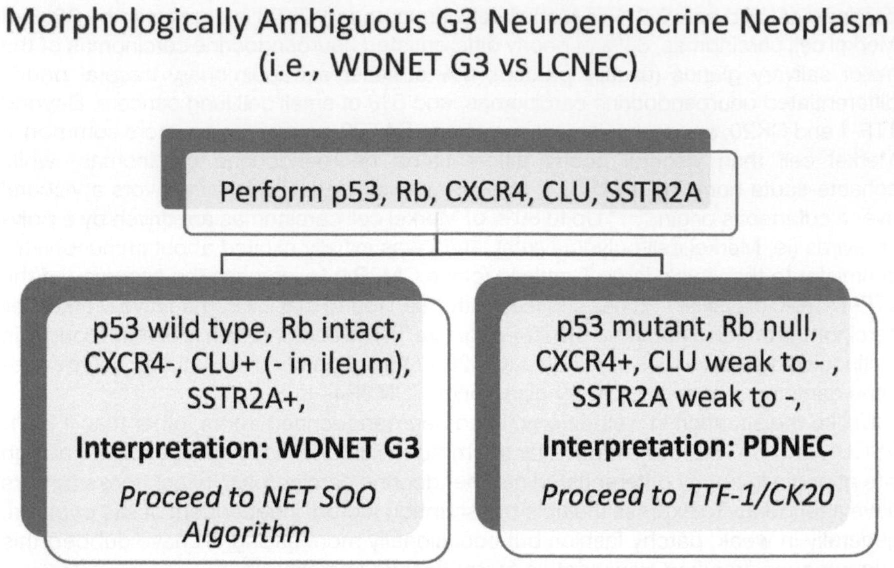

Morphologically Ambiguous G3 Neuroendocrine Neoplasm (i.e., WDNET G3 vs LCNEC)

Perform p53, Rb, CXCR4, CLU, SSTR2A

p53 wild type, Rb intact, CXCR4-, CLU+ (- in ileum), SSTR2A+,

Interpretation: WDNET G3

Proceed to NET SOO Algorithm

p53 mutant, Rb null, CXCR4+, CLU weak to - , SSTR2A weak to -,

Interpretation: PDNEC

Proceed to TTF-1/CK20

Fig. 10. Immunohistochemical algorithm for morphologically ambiguous G3 neuroendocrine epithelial neoplasms.

theranostic target in poorly differentiated neuroendocrine carcinomas. I recently found frequent, moderately strong (84%; average H-score 104) expression in 95 poorly differentiated neuroendocrine carcinomas and only rare, weak expression (4.5%; average H-score 3) in 66 well-differentiated gastroenteropancreatic tumors.[68] More

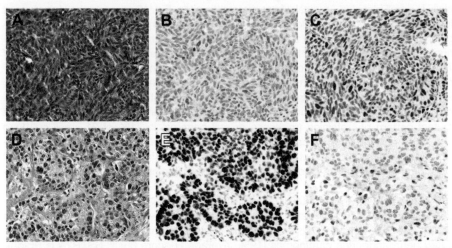

Fig. 11. p53 and Rb immunohistochemistry to distinguish well-differentiated neuroendocrine tumor G3 versus large cell neuroendocrine carcinoma. (*A*) This intermediate- to high-grade neuroendocrine epithelial neoplasm demonstrates (*B*) wild-type pattern p53 staining and (*C*) intact Rb expression, supporting the diagnosis of well-differentiated neuroendocrine tumor. (*D*) This high-grade neuroendocrine epithelial neoplasm demonstrates (*E*) missense-mutation pattern p53 staining (ie, diffuse, strong staining obscuring nuclear detail) and (*F*) loss of Rb expression, supporting the diagnosis of large cell neuroendocrine carcinoma.

Table 3
Required and recommended reporting elements for biopsies and resections of gastroenteropancreatic neuroendocrine epithelial neoplasms

	Associated Required or Recommended Immunohistochemistry
Required Data Element:	
Diagnosis: well-differentiated neuroendocrine tumor or poorly differentiated neuroendocrine carcinoma	• Synaptophysin and chromogranin A to establish neuroendocrine nature (required) • Broad-spectrum keratin to confirm epithelial nature (highly recommended in primary and regional disease and required in distant metastasis) • p53 and Rb are recommended in the distinction of well-differentiated neuroendocrine tumor G3 from poorly differentiated neuroendocrine carcinoma
Ki-67 proliferation index (proliferation index >20% is implied for poorly differentiated neuroendocrine carcinoma and performance is not mandatory)	• Ki-67 on at least 1 block of tumor (required) • Ki-67 on at least1 block of primary tumor and matched metastasis (recommended)
Mitotic count per 2mm² (in biopsies with <50 HPF to assess it is reasonable to express the total number of mitotic figures in the total number of microscopic fields; for poorly differentiated neuroendocrine carcinoma a mitotic count >20 per 2mm² is implied and performance is not mandatory)	
Grade: G1, G2, or G3 (G3 is implied for poorly differentiated neuroendocrine carcinoma and need not be explicitly stated)	
Data elements in College of American Pathologists Cancer Protocol: for resection specimens	
Recommend Data Element:	
Comment on site of origin (for metastasis of occult origin)	• Panel in a well-differentiated neuroendocrine tumor may include some combination of CDX2 for midgut origin; polyclonal PAX8 and/or PR (or islet 1 and PAX6) for pancreatic origin; TTF-1 (or OTP) for bronchopulmonary origin; and SATB2 for rectal origin • Panel in a poorly differentiated neuroendocrine carcinoma to include TTF-1 for visceral origin and CK20 for cutaneous origin; neurofilament and strong SATB2 expression also support a cutaneous origin

recently we have found that, among well-differentiated neuroendocrine tumors, CXCR4 positivity seems to be largely confined to atypical carcinoid tumor of lung origin (8 of 10 cases; average H-score 130).

REPORTING OF BIOPSY AND RESECTION SPECIMENS

Table 3 summarizes required and recommended reporting elements for biopsies and resections of gastroenteropancreatic neuroendocrine epithelial neoplasms. Reports of resection specimens should include all of the required data elements from the relevant College of American Pathologists Cancer Protocol.[69] These Cancer Protocols have been adapted from current staging criteria promulgated by the American Joint Committee on Cancer.[70] Of note, because of their especially poor prognosis, poorly differentiated neuroendocrine carcinomas are reported/staged based on protocols/criteria for nonneuroendocrine carcinomas.

DISCLOSURE

This work was supported by NIH grant P50 CA174521-01A1 (AMB).

REFERENCES

1. Ionescu DN, Treaba D, Gilks CB, et al. Nonsmall cell lung carcinoma with neuroendocrine differentiation–an entity of no clinical or prognostic significance. Am J Surg Pathol 2007;31(1):26–32.
2. Howe MC, Chapman A, Kerr K, et al. Neuroendocrine differentiation in non-small cell lung cancer and its relation to prognosis and therapy. Histopathology 2005; 46(2):195–201.
3. Graziano SL, Tatum AH, Newman NB, et al. The prognostic significance of neuroendocrine markers and carcinoembryonic antigen in patients with resected stage I and II non-small cell lung cancer. Cancer Res 1994;54(11):2908–13.
4. Bellizzi AM. Assigning site of origin in metastatic neuroendocrine neoplasms: a clinically significant application of diagnostic immunohistochemistry. Adv Anat Pathol 2013;20(5):285–314.
5. Bellizzi A. p53 and Rb immunohistochemistry as molecular surrogates show distinctive patterns in visceral and cutaneous poorly differentiated neuroendocrine carcinomas. Mod Pathol 2019;32(Supplement 2):540A.
6. Goto Y, De Silva MG, Toscani A, et al. A novel human insulinoma-associated cDNA, IA-1, encodes a protein with "zinc-finger" DNA-binding motifs. J Biol Chem 1992;267(21):15252–7.
7. Rosenbaum JN, Guo Z, Baus RM, et al. INSM1: a novel immunohistochemical and molecular marker for neuroendocrine and neuroepithelial neoplasms. Am J Clin Pathol 2015;144(4):579–91.
8. Rooper LM, Sharma R, Li QK, et al. INSM1 demonstrates superior performance to the individual and combined use of synaptophysin, chromogranin and CD56 for diagnosing neuroendocrine tumors of the thoracic cavity. Am J Surg Pathol 2017; 41(11):1561–9.
9. Al-Khafaji B, Noffsinger AE, Miller MA, et al. Immunohistologic analysis of gastrointestinal and pulmonary carcinoid tumors. Hum Pathol 1998;29(9):992–9.
10. So JS, Epstein JI. GATA3 expression in paragangliomas: a pitfall potentially leading to misdiagnosis of urothelial carcinoma. Mod Pathol 2013;26(10):1365–70.
11. Perrino CM, Ho A, Dall CP, et al. Utility of GATA3 in the differential diagnosis of pheochromocytoma. Histopathology 2017;71(3):475–9.

12. Barletta JA, Hornick JL. Succinate dehydrogenase-deficient tumors: diagnostic advances and clinical implications. Adv Anat Pathol 2012;19(4):193–203.

13. Huber K, Narasimhan P, Shtukmaster S, et al. The LIM-homeodomain transcription factor Islet-1 is required for the development of sympathetic neurons and adrenal chromaffin cells. Dev Biol 2013;380(2):286–98.

14. Rege TA, King EE, Barletta JA, et al. Ki-67 proliferation index in pancreatic endocrine tumors: comparison with mitotic count, interobserver variability, and impact on grading. Mod Pathol 2011;24(1S):372A.

15. McCall CM, Shi C, Cornish TC, et al. Grading of well-differentiated pancreatic neuroendocrine tumors is improved by the inclusion of both Ki67 proliferative index and mitotic rate. Am J Surg Pathol 2013;37(11):1671–7.

16. van Velthuysen ML, Groen EJ, van der Noort V, et al. Grading of neuroendocrine neoplasms: mitoses and Ki-67 are both essential. Neuroendocrinology 2014; 100(2–3):221–7.

17. Tang LH, Gonen M, Hedvat C, et al. Objective quantification of the Ki67 proliferative index in neuroendocrine tumors of the gastroenteropancreatic system: a comparison of digital image analysis with manual methods. Am J Surg Pathol 2012;36(12):1761–70.

18. Pelosi G, Rodriguez J, Viale G, et al. Typical and atypical pulmonary carcinoid tumor overdiagnosed as small-cell carcinoma on biopsy specimens: a major pitfall in the management of lung cancer patients. Am J Surg Pathol 2005;29(2):179–87.

19. Sorbye H, Welin S, Langer SW, et al. Predictive and prognostic factors for treatment and survival in 305 patients with advanced gastrointestinal neuroendocrine carcinoma (WHO G3): the NORDIC NEC study. Ann Oncol 2013;24(1):152–60.

20. Dhall D, Mertens R, Bresee C, et al. Ki-67 proliferative index predicts progression-free survival of patients with well-differentiated ileal neuroendocrine tumors. Hum Pathol 2012;43(4):489–95.

21. Zen Y, Heaton N. Elevated Ki-67 labeling index in 'synchronous liver metastases' of well differentiated enteropancreatic neuroendocrine tumor. Pathol Int 2013; 63(11):532–8.

22. Grillo F, Albertelli M, Brisigotti MP, et al. Grade increases in gastroenteropancreatic neuroendocrine tumor metastases compared to the primary tumor. Neuroendocrinology 2016;103(5):452–9.

23. Shi C, Gonzalez RS, Zhao Z, et al. Liver metastases of small intestine neuroendocrine tumors: Ki-67 heterogeneity and World Health Organization grade discordance with primary tumors. Am J Clin Pathol 2015;143(3):398–404.

24. Keck KJ, Choi A, Maxwell JE, et al. Increased grade in neuroendocrine tumor metastases negatively impacts survival. Ann Surg Oncol 2017;24(8):2206–12.

25. Basturk O, Yang Z, Tang LH, et al. The high-grade (WHO G3) pancreatic neuroendocrine tumor category is morphologically and biologically heterogenous and includes both well differentiated and poorly differentiated neoplasms. Am J Surg Pathol 2015;39(5):683–90.

26. Tang LH, Untch BR, Reidy DL, et al. Well-differentiated neuroendocrine tumors with a morphologically apparent high-grade component: a pathway distinct from poorly differentiated neuroendocrine carcinomas. Clin Cancer Res 2016; 22(4):1011–7.

27. Milione M, Maisonneuve P, Spada F, et al. The clinicopathologic heterogeneity of grade 3 gastroenteropancreatic neuroendocrine neoplasms: morphological differentiation and proliferation identify different prognostic categories. Neuroendocrinology 2017;104(1):85–93.

28. Travis WD, Brambilla E, Burke AP, et al, editors. WHO classification of Tumours of the lung, Pleura, Thymus and Heart. 4th edition. Lyon (France): IARC; 2015.

29. Pelosi G, Rindi G, Travis WD, et al. Ki-67 antigen in lung neuroendocrine tumors: unraveling a role in clinical practice. J Thorac Oncol 2014;9(3):273–84.

30. Rindi G, Klersy C, Inzani F, et al. Grading the neuroendocrine tumors of the lung: an evidence-based proposal. Endocr Relat Cancer 2014;21(1):1–16.

31. Quinn AM, Chaturvedi A, Nonaka D. High-grade neuroendocrine carcinoma of the lung with carcinoid morphology: a study of 12 cases. Am J Surg Pathol 2017;41(2):263–70.

32. La Rosa S, Inzani F, Vanoli A, et al. Histologic characterization and improved prognostic evaluation of 209 gastric neuroendocrine neoplasms. Hum Pathol 2011;42(10):1373–84.

33. Vanoli A, La Rosa S, Klersy C, et al. Four neuroendocrine tumor types and neuroendocrine carcinoma of the duodenum: analysis of 203 cases. Neuroendocrinology 2017;104(2):112–25.

34. Keck KJ, Maxwell JE, Utria AF, et al. The distal predilection of small bowel neuroendocrine tumors. Ann Surg Oncol 2018;25(11):3207–13.

35. Sei Y, Zhao X, Forbes J, et al. A hereditary form of small intestinal carcinoid associated with a germline mutation in inositol polyphosphate multikinase. Gastroenterology 2015;149(1):67–78.

36. Burke AP, Thomas RM, Elsayed AM, et al. Carcinoids of the jejunum and ileum: an immunohistochemical and clinicopathologic study of 167 cases. Cancer 1997; 79(6):1086–93.

37. Boudreaux JP, Klimstra DS, Hassan MM, et al. The NANETS consensus guideline for the diagnosis and management of neuroendocrine tumors: well-differentiated neuroendocrine tumors of the jejunum, ileum, appendix, and cecum. Pancreas 2010;39(6):753–66.

38. Pape UF, Niederle B, Costa F, et al. ENETS consensus guidelines for neuroendocrine neoplasms of the appendix (excluding goblet cell carcinomas). Neuroendocrinology 2016;103(2):144–52.

39. Federspiel BH, Burke AP, Sobin LH, et al. Rectal and colonic carcinoids. A clinicopathologic study of 84 cases. Cancer 1990;65(1):135–40.

40. Ramage JK, De Herder WW, Delle Fave G, et al. ENETS consensus guidelines update for colorectal neuroendocrine neoplasms. Neuroendocrinology 2016; 103(2):139–43.

41. Yao JC, Hassan M, Phan A, et al. One hundred years after "carcinoid": epidemiology of and prognostic factors for neuroendocrine tumors in 35,825 cases in the United States. J Clin Oncol 2008;26(18):3063–72.

42. Wang SC, Parekh JR, Zuraek MB, et al. Identification of unknown primary tumors in patients with neuroendocrine liver metastases. Arch Surg 2010;145(3):276–80.

43. Keck KJ, Maxwell JE, Menda Y, et al. Identification of primary tumors in patients presenting with metastatic gastroenteropancreatic neuroendocrine tumors. Surgery 2017;161(1):272–9.

44. Lorenzo PI, Jimenez Moreno CM, Delgado I, et al. Immunohistochemical assessment of Pax8 expression during pancreatic islet development and in human neuroendocrine tumors. Histochem Cell Biol 2011;136(5):595–607.

45. Bellizzi AM. SATB2 in neuroendocrine neoplasms: strong expression is restricted to well-differentiated tumors of lower gastrointestinal tract origin and is more frequent in Merkel cell carcinoma among poorly differentiated carcinomas. Histopathology 2020;76(2):251–64.

46. Agaimy A, Erlenbach-Wunsch K, Konukiewitz B, et al. ISL1 expression is not restricted to pancreatic well-differentiated neuroendocrine neoplasms, but is also commonly found in well and poorly differentiated neuroendocrine neoplasms of extrapancreatic origin. Mod Pathol 2013;26(7):995–1003.

47. Papaxoinis G, Lamarca A, Quinn AM, et al. Clinical and pathologic characteristics of pulmonary carcinoid tumors in central and peripheral locations. Endocr Pathol 2018;29(3):259–68.

48. Pelletier D, Sachs CR, Czeczok T, et al. Orthopedia homeobox (OTP) expression in a well-differentiated neuroendocrine tumor supports a bronchopulmonary origin. Lab Invest 2018;98(Supplement 1):236A.

49. Scarpa A, Chang DK, Nones K, et al. Whole-genome landscape of pancreatic neuroendocrine tumours. Nature 2017;543(7643):65–71.

50. Banck MS, Kanwar R, Kulkarni AA, et al. The genomic landscape of small intestine neuroendocrine tumors. J Clin Invest 2013;123(6):2502–8.

51. Simbolo M, Mafficini A, Sikora KO, et al. Lung neuroendocrine tumours: deep sequencing of the four World Health Organization histotypes reveals chromatin-remodelling genes as major players and a prognostic role for TERT, RB1, MEN1 and KMT2D. J Pathol 2017;241(4):488–500.

52. Singhi AD, Liu TC, Roncaioli JL, et al. Alternative lengthening of telomeres and loss of DAXX/ATRX expression predicts metastatic disease and poor survival in patients with pancreatic neuroendocrine tumors. Clin Cancer Res 2017;23(2):600–9.

53. Kim JY, Brosnan-Cashman JA, An S, et al. Alternative lengthening of telomeres in primary pancreatic neuroendocrine tumors is associated with aggressive clinical behavior and poor survival. Clin Cancer Res 2017;23(6):1598–606.

54. Fishbein L, Khare S, Wubbenhorst B, et al. Whole-exome sequencing identifies somatic ATRX mutations in pheochromocytomas and paragangliomas. Nat Commun 2015;6:6140.

55. Czeczok TW, Stashek KM, Maxwell JE, et al. Clusterin in neuroendocrine epithelial neoplasms: absence of expression in a well-differentiated tumor suggests a jejunoileal origin. Appl Immunohistochem Mol Morphol 2018;26(2):94–100.

56. Roquiz W, Maxwell JE, Pelletier D, et al. Comparison of serotonin to the midgut marker CDX2 to assign site of origin in a well-differentiated neuroendocrine tumor. Lab Invest 2018;98(Supplement 1):237A.

57. Viale G, Doglioni C, Gambacorta M, et al. Progesterone receptor immunoreactivity in pancreatic endocrine tumors. An immunocytochemical study of 156 neuroendocrine tumors of the pancreas, gastrointestinal and respiratory tracts, and skin. Cancer 1992;70(9):2268–77.

58. Stashek KM, Czeczok TW, Bellizzi AM. Extensive evaluation of immunohistochemistry to assign site of origin in well-differentiated neuroendocrine tumors: a study of 10 markers in 265 tumors. Mod Pathol 2014;27(Supplement 2):160A.

59. Ralston J, Chiriboga L, Nonaka D. MASH1: a useful marker in differentiating pulmonary small cell carcinoma from Merkel cell carcinoma. Mod Pathol 2008;21(11):1357–62.

60. Shuda M, Arora R, Kwun HJ, et al. Human Merkel cell polyomavirus infection I. MCV T antigen expression in Merkel cell carcinoma, lymphoid tissues and lymphoid tumors. Int J Cancer 2009;125(6):1243–9.

61. Busam KJ, Jungbluth AA, Rekthman N, et al. Merkel cell polyomavirus expression in merkel cell carcinomas and its absence in combined tumors and pulmonary neuroendocrine carcinomas. Am J Surg Pathol 2009;33(9):1378–85.

62. Czeczok TW, Gailey MP, Hornick JL, et al. High-grade neuroendocrine carcinomas are characterized by marked transcription factor lineage infidelity: an evaluation of 36 diagnostic markers in 83 tumors. Mod Pathol 2014; 27(Supplement 2):152A.

63. George J, Lim JS, Jang SJ, et al. Comprehensive genomic profiles of small cell lung cancer. Nature 2015;524(7563):47–53.

64. Rekhtman N, Pietanza MC, Hellmann MD, et al. Next-generation sequencing of pulmonary large cell neuroendocrine carcinoma reveals small cell carcinoma-like and non-small cell carcinoma-like subsets. Clin Cancer Res 2016;22(14): 3618–29.

65. Yachida S, Vakiani E, White CM, et al. Small cell and large cell neuroendocrine carcinomas of the pancreas are genetically similar and distinct from well-differentiated pancreatic neuroendocrine tumors. Am J Surg Pathol 2012;36(2):173–84.

66. Alkapalan D, Maxwell JE, O'Dorisio TM, et al. Prospective experience with routine SSTR2A immunohistochemistry in neuroendocrine epithelial neoplasms. Mod Pathol 2016;29(Suppl 2):145A.

67. Bellizzi A, Czeczok T, McMullen E. Somatostatin receptor subtype 2a is frequently expressed by poorly differentiated neuroendocrine carcinomas: a potential novel therapeutic target. Mod Pathol 2015;28(Supplement 2):132A.

68. Pelletier D, Mott SL, O'Dorisio MS, et al. CXCR4 is highly expressed by poorly differentiated neuroendocrine carcinoma: a novel diagnostic, prognostic, and potential therapeutic target. Lab Invest 2018;98(Supplement 1):236A.

69. College of American Pathologists Cancer Protocols. Available at: https://www.cap.org/protocols-and-guidelines/cancer-reporting-tools/cancer-protocol-templates. Accessed July 29, 2019.

70. Bergsland EK, Woltering EA, Rindi G, et al. Neuroendocrine tumors of the pancreas. In: Amin MB, editor. AJCC cancer staging manual. 8th edition. New York: Springer; 2017. p. 407–19.

Nuclear Imaging of Neuroendocrine Tumors

Janet Pollard, MD*, Parren McNeely, MD, Yusuf Menda, MD

KEYWORDS

- Nuclear imaging • Neuroendocrine tumors • NET
- Somatostatin receptor analog, Gallium Ga-68

KEY POINTS

- Multiple consensus guidelines acknowledge the role of gallium Ga-68 (^{68}Ga)–1,4,7,10-tet-raazacyclododecane-N,N',N'',N'''-tetraacetic (DOTA)–somatostatin receptor (SSTR) positron emission tomography/computed tomography (PET/CT) at multiple points along the management path of neuroendocrine tumor (NET) patients.
- ^{68}Ga-DOTA-SSTR PET/CT demonstrates superior performance to conventional imaging in the setting of initial detection, staging, detection of recurrent tumor, and detection of unknown primary in the setting of known metastatic disease.
- ^{68}Ga-DOTA-SSTR PET/CT has a low yield in diagnosis of NETs in the setting of symptoms and biochemical suspicion of NET. It still may play a role, however, in guiding management in this patient population.
- Familiarity with normal distribution and causes of false positives on ^{68}Ga-DOTA-SSTR PET/CT, such as inflammatory conditions and other neoplasms, is essential for optimal imaging.
- The role of ^{68}Ga-DOTA-SSTR PET/CT is not established in monitoring response to systemic therapy but may identify suspected progression through detection of new sites of disease.

Somatostatin receptor (SSTR) imaging has been of interest since the 1980s, when SSTR overexpression was identified on neuroendocrine tumor (NET) cells (specifically subtype 2).[1] SSTR imaging has been in clinical use for more than 20 years since the initial approval of indium In-111 (^{111}In)-pentetreotide (known by the trade name OctreoScan) for whole-body planar and single-photon emission computed tomography/computed tomography (SPECT/CT) in 1994. Recently, ^{111}In-pentetreotide has been largely superseded by the ^{68}Ga-labeled SSTR analog (^{68}Ga-DOTA-SSTR) PET/CT agents. ^{68}Ga-DOTA-Tyr(3)-Thr(8)-octreotate(DOTATATE) was approved in 2016 and [68]Ga-(DOTA(0)-Phe(1)-Tyr(3))octreotide (DOTATOC) in August 2019. In addition to the higher resolution offered by PET over SPECT, ^{68}Ga-DOTA-SSTR agents

Department of Radiology, Roy J. and Lucille A. Carver College of Medicine, University of Iowa Hospitals and Clinics, 200 Hawkins Drive, Iowa City, IA 52242, USA
* Corresponding author.
E-mail address: janet-pollard@uiowa.edu

Surg Oncol Clin N Am 29 (2020) 209–221
https://doi.org/10.1016/j.soc.2019.11.007
1055-3207/20/Published by Elsevier Inc.

surgonc.theclinics.com

have significantly higher affinity for SSTR subtype 2 compared with ^{111}In-pentetreotide which results in significantly higher detection rates of NETs with ^{68}Ga-DOTA-SSTR compared with ^{111}In-pentetreotide.[2,3] A prospective intrapatient comparison of ^{68}Ga-DOTATATE and ^{111}In-pentetreotide in 130 patients with known or suspected NET demonstrated sensivities of 95.1% for ^{68}Ga-DOTATATE versus 30.9% for ^{111}In-pentetreotide.[4] The radiation dose also is significantly lower from ^{68}Ga-DOTA-SSTR agents compared with ^{111}In-pentetreotide, with an adult dose of 4.3 mSv to 4.8 mSv for 185 MBq of ^{68}Ga-DOTA-SSTR agents versus 17.7 mSv for a typical 222-MBq administration of ^{111}In-pentetreotide.[5–7] ^{68}Ga-DOTA-SSTR PET/CT is best suited for well-differentiated (grade 1 and grade 2) gastroenteropancreatic (GEP) NETs, given their high expression of SSTRs, whereas fluorine F-18 fluorodeoxyglucose (^{18}F-FDG) PET is better suited for imaging less well-differentiated and poorly differentiated (high Ki-67 grade 2 and grade 3) GEP-NETs due to higher glucose metabolism and relatively lower or absent SSTRs.[8,9]

Guidelines for the appropriate clinical use of ^{68}Ga-DOTA-SSTRs have been published. Appropriate indications for SSTR PET imaging include (1) initial staging after histologic confirmation of NET; (2) identification of unknown primary tumor in patients with metastatic NET or elevation of certain serum biomarkers when a primary tumor cannot be identified on conventional imaging; (3) accurate staging prior to planned surgery; (4) detection, characterization, and staging in the setting of disease recurrence; (5) identification of patients who are likely to benefit from peptide receptor radiotherapy (PRRT); and (6) confirming the presence of SSTRs (presumptive diagnosis) in patients with anatomic lesions suspicious for NETs on conventional imaging or lesions that cannot undergo biopsy.[8–11]

GA-68 DOTA-SSTR PET/CT IN DIAGNOSIS OF GASTROENTEROPANCREATIC NEUROENDOCRINE TUMORS

Definitive diagnosis of GEP-NETs is based on histology, because imaging and circulating biomarkers alone are inadequate for diagnosis. Imaging, however, plays a critical role in detection and localization of primary and metastatic GEP-NETs for histologic diagnosis. The sensitivity, specificity, and accuracy of ^{68}Ga-DOTA-SSTRs have been studied. Four meta-analyses evaluating diagnostic performance of the ^{68}Ga-DOTA-SSTRs in NETs (all types) that have been published within the past 10 years are summarized. All of these meta-analyses suggest very high levels of sensitivity and specificity. Yang and colleagues[12] performed a meta-analysis of 10 individual studies (n = 415 patients) evaluating the diagnostic performance of ^{68}Ga-DOTATOC and ^{68}Ga-DOTATATE PET and with results based on histology or histology plus follow-up. The pooled sensitivity and specificity in the diagnosis of NETs on a per-patient basis were 93% and 85%, respectively, for ^{68}Ga-DOTATOC, and 96% and 100%, respectively, for ^{68}Ga-DOTATATE. The receiver operating characteristic (ROC) curves for ^{68}Ga-DOTATOC and ^{68}Ga-DOTATATE were 0.96 and 0.98, respectively.[12] Geijer and colleagues[13] performed a larger meta-analysis of 22 individual studies (n = 2105 patients), each evaluating 1 of the 3 ^{68}Ga-DOTA-SSTR radiotracers and a variety of NETs (such as GEP, lung, carcinoma with unknown primary, and thymus). Results were based on histology and/or imaging follow-up. The pooled sensitivity and specificity of ^{68}Ga-DOTA-SSTR were 93% and 96%, respectively, with area under the ROC 0.98.[13] Treglia and colleagues[14] reviewed 16 studies each evaluating 1 of the 3 ^{68}Ga-DOTA-SSTR (n = 567 patients), including a variety of NETs (such as GEP, lung, carcinoma with unknown primary, thymus, and others). Results were based on either histology or clinical/imaging follow-up. Pooled sensitivity and specificity were 93% and 91%, respectively, with area under the ROC 0.96.[14] John-beck and colleagues[15] reviewed the small number of head-to-head studies comparing the ^{68}Ga-DOTA-SSTRs to one another, as well as 21 other studies each focusing on an individual ^{68}Ga-DOTA-SSTR. They found relatively similar performances among the radiotracers, such that overall no one radiotracer could be advanced as outperforming the others. Summarizing their findings, ^{68}Ga-DOTATOC showed sensitivity 92% to 100% and specificity 83% to 92%; ^{68}Ga-DOTATATE showed sensitivity 72% to 96%, with specificity mostly unreported, except for a single study, where it was reported at 100%; and ^{68}Ga-DOTA-1-Nal(3)-octreotide (DOTANOC) showed sensitivity 68% to 100% and specificity 93% to 100%.[15]

Another situation in which ^{68}Ga-DOTA-SSTR PET may be used is suspected NET in the setting of symptoms (eg, flushing and diarrhea) and abnormal elevation of bio-markers suggestive of an underlying NET when a lesion cannot be identified on conventional imaging.[9] The yield for this modality in this patient group is low. Graham and colleagues[16] reviewed several articles reporting on ^{68}Ga-DOTATOC PET for this indication. Pooled results included 57 patients with 7 true-positive lesions (12%) and 1 false-positive result. The yield is higher in patients with positive conventional imaging.[17] Despite the low yield, this indication for ^{68}Ga-DOTA-SSTR PET is considered appropriate by consensus guidelines, because the results would substantially alter patient management.[9]

Despite its high specificity, there are several interpretive pitfalls with ^{68}Ga-DOTA-SSTR PET/CT imaging. Normal uptake of ^{68}Ga-DOTA-SSTR is seen in the pancreatic uncinate process and occasionally in the pancreatic tail; therefore, pancreatic findings in these areas should be generally correlated with cross-sectional imaging.[18] Areas of inflammation or infection and of reactive lymphadenopathy, recent surgery and radiotherapy, and granulomatous lesions also may show increased uptake of ^{68}Ga-DOTA-SSTR due to SSTR expression on activated lymphocytes and macrophages.[19] Benign bone lesions, such as vertebral hemangiomas, degenerative changes, and fractures, also have been reported to show increased uptake on ^{68}Ga-DOTA-SSTR PET/CT scan.[20]

Multiple neoplasms besides NETs are known to express SSTRs and show variable ^{68}Ga-DOTA-SSTR uptake. These include meningioma and multiple other types of brain tumors, breast carcinoma, melanoma, lymphoma, prostate carcinoma, non–small cell lung cancer, esophageal cancer, colorectal cancer, head and neck cancer, sarcoma, renal cell carcinoma, ovarian cancer, testicular cancer, and differentiated thyroid carcinoma.[8,21]

GA-68 DOTA-SSTR PET/CT IN STAGING OF GASTROENTEROPANCREATIC NEUROENDOCRINE TUMORS

Complete and accurate staging of GEP-NETs is important for therapeutic considerations. Five-year survival is directly related to the localization of disease and development of metastases: 96% (localized), 77% (nodal), 73% (liver), and 50% (extrahepatic metastases).[22] Surgery is the only curative treatment of NETs. Patients with stages I to III NET undergo small bowel resection and lymphadenectomy; however, most patients (75%) have metastatic liver disease at presentation.[23] Patients with stage IV NET may be eligible to undergo additional debulking of hepatic and peritoneal metastases depending on the extent of disease.[24]

Conventional imaging with contrast-enhanced (ce) CT or magnetic resonance imaging (MRI) is the first-line staging modality for NETs. Advantages of CT are its wide availability, short scan time, and capability of scanning extended fields of view. CT has relatively low sensitivity for detection of bone metastases, because there may be no accompanying osteosclerosis or osteolysis. Liver/pancreas MRI demonstrates higher rates of detection for liver metastases and pancreatic primary lesions compared with CT. Detection of bone metastases by MRI also is superior to CT. Due to the time-intensive nature of this scanning modality and its small field of view, however, MRI is used more often as a tool for evaluation of a specific body part rather than whole-body skeletal staging. Whole-body protocols have been developed, but to achieve the necessary extended field of view within an acceptable time frame, scan time is shortened at the expense of image detail. Both CT and MRI are limited in their detection of small nodal metastases based on short-axis size criteria. MRI also is less sensitive for lung lesions.[25]

Some of the shortcomings of conventional imaging for staging NET may be addressed with whole-body PET. Multiple studies have demonstrated the superiority of ^{68}Ga-DOTA-SSTR PET over conventional imaging in staging of NETs. **Fig. 1** demonstrates a patient with NET with widespread metastases in liver, bone, and lungs; the extended field of view and sensitivity of the ^{68}Ga-DOTATATE PET/CT are essential to identifying all sites of metastatic tumor.

For detection of NET in the liver, bowel, lymph node, and bones, Sadowski and colleagues[4] reported a detection rate between 94% and 97% for ^{68}Ga-DOTATATE, all of which were significantly better compared with ^{111}In-pentetreotide and CT scan. Frilling and colleagues[26] were able to identify larger numbers of liver and nodal metastases in a group of NET patients with ^{68}Ga-DOTATOC PET/CT compared with conventional imaging with CT or MRI. Albanus and colleagues[27] reported higher sensitivity and specificity on a per-patient basis for ^{68}Ga-DOTATATE PET plus contrast enhanced CT (ceCT) versus ceCT alone with bone lesions (sensitivity 100% vs 47%, respectively; specificity 89% vs 49%, respectively) and nodal lesions (sensitivity 92% vs 64%, respectively; specificity 83% vs 59% respectively). For lung lesions, both PET/ceCT and ceCT showed equal sensitivity (100%) and slightly better specificity with PET/ceCT (95% vs 82%, respectively).[27] Ambrosini and colleagues[28] reported higher sensitivity (100% vs 80%, respectively) and similar specificity (100% vs 98%, respectively) for bone metastases on a per-patient basis for ^{68}Ga-DOTANOC PET/CT versus CT. Whole-body PET also has proved useful in uncovering sites of NET metastases beyond liver, bone, and lymph nodes, including atypical sites, such as cardiac and breast metastases.[29]

An important question to ask in assessing performance of ^{68}Ga-DOTA-SSTR PET/CT in diagnosis and staging compared with conventional imaging is whether detection of more lesions is clinically meaningful, that is, does it affect patient care? Several studies have assessed clinical impact of this imaging modality. Barrio and colleagues[30] performed a meta-analysis of studies dealing with change in management for ^{68}Ga-DOTATATE, ^{68}Ga-DOTATOC, and ^{68}Ga-DOTANOC, with the conclusion that change in management was seen in 44% of patients undergoing the ^{68}Ga-DOTA-SSTR PET/CT. Based on 5 studies evaluating change in management in patients in whom ^{111}In-pentetreotide (OctreoScan) SPECT/CT was previously done, ^{68}Ga-DOTA-SSTR PET/CT resulted in change in management an average of 39% of the time (range of 16%–71%).[30] Recognizing that change in management is not the same thing as implementation of those changes, Calais and colleagues[31] examined the rate of clinical follow-through. Their prospective study of ^{68}Ga-DOTATATE PET/CT (n = 96 patients) showed an intended change in management in 50% of cases and a high implementation rate (75%).

In summary, ^{68}Ga-DOTA-SSTR PET/CT is clearly superior to conventional imaging and SSTR scintigraphy for detection of hepatic and extrahepatic metastases. Therefore, ^{68}Ga-DOTA-SSTR PET/CT plays an important role in localizing all sites of disease

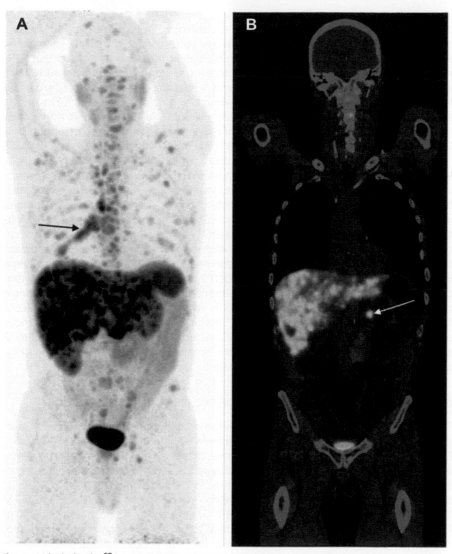

Fig. 1. Whole-body ^{68}Ga-DOTATATE PET/CT in a patient with NET of unknown primary. Maximum intensity projection image (*A*) shows numerous liver and bone metastases as well as bronchopulmonary involvement (*black arrow*). In addition, the fused coronal PET/CT image (*B*) shows the primary pancreatic tumor (*white arrow*).

for the purposes of guiding the appropriate course of treatment, and its use for this indication is supported by published guidelines.

GA-68 DOTA-SSTR PET/CT IN IDENTIFICATION OF UNKNOWN PRIMARY NEUROENDOCRINE TUMOR IN PATIENTS PRESENTING WITH METASTASES

Between 9% and 19% of NET patients present with metastatic disease with an unknown primary tumor site.[32] Localization of the primary tumor is important in the management of this patient population because resection of the primary tumor and metastases significantly improves survival and is the treatment goal for patients with well-differentiated NET metastases.[33] Even if the disease is not completely resectable, debulking surgery can significantly improve symptom control in patients with severe endocrine manifestations.[33] In patients with metastatic liver disease from midgut NET, resection of the primary tumor was found to be an independent predictor of survival with a median survival of 9.92 years for patients who underwent resection of the primary NET versus 4.68 years for patients with no resection of the primary tumor.[34] The benefit of resection of the primary NET also was demonstrated in pancreatic NETs with metastases, with a median survival of 5.42 years for patients who had resection of the nonfunctional pancreatic primary lesion versus 0.83 years for patients without resection.[35]

Several studies have demonstrated the utility of ^{68}Ga-DOTA-SSTR PET in localization of the site of unknown primary NET in patients with liver metastasis. In a prospective study of patients with negative conventional imaging, Menda and colleagues[36] found ^{68}Ga-DOTATOC PET/CT detected 38% of confirmed unknown primary tumors, with a false-positive rate of 7%. In another study by Schreiter and colleagues,[37] 33 patients with metastatic NET underwent ^{68}Ga-DOTATOC PET/CT, with a detection rate of 46% of the unknown primary tumor site. Alonso and colleagues[38] reported a detection rate of 59% of primary tumors in 29 patients with metastatic NETs, with a change in management in 24% of patients. ^{68}Ga-DOTA-SSTR PET/CT has been recommended in this patient population because treatment options vary depending on the origin of the tumor.[9] Figs. 1 and 2 show patients in whom ^{68}Ga-DOTA-SSTR PET/CT was helpful for identification of the primary NET lesion. Fig. 1 shows a patient with widespread metastatic disease with the primary lesion identified in the pancreas. Fig. 2 shows a patient with liver metastases with a small primary tumor found in the distal small bowel with mesenteric nodal metastases.

GA-68 DOTA-SSTR PET/CT IN DETECTION OF RECURRENCE AND RESTAGING

^{68}Ga-DOTA-SSTR PET/CT is highly sensitive in detection of recurrent NETs.[39,40] Merola and colleagues[39] have followed 143 patients with metastatic NETs with CT every 6 months and SSTR imaging every 12 months. In this multicenter retrospective study, addition of SSTR imaging significantly improved the sensitivity for detection of recurrence with a change in management observed in 73% of patients as a result of SSTR imaging.[39] Haug and colleagues[40] also have reported a high accuracy for ^{68}Ga-DOTA-TATE PET/CT in the setting of recurrent NET. Their series of 63 patients consisted of individuals undergoing scans for routine surveillance (n = 30), increased serum tumor markers (n = 27), or clinical suspicion of recurrence (n = 6). Diagnosis was based on histopathologic confirmation (n = 25) and clinical follow-up (n = 38). Overall sensitivity and specificity for the modality in NETs were 90% and 82%, respectively.[40]

Despite these promising results for SSTR PET imaging in detection of recurrent NETs, there is no consensus on precise interval and duration of follow-up. Singh and colleagues[41] have reviewed and summarized guidelines from 5 different international organizations. Groups based in the United States (such as the National Comprehensive Cancer Network and North American Neuroendocrine Tumor Society) recommend interval surveillance imaging to be done with conventional imaging (CT or MRI) but recommend against routine interval surveillance with ^{68}Ga-DOTA-SSTR PET/CT.[8,40,42] SSTR PET/CT is not recommended routinely for restaging after curative surgery until evidence of biochemical or radiological progression because it is unlikely to change management. SSTR PET/CT is suggested for restaging at time of clinical or biochemical progression and for monitoring disease that is seen predominantly on SSTR PET/CT.[9]

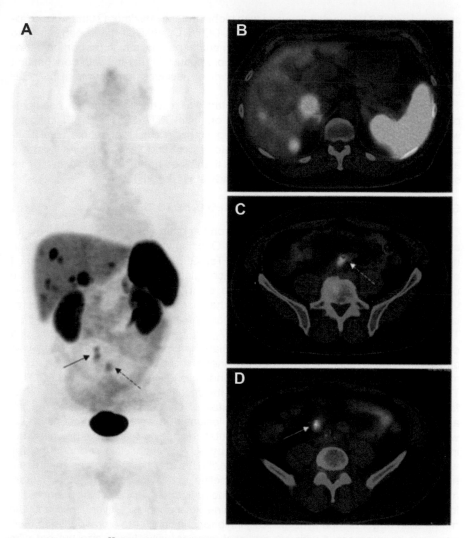

Fig. 2. Whole body ^{68}Ga-DOTATOC PET/CT in a patient with NET of unknown primary. (A) Maximum intensity projection whole body image shows liver metastases and foci of extra-hepatic uptake in the abdomen corresponding to lymphadenopathy (solid black arrow) and primary tumor in the distal small bowel (dashed black arrow). (B) Fused transaxial image shows multiple liver metastases. (C) Fused transaxial image shows primary tumor in the distal small bowel (white dashed arrow). (D) Fused transaxial image shows calcified mesenteric nodal metastasis (white solid arrow).

GA-68 DOTA-SSTR PET/CT TO DETERMINE ELIGIBILITY FOR PEPTIDE RECEPTOR RADIONUCLIDE THERAPY

SSTR-based PRRT with lutetium Lu-177 (^{177}Lu)-DOTATATE is indicated for treatment of metastatic and unresectable GEP-NETs and has been shown to significantly improve progression-free survival and overall survival compared with octreotide treatment.[43] Ideal candidates for PRRT should exhibit high SSTR expression, which is assessed with SSTR imaging. Lesions with higher uptake (maximum standardized uptake value [SUV_{max}] of 16.4 or higher) of ^{68}Ga-DOTATOC PET/CT have been shown to have more favorable response to PRRT.[44] In another study, a high proportion of patients responded to ^{177}Lu-DOTATATE chemoradionuclide therapy with concomitant fluorouracil chemotherapy when selection criteria included tumor uptake of ^{68}Ga-DOTA-SSTR greater than liver.[45]

For ^{68}Ga-DOTA-SSTR PET, a 3-point qualitative assessment scoring has been proposed to measure SSTR-expression based on ^{68}Ga-DOTA-SSTR PET/CT imaging, with level 3 uptake indicating tumor uptake higher than normal liver uptake, level 2 uptake describing uptake intensity between blood pool and liver, and level 1 uptake assigned to lesions with uptake equal or less than blood pool.[46] Patients with NET lesions with level 3 uptake are considered candidates for PRRT.[46]

GA-68 DOTA-SSTR PET/CT IN MONITORING RESPONSE TO THERAPY

Conventional imaging techniques that focus on tumor size based on response evaluation criteria in solid tumors and Southwest Oncology Group criteria risk underestimating response to treatment in GEP-NETs. GEP-NETs tend to show modest morphologic change in response to pharmacologic therapy or PRRT, even in those patients in whom these therapies improve symptoms and progression-free survival.[47,48] Haug and colleagues[47] evaluated the change in tumor-to-spleen standardized uptake value ($SUV_{T/S}$) in 33 patients at baseline and after a single cycle of PRRT. They found that the 23 patients in whom $SUV_{T/S}$ decreased any amount after the first cycle had longer progression-free survival than the 8 patients in whom $SUV_{T/S}$ was stable or increased after the first cycle. They noted that SUV_{max} alone did not demonstrate the same predictive value.[47] Gabriel and colleagues[49] compared ^{68}Ga-DOTA-TOC PET/CT with conventional imaging in the monitoring effects of therapy. They found that PET was useful in identifying sites of early progression based on the appearance of new lesions, because some lesions that were inconspicuous on CT were readily identifiable on PET. As a quantitative imaging technique, however, the intrinsic tumor activity on PET as measured by SUV_{max} at baseline or during therapy was not useful in predicting patient outcome.[49] This may have been due to inherent heterogeneity of tumor avidity both at baseline and follow-up and other factors affecting repeatability and reproducibility of the radiotracer. In the setting of nonradiologic targeted therapies, such as the tyrosine kinase inhibitor everolimus and the mammalian target of rapamycin (mTOR) inhibitor sunitinib, data on response to therapy have been assessed with conventional imaging using lesion size but not with receptor-based imaging, such as ^{68}Ga-DOTA-SSTR PET/CT.[50]

At present, there is a need to identify optimal methods for monitoring response to treatment in NETs. ^{68}Ga-DOTA-SSTR PET/CT shows utility in detection of disease progression based on development of new lesions; however, change in intrinsic tumor activity based on standardized uptake value measures has not yet shown reliability in monitoring response to therapy. Nonimaging biomarkers based on the circulating mRNA transcriptome (eg, the liquid biopsy NETest [Wren Laboratories, Branford, Connecticut]) may be useful as a method of response assessment. The NET liquid biopsy has shown utility in predicting response to somatostatin analogs, and when integrated with tumor grade information, also predicts and monitors PRRT efficacy.[51]

GA-68 DOTA-SSTR PET/MRI IN NEUROENDOCRINE TUMORS

Currently, ^{68}Ga-DOTA-SSTR PET/MRI in NETs is not widely available for clinical use. MRI exhibits better tissue contrast than CT for organs, such as liver, pancreas, bone, and brain. MRI is particularly helpful in detecting liver metastases and, given the tendency of NETs to metastasize to the liver, combination of ^{68}Ga-DOTA-SSTR PET with MRI may be useful. At this time, there are no data to suggest superiority of ^{68}Ga-DOTA-SSTR PET/MRI versus ^{68}Ga-DOTA-SSTR PET/CT in regard to disease detection. Two prospective studies comparing ^{68}Ga-DOTATOC PET/MRI (n = 8) and ^{68}Ga-DOTA-NOC PET/MRI (n = 28) with PET/CT, with the same radiotracers, showed comparable performance between the PET/MRI and PET/CT in terms of lesion detection.[52,53] Whether or not the PET/MRI modality will play a role in prediction of response to therapy and assessment of treatment response is an ongoing topic of research interest.[48]

Challenges of PET/MRI that slow its adoption include length of time for acquisition of multiple MRI pulse sequences (which can add up to an hour or more), attenuation correction, claustrophobia from longer narrower gantry, lack of familiarity with MRI acquisition and interpretation, issues with reimbursement, and lack of consensus about where PET/MRI adds value.[54] MRI also is limited in its evaluation of lung tissue. Sawicki and colleagues[55] observed that ^{18}F-FDG PET/MRI missed more pulmonary nodules less than 5 mm to 10 mm compared with PET/CT in a series of oncologic patients. Although most of these missed nodules turned out to be benign, some relevant metastatic lesions were missed, suggesting that PET/MRI with current available techniques may be problematic for accurate staging.[55] Conventional MRI is the most sensitive technique for identification of liver metastases.[48] These scans are performed with multiphase contrast enhancement, which some imagers also advocate for PET/MRI for these patients.[56] Given that it is the MRI rather than PET that contributes the most to the long imaging times of PET/MRI, there are pressures to minimize MRI pulse sequences to shorten the overall time of imaging acquisition. To that end, Seith and colleagues[57] reported that eliminating the intravenous contrast and performing nonenhanced ^{68}Ga-DOTA-SSTR PET/MRI comprised of only 3 MRI sequences (T2 half-Fourier acquisition single-shot turbo spin-echo, T2-weighted fast spin-echo sequence, and diffusion-weighted imaging) resulted in a shorter acquisition time (35 min) and comparable performance in lesion detection compared with PET/CT.

SUMMARY

- Multiple consensus guidelines acknowledge the role of ^{68}Ga-DOTA-SSTR PET at multiple points along the management path of NET patients.
- ^{68}Ga-DOTA-SSTR PET demonstrates superior performance to conventional imaging in the setting of initial detection, staging, detection of recurrent tumor, and detection of unknown primary in the setting of known metastatic disease.
- ^{68}Ga-DOTA-SSTR PET has a low yield in diagnosis of NETs in the setting of symptoms and biochemical suspicion of NET. It still may play a role, however, in guiding management in this patient population.
- Familiarity with normal distribution and causes of false positives on ^{68}Ga-DOTA-SSTR PET, such as inflammatory conditions and other neoplasms, is essential for optimal imaging.
- The role of ^{68}Ga-DOTA-SSTR PET/CT is not established in monitoring response to systemic therapy but may identify suspected progression through detection of new sites of disease.

REFERENCES

1. Reubi JC, Häcki WH, Lamberts SWJ. Hormone-producing gastrointestinal tumors contain a high density of somatostatin receptors. J Clin Endocrinol Metab 1987; 65(6):1127–34.

2. Antunes P, Ginj M, Zhang H, et al. Are radiogallium-labelled DOTA-conjugated somatostatin analogues superior to those labelled with other radiometals? Eur J Nucl Med Mol Imaging 2007;34(7):982–93.

3. Reubi JC, Schar JC, Waser B, et al. Affinity profiles for human somatostatin receptor subtypes SST1-SST5 of somatostatin radiotracers selected for scintigraphic and radiotherapeutic use. Eur J Nucl Med 2000;27(3):273–82.

4. Sadowski SM, Neychev V, Millo C, et al. Prospective study of 68Ga-DOTATATE positron emission tomography/computed tomography for detecting gastro-entero-pancreatic neuroendocrine tumors and unknown primary sites. J Clin Oncol 2016;34(6):588–96.

5. Hartmann H, Zophel K, Freudenberg R, et al. Radiation exposure of patients during 68Ga-DOTATOC PET/CT examinations. Nuklearmedizin 2009;48(5):201–7 [in German].

6. Krenning EP, Bakker WH, Kooij PP, et al. Somatostatin receptor scintigraphy with indium-111-DTPA-D-Phe-1-octreotide in man: metabolism, dosimetry and comparison with iodine-123-Tyr-3-octreotide. J Nucl Med 1992;33(5):652–8.

7. Walker RC, Smith GT, Liu E, et al. Measured human dosimetry of 68Ga-DOTATATE. J Nucl Med 2013;54(6):855–60.

8. Bozkurt MF, Virgolini I, Balogova S, et al. Guideline for PET/CT imaging of neuroendocrine neoplasms with (68)Ga-DOTA-conjugated somatostatin receptor targeting peptides and (18)F-DOPA. Eur J Nucl Med Mol Imaging 2017;44(9):1588–601.

9. Hope TA, Bergsland EK, Bozkurt MF, et al. Appropriate use criteria for somatostatin receptor PET imaging in neuroendocrine tumors. J Nucl Med 2018;59(1):66–74.

10. American College of Radiology. ACR practice parameter for the performance of gallium-68 dotatate PET/CT for neuroendocrine tumors. 2018; Available at: https://www.acr.org/-/media/ACR/Files/Practice-Parameters/DOTATATE_PET_CT.pdf?la=en. Accessed October 20, 2019.

11. Virgolini I, Ambrosini V, Bomanji JB, et al. Procedure guidelines for PET/CT tumour imaging with 68Ga-DOTA-conjugated peptides: 68Ga-DOTA-TOC, 68Ga-DOTA-NOC, 68Ga-DOTA-TATE. Eur J Nucl Med Mol Imaging 2010;37(10):2004–10.

12. Yang J, Kan Y, Ge BH, et al. Diagnostic role of Gallium-68 DOTATOC and Gallium-68 DOTATATE PET in patients with neuroendocrine tumors: a meta-analysis. Acta Radiol 2014;55(4):389–98.

13. Geijer H, Breimer LH. Somatostatin receptor PET/CT in neuroendocrine tumours: update on systematic review and meta-analysis. Eur J Nucl Med Mol Imaging 2013;40(11):1770–80.

14. Treglia G, Castaldi P, Rindi G, et al. Diagnostic performance of Gallium-68 somatostatin receptor PET and PET/CT in patients with thoracic and gastroenteropancreatic neuroendocrine tumours: a meta-analysis. Endocrine 2012;42(1):80–7.

15. Johnbeck CB, Knigge U, Kjaer A. PET tracers for somatostatin receptor imaging of neuroendocrine tumors: current status and review of the literature. Future Oncol 2014;10(14):2259–77.

16. Graham MM, Gu X, Ginader T, et al. (68)Ga-DOTATOC imaging of neuroendocrine tumors: a systematic review and metaanalysis. J Nucl Med 2017;58(9):1452–8.

17. Ambrosini V, Campana D, Nanni C, et al. Is (6)(8)Ga-DOTA-NOC PET/CT indicated in patients with clinical, biochemical or radiological suspicion of neuroendocrine tumour? Eur J Nucl Med Mol Imaging 2012;39(8):1278–83.

18. Jacobsson H, Larsson P, Jonsson C, et al. Normal uptake of 68Ga-DOTA-TOC by the pancreas uncinate process mimicking malignancy at somatostatin receptor PET. Clin Nucl Med 2012;37(4):362–5.

19. Bodei L, Ambrosini V, Herrmann K, et al. Current concepts in (68)Ga-DOTATATE imaging of neuroendocrine neoplasms: interpretation, biodistribution, dosimetry, and molecular strategies. J Nucl Med 2017;58(11):1718–26.

20. Hofman MS, Lau WF, Hicks RJ. Somatostatin receptor imaging with 68Ga DOTA-TATE PET/CT: clinical utility, normal patterns, pearls, and pitfalls in interpretation. Radiographics 2015;35(2):500–16.

21. Sharma P, Mukherjee A, Bal C, et al. Somatostatin receptor–based PET/CT of intracranial tumors: a potential area of application for 68Ga-DOTA peptides? AJR Am J Roentgenol 2013;201(6):1340–7.

22. Panzuto F, Nasoni S, Falconi M, et al. Prognostic factors and survival in endocrine tumor patients: comparison between gastrointestinal and pancreatic localization. Endocr Relat Cancer 2005;12(4):1083–92.

23. Steinmuller T, Kianmanesh R, Falconi M, et al. Consensus guidelines for the management of patients with liver metastases from digestive (neuro)endocrine tumors: foregut, midgut, hindgut, and unknown primary. Neuroendocrinology 2008;87(1):47–62.

24. Scott AT, Howe JR. Management of small bowel neuroendocrine tumors. J Oncol Pract 2018;14(8):471–82.

25. Sundin A, Arnold R, Baudin E, et al. ENETS consensus guidelines for the standards of care in neuroendocrine tumors: radiological, nuclear medicine & hybrid imaging. Neuroendocrinology 2017;105(3):212–44.

26. Frilling A, Sotiropoulos GC, Radtke A, et al. The impact of 68Ga-DOTATOC positron emission tomography/computed tomography on the multimodal management of patients with neuroendocrine tumors. Ann Surg 2010;252(5):850–6.

27. Albanus DR, Apitzsch J, Erdem Z, et al. Clinical value of (6)(8)Ga-DOTATATE-PET/CT compared to stand-alone contrast enhanced CT for the detection of extra-hepatic metastases in patients with neuroendocrine tumours (NET). Eur J Radiol 2015;84(10):1866–72.

28. Ambrosini V, Nanni C, Zompatori M, et al. (68)Ga-DOTA-NOC PET/CT in comparison with CT for the detection of bone metastasis in patients with neuroendocrine tumours. Eur J Nucl Med Mol Imaging 2010;37(4):722–7.

29. Carreras C, Kulkarni HR, Baum RP. Rare metastases detected by (68)Ga-somatostatin receptor PET/CT in patients with neuroendocrine tumors. Recent Results Cancer Res 2013;194:379–84.

30. Barrio M, Czernin J, Fanti S, et al. The impact of somatostatin receptor-directed pet/ct on the management of patients with neuroendocrine tumor: a systematic review and meta-analysis. J Nucl Med 2017;58(5):756–61.

31. Calais J, Czernin J, Eiber M, et al. Most of the intended management changes after (68)Ga-DOTATATE PET/CT are implemented. J Nucl Med 2017;58(11):1793–6.

32. Bellizzi AM. Assigning site of origin in metastatic neuroendocrine neoplasms: a clinically significant application of diagnostic immunohistochemistry. Adv Anat Pathol 2013;20(5):285–314.

33. Pavel M, Baudin E, Couvelard A, et al. ENETS consensus guidelines for the management of patients with liver and other distant metastases from neuroendocrine

neoplasms of foregut, midgut, hindgut, and unknown primary. Neuroendocrinology 2012;95(2):157–76.

34. Ahmed A, Turner G, King B, et al. Midgut neuroendocrine tumours with liver metastases: results of the UKINETS study. Endocr Relat Cancer 2009;16(3):885–94.

35. Keutgen XM, Nilubol N, Glanville J, et al. Resection of primary tumor site is associated with prolonged survival in metastatic nonfunctioning pancreatic neuroendocrine tumors. Surgery 2016;159(1):311–9.

36. Menda Y, O'Dorisio TM, Howe JR, et al. Localization of unknown primary site with (68)Ga-DOTATOC PET/CT in patients with metastatic neuroendocrine tumor. J Nucl Med 2017;58(7):1054–7.

37. Schreiter NF, Bartels AM, Froeling V, et al. Searching for primaries in patients with neuroendocrine tumors (NET) of unknown primary and clinically suspected NET: evaluation of Ga-68 DOTATOC PET/CT and In-111 DTPA octreotide SPECT/CT. Radiol Oncol 2014;48(4):339–47.

38. Alonso O, Rodriguez-Taroco M, Savio E, et al. (68)Ga-DOTATATE PET/CT in the evaluation of patients with neuroendocrine metastatic carcinoma of unknown origin. Ann Nucl Med 2014;28(7):638–45.

39. Merola E, Pavel ME, Panzuto F, et al. Functional imaging in the follow-up of enteropancreatic neuroendocrine tumors: clinical usefulness and indications. J Clin Endocrinol Metab 2017;102(5):1486–94.

40. Haug AR, Cindea-Drimus R, Auernhammer CJ, et al. Neuroendocrine tumor recurrence: diagnosis with 68Ga-DOTATATE PET/CT. Radiology 2014;270(2): 517–25.

41. Singh S, Moody L, Chan DL, et al. Follow-up recommendations for completely resected gastroenteropancreatic neuroendocrine tumors. JAMA Oncol 2018;4(11): 1597–604.

42. Kayani I, Bomanji JB, Groves A, et al. Functional imaging of neuroendocrine tumors with combined PET/CT using 68Ga-DOTATATE (DOTA-DPhe1,Tyr3-octreotate) and 18F-FDG. Cancer 2008;112(11):2447–55.

43. Strosberg J, El-Haddad G, Wolin E, et al. Phase 3 trial of 177Lu-Dotatate for midgut neuroendocrine tumors. N Engl J Med 2017;376(2):125–35.

44. Kratochwil C, Stefanova M, Mavriopoulou E, et al. SUV of [68Ga]DOTATOC-PET/CT predicts response probability of PRRT in neuroendocrine tumors. Mol Imaging Biol 2015;17(3):313–8.

45. Kong G, Thompson M, Collins M, et al. Assessment of predictors of response and long-term survival of patients with neuroendocrine tumour treated with peptide receptor chemoradionuclide therapy (PRCRT). Eur J Nucl Med Mol Imaging 2014; 41(10):1831–44.

46. Werner RA, Solnes LB, Javadi MS, et al. SSTR-RADS version 1.0 as a reporting system for SSTR PET imaging and selection of potential PRRT candidates: a proposed standardization framework. J Nucl Med 2018;59(7):1085–91.

47. Haug AR, Auernhammer CJ, Wangler B, et al. 68Ga-DOTATATE PET/CT for the early prediction of response to somatostatin receptor-mediated radionuclide therapy in patients with well-differentiated neuroendocrine tumors. J Nucl Med 2010; 51(9):1349–56.

48. Bodei L, Sundin A, Kidd M, et al. The status of neuroendocrine tumor imaging: from darkness to light? Neuroendocrinology 2015;101(1):1–17.

49. Gabriel M, Oberauer A, Dobrozemsky G, et al. 68Ga-DOTA-Tyr3-octreotide PET for assessing response to somatostatin-receptor-mediated radionuclide therapy. J Nucl Med 2009;50(9):1427–34.

50. Merino-Casabiel X, Aller J, Arbizu J, et al. Consensus document on the progression and treatment response criteria in gastroenteropancreatic neuroendocrine tumors. Clin Transl Oncol 2018;20(12):1522–8.
51. Modlin IM, Kidd M, Malczewska A, et al. The NETest: the clinical utility of multi-gene blood analysis in the diagnosis and management of neuroendocrine tumors. Endocrinol Metab Clin North Am 2018;47(3):485–504.
52. Beiderwellen KJ, Poeppel TD, Hartung-Knemeyer V, et al. Simultaneous 68Ga-DOTATOC PET/MRI in patients with gastroenteropancreatic neuroendocrine tumors: initial results. Invest Radiol 2013;48(5):273–9.
53. Berzaczy D, Giraudo C, Haug AR, et al. Whole-body 68Ga-DOTANOC PET/MRI versus 68Ga-DOTANOC PET/CT in patients with neuroendocrine tumors: a prospective study in 28 patients. Clin Nucl Med 2017;42(9):669–74.
54. Ehman EC, Johnson GB, Villanueva-Meyer JE, et al. PET/MRI: where might it replace PET/CT? J Magn Reson Imaging 2017;46(5):1247–62.
55. Sawicki LM, Grueneisen J, Buchbender C, et al. Evaluation of the outcome of lung nodules missed on 18F-FDG PET/MRI compared with 18F-FDG PET/CT in patients with known malignancies. J Nucl Med 2016;57(1):15–20.
56. Sundin A. Novel functional imaging of neuroendocrine tumors. Endocrinol Metab Clin North Am 2018;47(3):505–23.
57. Seith F, Schraml C, Reischl G, et al. Fast non-enhanced abdominal examination protocols in PET/MRI for patients with neuroendocrine tumors (NET): comparison to multiphase contrast-enhanced PET/CT. Radiol Med 2018;123(11):860–70.

Management of Small Bowel Neuroendocrine Tumors

Aaron T. Scott, MD[a], James R. Howe, MD[a,b],*

KEYWORDS

- Small bowel • Neuroendocrine tumor • Carcinoid • SBNET • Surgery

KEY POINTS

- Small bowel neuroendocrine tumors (SBNETS) are the most common primary tumors of the small bowel.
- SBNETs most commonly present with abdominal pain or obstruction, which may necessitate emergency surgery.
- Distant metastases are present in approximately 30% of patients at diagnosis, and regional lymph node metastases are seen in another 40%.
- Treatment of metastatic SBNETs is multimodal and includes primary resection, cytoreductive surgery, liver-directed therapy, and a variety of systemic treatments.
- SBNETs have an excellent prognosis, and patients may live for a decade or more even after the development of metastasis.

INTRODUCTION

The first description of a small bowel neuroendocrine tumor (SBNET) was by Theodor Langhans, who in 1867 reported a polypoid tumor of the small bowel discovered on autopsy.[1] This was followed in 1888 by Otto Lubarsch's description of 2 additional patients found to have multiple small bowel tumors.[2] The first English-language report of an SBNET was in 1890 by William Ransom, who gives an excellent description of a patient suffering from what would later come to be known as carcinoid syndrome, and who was found on autopsy to have a small bowel tumor with extensive liver metastases.[3] In 1907, Siegfried Oberndorfer coined the term *karzinoide*, meaning "carcinoma-like," in description of 6 patients with submucosal tumors of the small intestine.[4] Over the following hundred years, the term "carcinoid" would be expanded to refer to a group of diverse neoplasms from a wide variety of primary sites that are now known as neuroendocrine tumors (NETs). Although the term "NET" has largely supplanted

a Department of Surgery, University of Iowa Carver College of Medicine, Iowa City, IA, USA;
b Division of Surgical Oncology and Endocrine Surgery, University of Iowa Carver College of Medicine, Iowa City, IA, USA
* Corresponding author. University of Iowa Hospitals and Clinics, 200 Hawkins Drive, 4644 JCP, Iowa City, IA 52242.
E-mail address: james-howe@uiowa.edu

Surg Oncol Clin N Am 29 (2020) 223–241
https://doi.org/10.1016/j.soc.2019.11.006
surgonc.theclinics.com

"carcinoid," the older term is still variably used to refer to NETs arising from the lung or small bowel, and it persists in the clinical entity known as carcinoid syndrome.

SBNETs are, by definition, located between the ligament of the Treitz and the ileo-cecal valve. Although duodenal NETs are sometimes included with jejunal and ileal NETs under the umbrella term "SBNET," these tumors are clinically and biologically distinct and should not be considered to represent the same entity.[5] Similarly, SBNETs are sometimes grouped together with NETs arising in the proximal colon and appendix as "midgut NETs" based on the classification system proposed by Williams and Sandler, but these tumors are likewise outside the scope of this article.[6] The management of duodenal, appendiceal, and colonic NETs are discussed elsewhere in this issue.

EPIDEMIOLOGY

The incidence of SBNETs in the United States has increased roughly 6-fold since the 1970s, to a rate of 1.3 cases per year per 100,000 persons, making the small bowel the second most common primary site for NETs, behind the lung.[7] Although the incidence varies internationally, studies from Europe, Canada, and Japan show similar increases.[8,9] As a result of this pronounced increase, SBNETs are now the most common primary malignancies of the small bowel.[10] In addition, although SBNETs are classically thought of as rare cancers, their increasing incidence combined with their comparatively favorable prognosis results in a prevalence that exceeds many other common gastrointestinal (GI) cancers, including esophageal, gastric, pancreatic, and hepatobiliary cancers.[11,12] The mean and median ages at diagnosis are in the 6th decade, whereas the peak incidence is between 70 and 80 years.[9,10,12,13]

PRESENTATION

SBNETs present in many ways depending on the disease stage and tumor burden at the time of diagnosis. Population-based studies have shown that roughly 30% of patients with SBNETs will have distant metastases at the time of diagnosis, and another 40% will have regional lymph node involvement.[9,11–13] However, the incidence of distant metastasis is significantly higher, upward of 60%, in institutional series from tertiary referral centers.[14–17]

Almost all SBNETs produce a wide variety of biologically active peptides, including serotonin, neurokinin A, and histamine, which are responsible for carcinoid syndrome.[18,19] However, for tumors confined to the small bowel and regional lymph nodes, these compounds are inactivated by the liver, and hormonal symptoms are uncommon.[15,18–20] The primary tumors are characteristically small, but have a tendency to induce an extensive fibrotic reaction in the small bowel and mesentery, resulting in narrowing or kinking of the bowel, and potentially mesenteric ischemia (**Fig. 1**).[21] The most common presenting symptoms are abdominal pain followed by partial or complete bowel obstruction and diarrhea.[13,15,17] As many as half of patients undergo resection before diagnosis on an urgent or emergent basis due to bowel obstruction.[17,22] In addition, around 15% to 20% of SBNETs do not cause symptoms and are detected incidentally, which is more common in patients with localized disease.[13,15]

The liver is the overwhelmingly favored site of metastasis for SBNETs, with 80% of distant stage patients having hepatic involvement, but metastases to distant lymph nodes, bone, and the peritoneal cavity are also frequently observed (**Fig. 2**).[13,23,24] With the development of distant metastases, hormones secreted by SBNETs are able to bypass the portal circulation, leading to the development of carcinoid syndrome. This syndrome was first described by Thorson and colleagues[25] in 1954 and consists of flushing, diarrhea, valvular heart disease, and bronchospasm. Despite

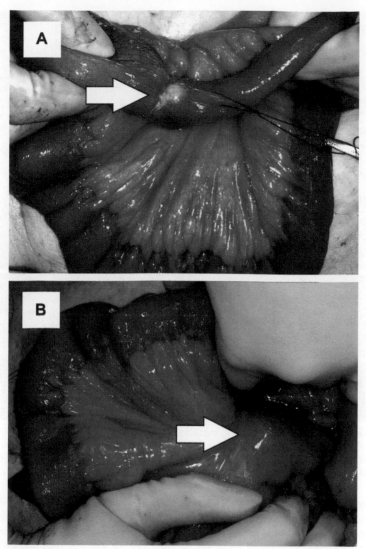

Fig. 1. Intraoperative images of a primary tumor (*A, arrow*) and the associated mesenteric mass (*B, arrow*) in a patient undergoing resection of an SBNET.

the common nomenclature used to describe carcinoid tumors and carcinoid syndrome, even among patients with metastases the most common presenting symptom is vague abdominal pain, and only a minority will have all components of the carcinoid syndrome at the time of diagnosis.[15,18] Flushing associated with carcinoid syndrome is typically transient and involves the face and upper trunk. Carcinoid symptoms may be spontaneous or be provoked by stress, exercise, or ingestion of ethanol and amine-rich foods such as chocolate or cheese.[18,19]

The cardiac manifestations of carcinoid syndrome, termed "carcinoid heart disease," consist of valvular fibrosis primarily affecting the right side of the heart.[18,26–28] Cardiac involvement is seen in at least 20% of patients with carcinoid syndrome, and the incidence is decreasing, possibly due to widespread use of somatostatin analogues (SSAs).[26–28]

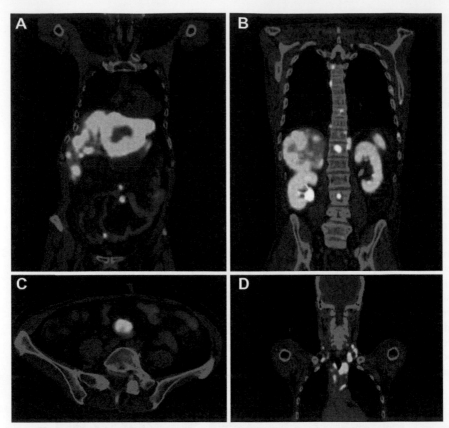

Fig. 2. ^{68}Ga-PET images demonstrating metastatic disease in patients with SBNETs. (*A*) Multifocal, small primary tumors and extensive liver involvement. (*B*) Multiple skeletal metastases to the spine, ribs, and left scapula along with extensive liver involvement. (*C*) Large mesenteric nodal metastasis. (*D*) Supraclavicular and mediastinal lymph node metastases.

The cause is thought to be related to high circulating levels of serotonin that induce a fibrotic reaction in the right heart, similar to the mesenteric fibrosis observed near the primary tumors. The presence of carcinoid heart disease portends a significantly worse prognosis, but clinical signs of heart failure may not be evident until severe valvular compromise has occurred, and thus a high index of suspicion is indicated in patients with elevated serotonin levels or other signs of carcinoid syndrome.[18,26–28]

The presentation of SBNETs runs the gamut from asymptomatic to debilitating flushing and diarrhea associated with carcinoid syndrome or complete bowel obstruction necessitating emergency surgery. This variety in presentation, combined with the relative rarity of the tumors and the nonspecific nature of the symptoms, complicates the diagnosis of these tumors. Although the median duration of symptoms before diagnosis is 4 to 5 months, misdiagnosis is not uncommon and delays of up to a decade are well described in the literature.[9,13,15,29]

DIAGNOSIS

The diagnostic sequence for patients suspected to have SBNETs should be tailored to the individual. Those who present with flushing and diarrhea will likely undergo biochemical testing first, whereas those with abdominal pain or obstructive symptoms may be investigated initially with anatomic imaging such as computed tomography (CT) or be diagnosed only after emergent operation. Still others present with an incidentally discovered liver mass and undergo biopsy as the initial step in the diagnostic workup. Ultimately, the diagnosis of SBNET is made by immunohistochemical examination of the tumor, but for most patients, biochemical testing and anatomic or functional imaging will precede this step.

Biochemical Evaluation

In addition to the hormones and neuroamines responsible for carcinoid syndrome, SBNETs secrete several different compounds that can be used as biomarkers for diagnosis and surveillance. These include chromogranin A (CgA), pancreastatin, and serotonin. Among these, CgA, an acidic glycoprotein that is secreted by a wide variety of NETs, is the best studied.[18,19,27,28] CgA is both sensitive and specific for the diagnosis of NETs, correlates with disease burden, and is predictive of survival. However, several conditions can cause false elevations of CgA, including proton pump inhibitor therapy, severe hypertension, or renal failure.[19,27,30] Pancreastatin is a breakdown product of CgA that may be less susceptible to nonspecific elevation and is frequently elevated in patients with SBNETs.[19,27] In addition to its role in the diagnosis of SBNETs, serial measurements of pancreastatin are useful for prognostication and monitoring response to therapy. Preoperative levels of pancreastatin are predictive of progression-free survival (PFS) and overall survival (OS) in surgically treated patients with SBNET,[31] and in patients undergoing surgical cytoreduction or chemoembolization, normalization or greater than 50% decrease in pancreastatin following treatment was associated with improved OS.[32,33]

Although serotonin is thought to be responsible for many of the symptoms of carcinoid syndrome, including carcinoid heart disease, serum levels vary significantly throughout the day, and thus its utility as a biomarker is limited.[19] The serotonin breakdown product, 5-hydroxyindole acetic acid (5-HIAA) is commonly measured in a 24 hour urine collection as a marker for serotonin-secreting tumors. This test is highly specific for the diagnosis of SBNETs, but patients must be advised to avoid several serotonin-rich foods during the collection.[18,19,34]

Several other markers have been studied and are variably elevated in patients with SBNETs including neurokinin A, substance P, chromogranin B, and neuron-specific enolase, but there is insufficient evidence to draw strong conclusions on their utility. Biochemical testing is widely used both for the diagnosis of SBNETs and for monitoring the disease course, but agreement is lacking on how frequently they should be measured or how their measurement should influence treatment decisions.[19,27]

Imaging

Imaging of SBNETs includes both anatomic and functional studies. The former includes CT, MR imaging, and ultrasound (US), whereas the latter includes somatostatin receptor–based single-photon emission CT (SPECT) and PET as well as conventional fluorodeoxyglucose (FDG) PET. Anatomic imaging is useful for localizing tumors and for surgical planning, whereas functional imaging has a higher sensitivity and is useful for identifying occult metastases or equivocal evidence of recurrence.

Anatomic imaging
Computed tomography is the most common imaging test for evaluating SBNETs (**Fig. 3**).[35] This modality is widely available, has quick acquisition time, provides great anatomic information regarding lymph node and liver metastases, and allows for

accurate staging and operative planning.[28,35,36] Primary SBNET tumors are frequently small and mesenteric fibrosis or nodal metastasis may be the only evidence of the primary tumor.[37] Liver metastases are hyperenhancing and usually appear as hypervascular lesions on the arterial phase; occasionally these tumors are hypovascular and are better seen as darker lesions on the venous phase.[38,39] With this in mind, it is critically important to obtain a multiphase CT scan when evaluating patients with SBNET for liver metastases.[40] Notably, CT tends to underestimate the degree of liver replacement, particularly when compared with MR imaging.[36,39] The mean reported CT sensitivity for the detection of NET disease is 82%.[38]

MR imaging has several advantages over CT for the evaluation of SBNETs, most notably the avoidance of ionizing radiation and improved detection of liver metastases (see **Fig. 3**).[35,36,38,39] These tumors generally show up as low-intensity lesions on T1-weighted images and as hyperintense on T2- or diffusion-weighted images.[38] A study comparing CT with MR imaging found that the sensitivities for the detection of liver metastases were 78.5% and 95.2%, respectively, with MR imaging also demonstrating significantly more lesions on average.[39] The sensitivity for liver metastases can be improved further through the use of hepatocyte-specific contrast agents and acquisition of hepatocellular phase imaging.[38,41]

Ultrasound plays a limited role in the diagnosis of SBNETs, owing to its inability to image the entire abdomen and operator-dependent results. Liver metastases are

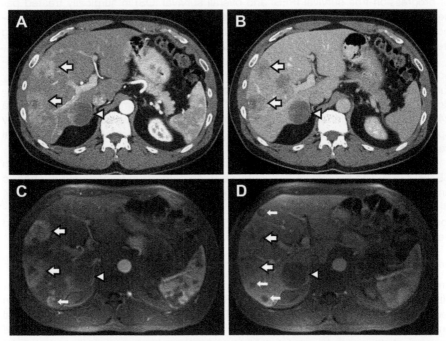

Fig. 3. A comparison of contrast-enhanced CT and MR imaging for the evaluation of liver metastases in a single patient: (A) arterial phase CT scan, (B) venous phase CT scan, (C) arterial phase MR imaging, (D) portal venous phase MR imaging. Large arrows indicate 2 dominant liver metastases that are hyperenhancing on the arterial phase and hypoenhancing on the venous phase. The arrowhead indicates a metastatic lesion that is hypoenhancing on both the arterial and venous phases. Smaller arrows indicate smaller metastases that were apparent on MR imaging but not on CT.

sometimes discovered in patients with pain mimicking biliary pathology prompting right upper quadrant US. In addition, biopsy of hepatic metastases and operative or percutaneous ablation is commonly performed under US guidance.[28,35,38] Finally, in patients with clinical or biochemical evidence of serotonin hypersecretion, echocardiography should be obtained to evaluate for carcinoid heart disease.[26–28]

Functional imaging

SBNETs express somatostatin receptors at high density in 80% to 100% of cases that can be targeted using SSAs for the treatment and imaging of these tumors.[42] In the same way that conventional FDG-PET uses radiolabeled glucose to localize metabolically active tumors, radiolabeled SSAs are used to localize NETs. The first such compound to be widely used clinically was ^{111}In-octreotide, in which the gamma-emitter indium-111 is chelated to an SSA and used in a test known as indum-111 somatostatin receptor scintigraphy (^{111}In-SRS, Octreoscan).[43] Tumors were localized using ^{111}In-SRS initially using planar scintigraphy and later with SPECT, which incorporates CT imaging for improved localization. Modern ^{111}In-SRS has an overall sensitivity of 60% to 80% for the detection of NETs,[38] but the sensitivity is significantly lower for primary SBNETs.[36,37]

In the last 2 decades, gallium-68–based imaging has replaced ^{111}In-SRS as the modality of choice for functional imaging of SBNETs (see **Fig. 2**).[35,36,38,44,45] Several ^{68}Ga-labeled ligands are available for this purpose, including ^{68}Ga-DOTATATE, ^{68}Ga-DOTATOC, and ^{68}Ga-DOTANOC, which differ slightly in their affinities for the various somatostatin receptor subtypes.[35,45] ^{68}Ga-PET is superior to ^{111}In-SRS imaging by a variety of measures, including lower radiation dose, quicker acquisition time, better spatial resolution, and improved accuracy.[35,38,44] In a direct, lesion-by-lesion comparison of ^{111}In-SRS and ^{68}Ga-PET, the latter detected significantly more lesions and was more sensitive, particularly for metastases to the skeleton or liver.[44] Meta-analyses have shown the mean sensitivity of ^{68}Ga-PET for the detection of NETs to be between 88% and 93%.[38] Despite the improved resolution of ^{68}Ga-PET compared with ^{111}In-SRS, the noncontrast-enhanced CT scan that accompanies it is inadequate for surgical planning, and dedicated, contrast-enhanced imaging with CT or MR imaging is indicated for this purpose.

Because well-differentiated SBNETs do not typically show avid uptake of radiolabeled glucose, the role for conventional [18]FDG-PET in the diagnosis of these tumors is limited. The overall sensitivity for any NET disease has been reported from 37% to 72%.[38] However, because poorly differentiated tumors are more metabolically active and less likely to express somatostatin receptors, [18]FDG-PET is useful for the diagnosis of these tumors.[42] In a study comparing [18]FDG-PET with ^{111}In-SRS, the sensitivity of PET increased with grade to 100% in high- grade tumors, whereas an inverse relationship was seen for the sensitivity of ^{111}In-SRS.[46] In addition, there is evidence that combined imaging with [18]FDG-PET and ^{68}Ga-PET provides important prognostic information, with increased uptake on the former and decreased uptake on the latter indicating more aggressive tumor behavior.[47]

Pathology

The diagnosis of SBNET is established by pathologic examination of the tumor. Tissue may be obtained either at the time of surgery or by percutaneous biopsy in patients who present with liver metastases.[20] Immunohistochemistry is used to confirm the diagnosis, with low-molecular-weight keratins, chromogranin, and synaptophysin serving as general NET markers, irrespective of primary site.[20,27,28,34,48] Once the neuroendocrine nature of the tumor is established, the tumor should be graded according to the fifth edition of *Digestive System Tumors: WHO Classification of Tumors* published in 2019 (**Table 1**).[49] New to the most recent edition is the adoption of a unified classification framework for NETs from any anatomic location, which recognizes well-differentiated G3 NETs as distinct from poorly differentiated neuroendocrine carcinoma (NEC), based on the proposal consensus meeting of the WHO and International Agency for Research on Cancer.[50] Under this framework, neuroendocrine neoplasms are divided into well-differentiated NET and poorly differentiated NEC. Based on the proliferative index, assessed by staining for Ki-67 and the mitotic rate (expressed as mitoses per 10 high-power fields), NETs are further subdivided into grade G1 through G3. NECs are considered high grade by definition and are further classified as either small cell or large cell type.[49] Immunohistochemistry should be performed for Ki-67 on both the primary tumor and metastatic tumors, as discrepancies can be seen in up to one-third of patients, with increased grade in the metastasis associated with worse prognosis.[51] For metastatic NETs with unknown primary, additional immunohistochemical staining can be used to suggest the site of origin. Strong positive staining for CDX2 indicates a small bowel primary, whereas TTF-1 positivity suggests pulmonary origin, and staining for ISL1 or PAX6/PAX8 suggests pancreatic origin.[48] The eighth edition of the *AJCC Cancer Staging Manual* is used to stage SBNETs (available at https://www.cancer.org/cancer/gastrointestinal-carcinoid-tumor/detection-diagnosis-staging/staged.html).[52]

SURGICAL MANAGEMENT
Stage I to Stage III Tumors

Surgery is the cornerstone of treatment of locoregional SBNETs and is potentially curative.[20,28,34,36] Primary SBNET tumors are usually small, commonly located within 100 cm of the ileocecal valve and are multifocal in more than half of the cases.[17,53] Because of this, the small bowel should be carefully palpated in its entirety, as additional tumors can easily be missed.[36] Resection of SBNETs consists of segmental small bowel resection or ileocolic resection for distal tumors. For multifocal tumors that are in close proximity to each other, a single segment incorporating all tumors is resected, whereas widely separated tumors may be resected separately.

Table 1
2019 WHO classification of neuroendocrine neoplasms of the gastrointestinal tract

Classification	Ki-67 Index	Mitotic Rate
Well-differentiated NET		
Grade 1	<3%	<2
Grade 2	3%–20%	2–20
Grade 3	>20%	>20
Poorly differentiated NEC		
Small Cell NEC	>20%	>20
Large Cell NEC	>20%	>20
MiNEN	Variable	Variable

Abbreviations: MiNEN, mixed neuroendocrine nonneuroendocrine neoplasm, mitotic rate expressed as mitoses per 10 high power fields; NEC, neuroendocrine carcinoma.

From Board WCoTE. *Digestive System Tumours.* Vol 1. 5th Edition ed: World Health Organization; 2019. With permission.

Metastases to the regional lymph nodes are seen in at least two-thirds of patients with SBNETs and are commonly more prominent than the primary tumors themselves.[11,16,17,22,54,55] In addition to removal of the primary tumor or tumors, optimal surgical treatment of SBNETs includes resection of the regional lymph nodes to the origin of the segmental branches of the superior mesenteric artery and vein, which has been shown to improve survival.[16,17,36,54] The optimal extent of lymphadenectomy in terms of lymph nodes harvested has not been conclusively established, but removal of at least 8 lymph nodes has been suggested as a target that facilitates accurate prognostication and may improve survival.[54,55] However, accurate node counts can be difficult in many cases because associated mesenteric masses may be a conglomeration of nodes not amenable to being counted. In some cases, the mesenteric nodal metastases and fibrosis are found to encase the root of the mesenteric vessels, complicating their removal.[21] Progressive tumor growth and fibrosis can lead to vascular damage and mesenteric ischemia, but the risk of attempted resection must be weighed against the possibility of catastrophic vascular injury from aggressive dissection.[36] Resection of these proximal lymph nodes can lead to significant, durable improvement in symptoms from mesenteric ischemia but is also dangerous, so may be best performed by surgeons specializing in the care of SBNETs.[17,34,36,56]

Complete resection of stage I to III tumors is potentially curative, but long-term recurrence rates of roughly 50% have been reported, with emergency surgery, tumor multifocality, stage, and grade predicting earlier relapse.[22,57] Because SBNETs can recur many years after surgery, surveillance should be continued for approximately 10 years following resection, at 6 to 12 month intervals. Follow-up should generally include cross-sectional imaging with CT or MR imaging, serum tumor markers, and physical examination, although there are significant variations in practice, and surveillance strategies should be tailored to the individual patient.[27,28,34,58]

Stage IV Tumors

The goals of surgery for metastatic SBNETs are to improve survival and palliate symptoms by primary tumor resection and debulking of metastatic disease.[28,34,36] Resection of the primary tumor is performed as described earlier irrespective of distant metastases. Techniques for liver debulking are varied and include formal hepatic resection, nonanatomic wedge resection, enucleation, and thermal ablation. Numerous retrospective surgical series have shown improved survival and symptomatic control in patients undergoing cytoreductive surgery for nodal or hepatic metastases.[16,17,56,59–65] However, despite these data, surgery for metastatic SBNETs is rarely, if ever, curative. Hepatic micrometastases can be observed in all patients with macrometastases, and long-term recurrence is nearly universal.[61,66] Moreover, there seems to be no survival benefit associated with R0 resection.[60,61,67] These data support an aggressive surgical approach, with an emphasis on balancing reduction of tumor bulk with preservation of normal hepatic parenchyma and suggest that curative resection is unlikely for metastatic SBNETs.

The feasibility of complete or greater than 90% cytoreduction has been proposed as the threshold for attempting hepatic debulking since the 1980s.[68,69] However, recent series have shown good results in terms of survival and symptomatic improvement when a lower goal of 70% cytoreduction is used.[59,60,63,64] The use of this less stringent cutoff to select patients for debulking surgery, along with the adoption of parenchyma-sparing surgical techniques including enucleation and ablation instead of formal resection, significantly increases the proportion of patients with SBNET who are eligible for surgery. Approximately three-quarters of patients will be eligible for cytoreductive surgery at the 70% cutoff, in contrast to fewer than a quarter when 90% is used.[36,64] Although the precise indications for and contraindications to debulking surgery continue to evolve, broadly speaking, patients with more than 50% to 70% hepatic replacement, numerous diffuse metastase, poor performance status, carcinoid heart disease, hepatic dysfunction, or high-grade disease should not undergo cytoreduction. Extrahepatic metastases are not a contraindication to cytoreduction and can be resected concurrently.[36] Liver transplantation is another treatment option for patients with SBNETs and hepatic metastases, which has been shown to improve survival in properly selected patients. However, the benefits of transplantation need to be balanced against the risks of lifelong immunosuppression and the shortage of suitable organs.[70] The indications for transplantation are defined by the Milan-NET criteria and are broadly similar to but more restrictive than those for hepatic cytoreduction. Patients must have had their primary tumor resected with no residual extrahepatic disease, have stable disease, and be younger than 55 years.[71] Liver transplantation is rarely performed, even in patients who qualify for it, and reported survival figures with transplant are not superior to those achieved with standard multimodal therapy.[72]

Peritoneal carcinomatosis is seen in 20% of patients with SBNETs and can lead to significant morbidity from bowel obstruction due to tumor implants and fibrosis and poor overall survival.[16,36,73-75] The abdominal cavity of any patient undergoing primary resection or hepatic cytoreduction should be thoroughly inspected for evidence of peritoneal disease. Limited areas of peritoneal seeding may be resected via localized peritoneal stripping or ablated with electrocautery or the argon beam with minimal additional morbidity.[36] However, more extensive cytoreduction of peritoneal metastases is associated with major postoperative complications in more than half of the cases. The addition of hyperthermic intraperitoneal chemotherapy to cytoreductive surgery likely increases the complication rate and has not been shown to improve survival.[75] The mechanism by which SBNETs develops into peritoneal nodules likely involves direct trans-serosal invasion by the primary tumor.[36,73] Thus, the best treatment of carcinomatosis is preemptive via resection of the primary tumor before the development of peritoneal disease.[36]

Resection of the primary tumor in the face of unresectable metastatic disease is performed for 2 reasons: to relieve symptoms due to the primary tumor and to improve survival. Primary resection has consistently been associated with improved survival in retrospective surgical series[16,17,76,77] and in meta-analyses of these series.[78,79] However, as for most surgical therapies in NETs, there are no randomized prospective trials comparing primary resection with observation. Primary resection is hypothesized to improve survival through several mechanisms including prevention of future bowel obstruction or peritoneal seeding and reduction in tumor burden and can be performed with acceptable surgical morbidity.

SURGICAL APPROACH

The standard surgical approach for SBNETs, whether localized or metastatic, is laparotomy. Open surgery facilities thorough inspection of the peritoneal cavity and palpation of the small bowel, which is critical for identifying small and possibly multifocal primary SBNETs. Laparoscopy has been successfully used to identify the primary site in patients with NETs of unknown primary; however, thorough palpation of the intestine, either through placement of a hand port or exteriorization of the bowel, is required.[36,80]

Cholecystectomy

The incidence of gallstones in patients receiving treatment with SSAs is approximately 50%, which is much higher than the general population.[81] The rate of symptomatic gallstone disease or cholecystitis remains low, and prophylactic cholecystectomy as a separate procedure is not generally recommended. However, for patients undergoing surgery for SBNETs, particularly those who are likely to receive long-term treatment with SSAs (eg, those with extensive nodal disease or distant metastases), concurrent cholecystectomy should be offered to potentially spare the need for future operation. Laparoscopic cholecystectomy may be more difficult later on after prior laparotomy.[20,36,81]

Perioperative Octreotide

Patients undergoing surgery are at risk for intraoperative hemodynamic instability, termed "carcinoid crisis," and are commonly given octreotide perioperatively to reduce this risk. Octreotide dosing in this setting is not standardized. The primary evidence for this practice comes from a single-institution, retrospective study of patients undergoing abdominal surgery with metastatic SBNETs, which found that the rate of intraoperative complications was 11% in patients who did not receive intraoperative octreotide, compared with 0% in those who did.[82] However, additional studies have failed to confirm the efficacy of octreotide to prevent intraoperative carcinoid crisis.[36,83] Nevertheless, prophylactic octreotide, either as a preoperative dose or as an intraoperative infusion, is relatively low risk and remains widely used.[36]

LIVER-DIRECTED THERAPY

In addition to surgical debulking, percutaneous ablation and hepatic artery embolization can be used for tumor debulking in patients with liver dominant disease.[20,27] NET metastases to the liver derive most of their blood supply from the hepatic arterial system; thus arterial embolization can be used to direct treatment toward these tumors while relatively sparing surrounding hepatic parenchyma that derives most of its blood flow from the portal vein.[84] Embolotherapy may be performed using inert particles to occlude the feeding arteries, known as bland embolization, or may incorporate locally delivered chemotherapy or radiotherapy with these beads. Currently, the choice of one modality over another is largely institution dependent, as none of these options has shown clearly superior outcomes.[20,84] Liver metastases can also be treated percutaneously using a wide variety of ablative technologies including microwave ablation, radiofrequency ablation, and cryoablation. As with hepatic artery embolization, none of these modalities has proved to be clearly superior for the treatment of NET metastases. The evidence supporting the use of percutaneous ablation is heterogenous and is usually limited to one or a few lesions, but reported symptomatic and radiologic response rates are favorable.[85,86] For patients with hepatic metastases who are not candidates for surgical resection, these other liver-directed therapies are good options for disease control.[20,27,84,86]

CARCINOID HEART DISEASE

Carcinoid heart disease is associated with significantly worse prognosis in patients with SBNETs, particularly those undergoing surgery.[16,26–28] All patients with carcinoid syndrome or with biochemical evidence of serotonin hypersecretion should undergo echocardiogram to evaluate for cardiac valvular disease, and screening by serum N-terminal-pro B-type natriuretic peptide or echocardiography should be considered in patients with metastatic disease, even in the absence of symptoms. Patients with severe valvular disease are treated with valve replacement. Although this is a high-risk surgical procedure that is associated with a 10% to 20% mortality rate, the survival benefits of surgery outweigh the risk in patients with an expected survival of more than 6 to 12 months.[26,27]

SYSTEMIC TREATMENT

Treatment of metastatic SBNETs is multimodal, and in the last several decades, several agents have emerged as promising therapies for SBNETs. Antiproliferative treatments include SSAs, targeted therapy, and peptide receptor radionuclide therapy (PRRT), whereas SSAs and telotristat are used for symptom control.[20,27] Although responses to systemic therapy are typically modest, several agents have been shown to improve PFS in randomized controlled trials. SSAs have long been used to decrease hormone secretion and treat the symptoms of carcinoid syndrome, but more recent studies have also demonstrated their antiproliferative activity.[20,27] In the PROMID trial, Octreotide long-acting release (LAR) was associated with a significantly longer median PFS than placebo (14.3 vs 6 months) in patients with metastatic midgut NETs.[87] In the CLARINET study, lanreotide was compared with placebo and was also associated with significantly improved median PFS (not reached vs 18 months).[88] Either of these SSAs can be used as first-line therapy in patients with metastatic SBNETs, and patients can be switched to the other agent if issues arise.[27] In the RADIANT-2 trial, the mammalian target of rapamycin inhibitor, everolimus, showed a trend toward improved PFS in a group of patients with NETs from a variety of primary sites, and although this did not reach statistical significance, the subsequent RADIANT-4 trial showed significantly longer median PFS in patients with NETs treated with everolimus compared with placebo (11 vs 3.9 months).[89,90] PRRT uses a radiolabeled SSA to deliver therapy selectively to cells expressing somatostatin receptors. In the NETTER-1 trial, ^{177}Lu-DOTATATE PRRT plus octreotide LAR was compared with octreotide LAR alone and was associated with significantly better PFS (not reached vs 8.4 months) in patients with advanced SBNETs.[91] Finally, for patients on SSAs with refractory carcinoid syndrome, the tryptophan hydroxylase inhibitor telotristat was shown to significantly reduce the frequency of bowel movements and urinary 5-HIAA levels in patients with carcinoid syndrome.[92,93]

PROGNOSIS

The prognosis for patients with SBNETs is favorable, particularly when compared with other malignancies arising from the GI tract and pancreas. For patients with completely resected, stage I through III SBNETs, the 20 year disease-specific survival is greater than 75%.[94] Even for patients diagnosed with metastatic disease, the median OS is approximately 8.5 years, and OS continues to improve.[7] Because of this and the increasing incidence of SBNETs, there are ever increasing numbers of patients living with these tumors, and one should be careful not to confuse their less aggressive biology with benign symptomatology. Patients with SBNETs receiving modern multimodal therapy report significantly decreased quality of life across a wide range of dimensions.[95]

HIGH-GRADE DISEASE

Formerly, all high-grade tumors were designated as poorly differentiated NEC by definition. In the most recent WHO system, high-grade tumors are classified as well-differentiated G3 NET or poorly differentiated NEC, and NECs are further subdivided into small-cell and large-cell types.[49,50] High-grade SBNETs and NECs originating in the small bowel are relatively rare, and owing to this, prognostication and treatment regimens in NECs are informed by data primarily derived from other primary sites.[36,96] The median survival for patients with gastroenteropancreatic NEC is 11 months.[97] First-line therapy for patients with NEC, regardless of primary site, is cisplatin or carboplatin plus etoposide or irinotecan.[96,98] Tumors with Ki-67 indices between 20% and 55% have better survival but are less likely to respond to platinum-based chemotherapy, whereas those with higher Ki-67 indices have better response rates but worse survival.[97] Several other agents have been used for second-line therapy, but none have been well validated and there is no standard second-line treatment.[96,98] Although surgical resection may be considered for patients with localized high-grade disease, the majority will present with or develop metastases and derive little benefit from cytoreductive surgery.[36,59]

SUMMARY

The incidence of NETs is increasing, and they are now the most common malignancy of the small intestine. They most commonly present with abdominal pain or other GI symptoms such as diarrhea, and because of the nonspecific nature of these symptoms, long delays in diagnosis are possible. In patients suspected to have SBNET, anatomic imaging with CT and MR imaging or functional imaging with ^{68}Ga-PET along with biochemical testing for tumor markers including CgA can lead to the correct diagnosis. Pathologic examination with immunohistochemistry for CgA and synaptophysin is required to confirm the diagnosis, but for patients without metastases, this is often performed only after surgery. For patients with localized disease, surgical resection is potentially curative, and although recurrence rates are high, long-term prognosis is generally excellent. Even for patients who present with or go on to develop metastases, survival of a decade or more is achievable with modern multimodal therapy, which includes SSAs, everolimus, surgical debulking, liver-directed therapy, and PRRT.

DISCLOSURE

The authors have no conflicts of interest to disclose. This work was supported by the T32 grant CA148062-0 (A.T. Scott) and SPORE grant P50 CA174521-01 (J.R. Howe).

REFERENCES

1. Langhans T. Ueber einen Drüsenpolyp im ileum. Virchows Arch 1867;38:559–60.

2. Lubarsch O. Ueber den primären Krebs des Ileum nebst Bemerkungen über das gleichzeitige Vorkommen von Krebs und Tuberculose. Virchows Arch 1888;111: 280–317.

3. Ransom WB. A case of primary carcinoma of the ileum. Lancet 1890;136(3507): 1020–3.

4. Oberndorfer S. Karzinoide Tumoren des Dünndarms. Frankf Z Pathol 1907;1: 425–32.

5. Kloppel G. Classification and pathology of gastroenteropancreatic neuroendocrine neoplasms. Endocr Relat Cancer 2011;18(Suppl 1):S1–16.

6. Williams ED, Sandler M. The classification of carcinoid tumours. Lancet 1963; 1(7275):238–9.

7. Dasari A, Shen C, Halperin D, et al. Trends in the incidence, prevalence, and survival outcomes in patients with neuroendocrine tumors in the United States. JAMA Oncol 2017;3(10):1335–42.

8. Fraenkel M, Kim M, Faggiano A, et al. Incidence of gastroenteropancreatic neuro-endocrine tumours: a systematic review of the literature. Endocr Relat Cancer 2014;21(3):R153–63.

9. Hallet J, Law CH, Cukier M, et al. Exploring the rising incidence of neuroendo-crine tumors: a population-based analysis of epidemiology, metastatic presenta-tion, and outcomes. Cancer 2015;121(4):589–97.

10. Bilimoria KY, Bentrem DJ, Wayne JD, et al. Small bowel cancer in the United States: changes in epidemiology, treatment, and survival over the last 20 years. Ann Surg 2009;249(1):63–71.

11. Yao JC, Hassan M, Phan A, et al. One hundred years after "carcinoid": epidemi-ology of and prognostic factors for neuroendocrine tumors in 35,825 cases in the United States. J Clin Oncol 2008;26(18):3063–72.

12. Lawrence B, Gustafsson BI, Chan A, et al. The epidemiology of gastroentero-pancreatic neuroendocrine tumors. Endocrinol Metab Clin North Am 2011; 40(1):1–18.

13. Landerholm K, Falkmer S, Jarhult J. Epidemiology of small bowel carcinoids in a defined population. World J Surg 2010;34(7):1500–5.

14. Dahdaleh FS, Calva-Cerqueira D, Carr JC, et al. Comparison of clinicopathologic factors in 122 patients with resected pancreatic and ileal neuroendocrine tumors from a single institution. Ann Surg Oncol 2012;19(3):966–72.

15. Ter-Minassian M, Chan JA, Hooshmand SM, et al. Clinical presentation, recur-rence, and survival in patients with neuroendocrine tumors: results from a pro-spective institutional database. Endocr Relat Cancer 2013;20(2):187–96.

16. Norlen O, Stalberg P, Oberg K, et al. Long-term results of surgery for small intes-tinal neuroendocrine tumors at a tertiary referral center. World J Surg 2012;36(6): 1419–31.

17. Hellman P, Lundstrom T, Ohrvall U, et al. Effect of surgery on the outcome of midgut carcinoid disease with lymph node and liver metastases. World J Surg 2002;26(8):991–7.

18. Modlin IM, Kidd M, Latich I, et al. Current status of gastrointestinal carcinoids. Gastroenterology 2005;128(6):1717–51.

19. Vinik AI, Chaya C. Clinical presentation and diagnosis of neuroendocrine tumors. Hematol Oncol Clin North Am 2016;30(1):21–48.

20. Singh S, Asa SL, Dey C, et al. Diagnosis and management of gastrointestinal neuroendocrine tumors: an evidence-based Canadian consensus. Cancer Treat Rev 2016;47:32–45.

21. Modlin IM, Shapiro MD, Kidd M. Carcinoid tumors and fibrosis: an association with no explanation. Am J Gastroenterol 2004;99(12):2466–78.

22. Le Roux C, Lombard-Bohas C, Delmas C, et al. Relapse factors for ileal neuroen-docrine tumours after curative surgery: a retrospective French multicentre study. Dig Liver Dis 2011;43(10):828–33.

23. Kunikowska J, Pawlak D, Kolasa A, et al. A frequency and semiquantitative anal-ysis of pathological 68Ga DOTATATE PET/CT uptake by primary site-dependent neuroendocrine tumor metastasis. Clin Nucl Med 2014;39(10):855–61.

24. Riihimaki M, Hemminki A, Sundquist K, et al. The epidemiology of metastases in neuroendocrine tumors. Int J Cancer 2016;139(12):2679–86.

25. Thorson A, Biorck G, Bjorkman G, et al. Malignant carcinoid of the small intestine with metastases to the liver, valvular disease of the right side of the heart (pulmo-nary stenosis and tricuspid regurgitation without septal defects), peripheral vaso-motor symptoms, bronchoconstriction, and an unusual type of cyanosis; a clinical and pathologic syndrome. Am Heart J 1954;47(5):795–817.

26. Luis SA, Pellikka PA. Carcinoid heart disease: diagnosis and management. Best Pract Res Clin Endocrinol Metab 2016;30(1):149–58.
27. Strosberg JR, Halfdanarson TR, Bellizzi AM, et al. The North American Neuroendocrine Tumor Society consensus guidelines for surveillance and medical management of midgut neuroendocrine tumors. Pancreas 2017;46(6):707–14.
28. Pape UF, Perren A, Niederle B, et al. ENETS consensus guidelines for the management of patients with neuroendocrine neoplasms from the jejuno-ileum and the appendix including goblet cell carcinomas. Neuroendocrinology 2012; 95(2):135–56.
29. Vinik AI, Silva MP, Woltering EA, et al. Biochemical testing for neuroendocrine tumors. Pancreas 2009;38(8):876–89.
30. Yang X, Yang Y, Li Z, et al. Diagnostic value of circulating chromogranin a for neuroendocrine tumors: a systematic review and meta-analysis. PLoS One 2015;10(4):e0124884.
31. Sherman SK, Maxwell JE, O'Dorisio MS, et al. Pancreastatin predicts survival in neuroendocrine tumors. Ann Surg Oncol 2014;21(9):2971–80.
32. Woltering EA, Voros BA, Beyer DT, et al. Plasma pancreastatin predicts the outcome of surgical cytoreduction in neuroendocrine tumors of the small bowel. Pancreas 2019;48(3):356–62.
33. Strosberg D, Schneider EB, Onesti J, et al. Prognostic impact of serum pancreastatin following chemoembolization for neuroendocrine tumors. Ann Surg Oncol 2018;25(12):3613–20.
34. Boudreaux JP, Klimstra DS, Hassan MM, et al. The NANETS consensus guideline for the diagnosis and management of neuroendocrine tumors: well-differentiated neuroendocrine tumors of the Jejunum, Ileum, Appendix, and Cecum. Pancreas 2010;39(6):753–66.
35. Maxwell JE, Howe JR. Imaging in neuroendocrine tumors: an update for the clinician. Int J Endocr Oncol 2015;2(2):159–68.
36. Howe JR, Cardona K, Fraker DL, et al. The surgical management of small bowel neuroendocrine tumors: consensus guidelines of the North American neuroendocrine tumor society. Pancreas 2017;46(6):715–31.
37. Keck KJ, Maxwell JE, Menda Y, et al. Identification of primary tumors in patients presenting with metastatic gastroenteropancreatic neuroendocrine tumors. Surgery 2017;161(1):272–9.
38. Sundin A, Arnold R, Baudin E, et al. ENETS consensus guidelines for the standards of care in neuroendocrine tumors: radiological, nuclear medicine & hybrid imaging. Neuroendocrinology 2017;105(3):212–44.
39. Dromain C, de Baere T, Lumbroso J, et al. Detection of liver metastases from endocrine tumors: a prospective comparison of somatostatin receptor scintigraphy, computed tomography, and magnetic resonance imaging. J Clin Oncol 2005;23(1):70–8.
40. Ruf J, Schiefer J, Furth C, et al. 68Ga-DOTATOC PET/CT of neuroendocrine tumors: spotlight on the CT phases of a triple-phase protocol. J Nucl Med 2011; 52(5):697–704.
41. Tirumani SH, Jagannathan JP, Braschi-Amirfarzan M, et al. Value of hepatocellular phase imaging after intravenous gadoxetate disodium for assessing hepatic metastases from gastroenteropancreatic neuroendocrine tumors: comparison with other MRI pulse sequences and with extracellular agent. Abdom Radiol (NY) 2018;43(9):2329–39.
42. Reubi JC. Somatostatin and other peptide receptors as tools for tumor diagnosis and treatment. Neuroendocrinology 2004;80(Suppl 1):51–6.

43. Krenning EP, Kwekkeboom DJ, Bakker WH, et al. Somatostatin receptor scintigraphy with [111In-DTPA-D-Phe1]- and [123I-Tyr3]-octreotide: the Rotterdam experience with more than 1000 patients. Eur J Nucl Med 1993;20(8):716–31.

44. Van Binnebeek S, Vanbilloen B, Baete K, et al. Comparison of diagnostic accuracy of (111)In-pentetreotide SPECT and (68)Ga-DOTATOC PET/CT: a lesion-by-lesion analysis in patients with metastatic neuroendocrine tumours. Eur Radiol 2016;26(3):900–9.

45. Bozkurt MF, Virgolini I, Balogova S, et al. Guideline for PET/CT imaging of neuroendocrine neoplasms with (68)Ga-DOTA-conjugated somatostatin receptor targeting peptides and (18)F-DOPA. Eur J Nucl Med Mol Imaging 2017;44(9): 1588–601.

46. Squires MH 3rd, Volkan Adsay N, Schuster DM, et al. Octreoscan versus FDG-PET for neuroendocrine tumor staging: a biological approach. Ann Surg Oncol 2015;22(7):2295–301.

47. Carideo L, Prosperi D, Panzuto F, et al. Role of combined [68Ga]Ga-DOTA-SST analogues and [18F]FDG PET/CT in the management of GEP-NENs: a systematic review. J Clin Med 2019;8(7) [pii:E1032].

48. Bellizzi AM. Assigning site of origin in metastatic neuroendocrine neoplasms: a clinically significant application of diagnostic immunohistochemistry. Adv Anat Pathol 2013;20(5):285–314.

49. WHO Classification of Tumors. 5th edition. Digestive system tumours. Lyon: International Agency for Research on Cancer(IARC); 2019.

50. Rindi G, Klimstra DS, Abedi-Ardekani B, et al. A common classification framework for neuroendocrine neoplasms: an International Agency for Research on Cancer (IARC) and World Health Organization (WHO) expert consensus proposal. Mod Pathol 2018;31(12):1770–86.

51. Keck KJ, Choi A, Maxwell JE, et al. Increased grade in neuroendocrine tumor metastases negatively impacts survival. Ann Surg Oncol 2017;24(8):2206–12.

52. Amin MB, Edge SB, Greene F, et al. AJCC cancer staging manual. 8th edition. New York: Springer; 2017.

53. Keck KJ, Maxwell JE, Utria AF, et al. The distal predilection of small bowel neuroendocrine tumors. Ann Surg Oncol 2018;25(11):3207–13.

54. Landry CS, Lin HY, Phan A, et al. Resection of at-risk mesenteric lymph nodes is associated with improved survival in patients with small bowel neuroendocrine tumors. World J Surg 2013;37(7):1695–700.

55. Zaidi MY, Lopez-Aguiar AG, Dillhoff M, et al. Prognostic role of lymph node positivity and number of lymph nodes needed for accurately staging small-bowel neuroendocrine tumors. JAMA Surg 2019;154(2):134–40.

56. Ohrvall U, Eriksson B, Juhlin C, et al. Method for dissection of mesenteric metastases in mid-gut carcinoid tumors. World J Surg 2000;24(11):1402–8.

57. Dieckhoff P, Runkel H, Daniel H, et al. Well-differentiated neuroendocrine neoplasia: relapse-free survival and predictors of recurrence after curative intended resections. Digestion 2014;90(2):89–97.

58. Arnold R, Chen YJ, Costa F, et al. ENETS consensus guidelines for the standards of care in neuroendocrine tumors: follow-up and documentation. Neuroendocrinology 2009;90(2):227–33.

59. Scott AT, Breheny PJ, Keck KJ, et al. Effective cytoreduction can be achieved in patients with numerous neuroendocrine tumor liver metastases (NETLMs). Surgery 2019;165(1):166–75.

60. Graff-Baker AN, Sauer DA, Pommier SJ, et al. Expanded criteria for carcinoid liver debulking: maintaining survival and increasing the number of eligible patients. Surgery 2014;156(6):1369–76.
61. Mayo SC, de Jong MC, Pulitano C, et al. Surgical management of hepatic neuroendocrine tumor metastasis: results from an international multi-institutional analysis. Ann Surg Oncol 2010;17(12):3129–36.
62. Sarmiento JM, Heywood G, Rubin J, et al. Surgical treatment of neuroendocrine metastases to the liver: a plea for resection to increase survival. J Am Coll Surg 2003;197(1):29–37.
63. Chambers AJ, Pasieka JL, Dixon E, et al. The palliative benefit of aggressive surgical intervention for both hepatic and mesenteric metastases from neuroendocrine tumors. Surgery 2008;144(4):645–51 [discussion: 651–3].
64. Maxwell JE, Sherman SK, O'Dorisio TM, et al. Liver-directed surgery of neuroendocrine metastases: what is the optimal strategy? Surgery 2016;159(1):320–33.
65. Boudreaux JP, Wang YZ, Diebold AE, et al. A single institution's experience with surgical cytoreduction of stage IV, well-differentiated, small bowel neuroendocrine tumors. J Am Coll Surg 2014;218(4):837–44.
66. Fossmark R, Balto TM, Martinsen TC, et al. Hepatic micrometastases outside macrometastases are present in all patients with ileal neuroendocrine primary tumour at the time of liver resection. Scand J Gastroenterol 2019;54(8):1003–7.
67. Glazer ES, Tseng JF, Al-Refaie W, et al. Long-term survival after surgical management of neuroendocrine hepatic metastases. HPB (Oxford) 2010;12(6):427–33.
68. Foster JH, Lundy J. Liver metastases. Curr Probl Surg 1981;18(3):157–202.
69. McEntee GP, Nagorney DM, Kvols LK, et al. Cytoreductive hepatic surgery for neuroendocrine tumors. Surgery 1990;108(6):1091–6.
70. Moris D, Tsilimigras DI, Ntanasis-Stathopoulos I, et al. Liver transplantation in patients with liver metastases from neuroendocrine tumors: a systematic review. Surgery 2017;162(3):525–36.
71. Mazzaferro V, Pulvirenti A, Coppa J. Neuroendocrine tumors metastatic to the liver: how to select patients for liver transplantation? J Hepatol 2007;47(4):460–6.
72. Norlen O, Daskalakis K, Oberg K, et al. Indication for liver transplantation in young patients with small intestinal NETs is rare? World J Surg 2014;38(3):742–7.
73. Vasseur B, Cadiot G, Zins M, et al. Peritoneal carcinomatosis in patients with digestive endocrine tumors. Cancer 1996;78(8):1686–92.
74. Norlen O, Edfeldt K, Akerstrom G, et al. Peritoneal carcinomatosis from small intestinal neuroendocrine tumors: clinical course and genetic profiling. Surgery 2014;156(6):1512–21 [discussion: 1521–2].
75. Elias D, David A, Sourrouille I, et al. Neuroendocrine carcinomas: optimal surgery of peritoneal metastases (and associated intra-abdominal metastases). Surgery 2014;155(1):5–12.
76. Givi B, Pommier SJ, Thompson AK, et al. Operative resection of primary carcinoid neoplasms in patients with liver metastases yields significantly better survival. Surgery 2006;140(6):891–7 [discussion: 897–8].
77. Lewis A, Raoof M, Ituarte PHG, et al. Resection of the primary gastrointestinal neuroendocrine tumor improves survival with or without liver treatment. Ann Surg 2019;270(6):1131–7.
78. Almond LM, Hodson J, Ford SJ, et al. Role of palliative resection of the primary tumour in advanced pancreatic and small intestinal neuroendocrine tumours: a systematic review and meta-analysis. Eur J Surg Oncol 2017;43(10):1808–15.
79. Tsilimigras DI, Ntanasis-Stathopoulos I, Kostakis ID, et al. Is resection of primary midgut neuroendocrine tumors in patients with unresectable metastatic liver

disease justified? A systematic review and meta-analysis. J Gastrointest Surg 2019;23(5):1044–54.

80. Massimino KP, Han E, Pommier SJ, et al. Laparoscopic surgical exploration is an effective strategy for locating occult primary neuroendocrine tumors. Am J Surg 2012;203(5):628–31.

81. Trendle MC, Moertel CG, Kvols LK. Incidence and morbidity of cholelithiasis in patients receiving chronic octreotide for metastatic carcinoid and malignant islet cell tumors. Cancer 1997;79(4):830–4.

82. Kinney MA, Warner ME, Nagorney DM, et al. Perianaesthetic risks and outcomes of abdominal surgery for metastatic carcinoid tumours. Br J Anaesth 2001;87(3): 447–52.

83. Massimino K, Harrskog O, Pommier S, et al. Octreotide LAR and bolus octreotide are insufficient for preventing intraoperative complications in carcinoid patients. J Surg Oncol 2013;107(8):842–6.

84. Kennedy AS. Hepatic-directed therapies in patients with neuroendocrine tumors. Hematol Oncol Clin North Am 2016;30(1):193–207.

85. Mohan H, Nicholson P, Winter DC, et al. Radiofrequency ablation for neuroendocrine liver metastases: a systematic review. J Vasc Interv Radiol 2015;26(7): 935–42.e1.

86. Lewis MA, Hobday TJ. Treatment of neuroendocrine tumor liver metastases. Int J Hepatol 2012;2012:973946.

87. Rinke A, Muller HH, Schade-Brittinger C, et al. Placebo-controlled, double-blind, prospective, randomized study on the effect of octreotide LAR in the control of tumor growth in patients with metastatic neuroendocrine midgut tumors: a report from the PROMID study group. J Clin Oncol 2009;27(28):4656–63.

88. Caplin ME, Pavel M, Cwikla JB, et al. Lanreotide in metastatic enteropancreatic neuroendocrine tumors. N Engl J Med 2014;371(3):224–33.

89. Pavel ME, Hainsworth JD, Baudin E, et al. Everolimus plus octreotide long-acting repeatable for the treatment of advanced neuroendocrine tumours associated with carcinoid syndrome (RADIANT-2): a randomised, placebo-controlled, phase 3 study. Lancet 2011;378(9808):2005–12.

90. Yao JC, Fazio N, Singh S, et al. Everolimus for the treatment of advanced, non-functional neuroendocrine tumours of the lung or gastrointestinal tract (RADIANT-4): a randomised, placebo-controlled, phase 3 study. Lancet 2016; 387(10022):968–77.

91. Strosberg J, El-Haddad G, Wolin E, et al. Phase 3 trial of (177)Lu-Dotatate for midgut neuroendocrine tumors. N Engl J Med 2017;376(2):125–35.

92. Kulke MH, Horsch D, Caplin ME, et al. Telotristat ethyl, a tryptophan hydroxylase inhibitor for the treatment of carcinoid syndrome. J Clin Oncol 2017;35(1):14–23.

93. Pavel M, Gross DJ, Benavent M, et al. Telotristat ethyl in carcinoid syndrome: safety and efficacy in the TELECAST phase 3 trial. Endocr Relat Cancer 2018; 25(3):309–22.

94. Chi W, Warner RRP, Chan DL, et al. Long-term outcomes of gastroenteropancreatic neuroendocrine tumors. Pancreas 2018;47(3):321–5.

95. Karppinen N, Linden R, Sintonen H, et al. Health-related quality of life in patients with small intestine neuroendocrine tumors. Neuroendocrinology 2018;107(4): 366–74.

96. Ilett EE, Langer SW, Olsen IH, et al. Neuroendocrine carcinomas of the gastroenteropancreatic system: a comprehensive review. Diagnostics (Basel) 2015;5(2): 119–76.

97. Sorbye H, Welin S, Langer SW, et al. Predictive and prognostic factors for treatment and survival in 305 patients with advanced gastrointestinal neuroendocrine carcinoma (WHO G3): the NORDIC NEC study. Ann Oncol 2013;24(1):152–60.
98. Garcia-Carbonero R, Rinke A, Valle JW, et al. ENETS consensus guidelines for the standards of care in neuroendocrine neoplasms. Systemic therapy 2: chemotherapy. Neuroendocrinology 2017;105(3):281–94.

Surgical Management of Pancreatic Neuroendocrine Tumors

Tanaz Vaghaiwalla, MD, Xavier M. Keutgen, MD*

KEYWORDS

- Pancreatic neuroendocrine tumor • Hepatic metastases • Liver debulking surgery
- Primary tumor resection

KEY POINTS

- Pancreatic neuroendocrine tumors (PNETs) originate from the islet cells of Langerhans, and their incidence is steadily increasing. Their prognosis is better than that of adenocarcinomas of the pancreas but worse than other gastrointestinal neuroendocrine tumors.
- PNETs can be classified according to their hormone production into functional and nonfunctional tumors. Common hormones secreted by PNETs include gastrin and insulin.
- Like other cancer types, PNETs need to be appropriately staged with anatomic and occasionally functional imaging modalities. However, additional information about tumor grade and biochemical markers also needs to be obtained.
- Localized PNETs greater than 2 cm should be resected surgically because this is the only chance for cure. PNETs less than 2 cm can be observed in certain circumstances.
- PNETs most commonly metastasize to the liver. Multiple therapies exist for liver metastases, and surgical debulking is one of them.

INCIDENCE, STAGING, DIAGNOSIS
Incidence and Prevalence

Pancreatic neuroendocrine tumors (PNETs) are a unique group of pancreatic neoplasms arising from the islets of Langerhans.[1,2] Historically they were thought to constitute only 2% to 3% of all pancreatic neoplasms, but more recent studies demonstrate that PNETs comprise nearly 10% of all pancreatic malignancies.[1] They exhibit a slight male predominance (55%) compared with women (45%) with an average age of diagnosis of 58 years. PNETs are most commonly diagnosed in white patients, whereas blacks and Asians seem to be less frequently affected.[2] In the

Department of Surgery, Division of General Surgery and Surgical Oncology, Endocrine Research Program, University of Chicago Medicine, 5841 South Maryland Avenue, MC4052, Chicago, IL 60637, USA
* Corresponding author.
E-mail address: xkeutgen@surgery.bsd.uchicago.edu

Surg Oncol Clin N Am 29 (2020) 243–252
https://doi.org/10.1016/j.soc.2019.11.008
1055-3207/20/© 2019 Elsevier Inc. All rights reserved.
surgonc.theclinics.com

United States, the estimated incidence for PNETs is less than 1 in 100,000; however, recent studies demonstrate that this incidence is increasing.[2–5] This increase may in part be due to technological advances in detection and the frequency of cross-sectional imaging being performed.[6] PNETs have the worse overall survival of all gastroenteropancreatic NETs (GEP-NETS), as demonstrated in a Surveillance, Epidemiology, and End Results (SEER) database analysis examining 49,012 GEP-NETS. In that study, patients with PNETs had a 5-year survival of only 36.5%, but survival is also stage dependent, and small, early-stage PNETs have an excellent prognosis. Unlike other GEP-NETs, PNETs are more often diagnosed at a higher stage with the presence of distant metastases in up to 40% at disease presentation, perhaps reflecting a more aggressive underlying biologic behavior than other abdominal NETs.[6] Poorly differentiated neuroendocrine carcinomas of the pancreas (PNECs) are aggressive tumors with tumor histology having a large- or small-cell pattern.[5] These tumors are often widely metastatic at diagnosis, and treatment very rarely involves surgical resection. Therefore, this review does not include PNECs but rather focuses on well- or moderately differentiated PNETs.

Functionality

PNETs can be classified as functional or nonfunctional tumors depending on whether they produce or secrete a particular hormone.[1] Nonfunctional tumors comprise most PNETs (>85%) and are often discovered either incidentally during cross-sectional imaging studies ordered for other diagnostic purposes or because of local symptoms.[2,7] Functional tumors on the other hand are often diagnosed because of a range of symptoms caused by the specific type of hormone secretion. Functional PNETs include insulinomas, glucagonomas, gastrinomas, VIPomas, and somatostatinomas and are named for the specific hormone produced in excess. Certain hormone-producing PNETs, such as those secreting pancreatic polypeptide, may not produce a clinical syndrome. The malignancy risk of functional PNETs varies widely between subtypes.[5]

Familial Syndromes

PNETS may arise either sporadically or be associated with familial syndromes. The most common familial syndromes that carry risk of developing PNETs are multiple endocrine neoplasia type 1 (MEN1) and Von Hippel–Lindau syndrome (VHL), mediated by inheritance and loss of the tumor suppressor genes Menin and VHL, respectively.[1,7–9] PNETs developing in patients with MEN1 syndrome can either be functional or nonfunctional. Insulinomas are most commonly resected surgically, whereas gastrinomas can either be managed surgically or medically depending on their size and stage. Nonfunctioning PNETs in patients with MEN1 are usually resected when they reach a tumor size of 2 cm, because larger tumors are more likely to metastasize. PNETs developing in patients with VHL are almost always nonfunctional and should be resected if they are equal or greater than 3 cm, with a tumor doubling time less than 500 days or with exon 3 mutations. Additional familial syndromes associated with the development of PNETs include tuberous sclerosis (TSC1 and TSC2) and neurofibromatosis type 1.[9]

Staging

Pancreatic NETs are staged according to the American Joint Committee on Cancer (AJCC) TNM staging system.[10] Although AJCC does not include tumor grade in the pathologic staging, it is one of the most important prognostic factors. Consequently, the grading of PNETs is of critical importance in determining therapeutic strategies. The tumor grade is determined by the tumor mitotic count and the Ki-67 proliferation index. In 2010, the World Health Organization (WHO) defined well-differentiated tumors to include low or intermediate grades with a mitotic count of ≤20 mitoses per high-power field and a Ki-67 index ≤20%. Poorly differentiated tumors were defined as those with greater than 20 mitoses per high-power field or a Ki-67 index greater than 20%.[11] This WHO classification was updated in 2017, with the recognition that grade 3 tumors with a Ki-67 index greater than 20% had different outcomes, depending on whether they had a well-differentiated or a poorly differentiated histopathology (now defined as neuroendocrine carcinoma) (Table 1).[12–14]

Diagnosis

The diagnostic evaluation of PNETs includes both biochemical workup and anatomic imaging. Additional diagnostic components may also include biopsies with pathologic confirmation or functional imaging, such as nuclear medicine studies. If the patient demonstrates hormone excess on biochemical workup (elevated gastrin, insulin, somatostatin, glucagon, or vasoactive intestinal peptide), medical therapies can be used for symptomatic relief, whereas surgery offers the chance for cure in patients with localized disease.[15] Serum tumor markers, such as Chromogranin A, can be performed at baseline, during, and after treatment but are not diagnostic on their own because false positive values are frequent.[8] Other markers such as pancreastatin for well-differentiated PNETs and neuron-specific enolase for poorly differentiated PNETs may be more accurate at diagnosing and monitoring these tumors.[16,17]

A careful assessment of the primary tumor should be performed with anatomic imaging, such as computed tomography (CT) or MRI with intravenous contrast, which is useful for determining the location of the primary tumor, the presence of involved regional nodes, and metastatic disease.[5] These tests can be performed with a pancreas protocol for primary tumor location and a triple-phase CT protocol, or MRI with gadoxetate disodium protocol to rule out metastatic disease to the liver. Endoscopic ultrasound (EUS) can be performed to identify the location of lesions within the pancreas, especially when anatomic imaging is nondiagnostic or indeterminate.[5] EUS can also be used to biopsy these lesions and determine their tumor grade, which may influence treatment.[5,8,18] Functional imaging with [68]Gallium-DOTATATE PET/CT is highly accurate at diagnosing well- or moderately differentiated PNETs when cross-sectional imaging is indeterminate or the primary tumor site is unknown. ^{111}In-DTPA-pentetreotide (Octreoscan) should be abandoned because [68]Gallium-DOTATATE PET/CT is more accurate, exposes patients to less radiation, and is faster to perform. Studies have demonstrated that performance of [68]Gallium-DOTATATE PET/CT changes therapeutic management in up to two-thirds of patients with NETs.[19]

Table 1
World Health Organization 2017 classification of neuroendocrine neoplasms

Differentiation	Definition	Grade	Ki67 (% of ≥500 Cells)	Mitotic Count (2 mm²)
Well differentiated	NET	G1	<3	<2
		G2	3–20	2–20
		G3	>20	>20
Poorly differentiated	NEC Small cell type Large cell type	G3 (default)	>20	>20

Abbreviations: NEC, neuroendocrine carcinoma; NEN, neuroendocrine neoplasm.
Data from Refs.[12–14]

TUMOR LOCATION

Insulinomas, glucagonomas, and VIPomas are found almost exclusively within the pancreatic parenchyma, but the location of these tumors within the pancreas varies as well. Insulinomas can be found anywhere in the pancreas and may arise as single or multiple tumors. Somatostatinomas are more often found in the pancreatic head or around the duodenal ampulla. VIPomas are most commonly found in the pancreatic tail. Gastrinomas may occur in the pancreas but are more common in the duodenum. Nonfunctional PNETs can be found in the head, body, or tail of the pancreas without a clear predilection.[5,20–22]

Localizing and staging the primary tumor play an important role in ensuring accurate diagnosis and appropriate surgical treatment. Surgical removal of PNETs consists of different operations depending on the location of the primary tumor, including pancreaticoduodenectomy for tumors localized to the pancreatic head, distal pancreatectomy with or without splenectomy for tumors localized in the body or tail, a central pancreatectomy for tumors in the body, and parenchymal-sparing enucleations with or without lymphadenectomy for smaller PNETs that do not involve the main pancreatic duct.[8,18,22] These cases can be performed open or via a minimal invasive approach depending on the surgeon's expertise.

RESECTION OF THE PRIMARY TUMOR

Although there are numerous treatment options for metastatic PNETs, such as somatostatin analogues, peptide receptor radionuclide therapy (PRRT), and chemotherapy, surgery remains the treatment of choice for localized PNETs.[5,21–23] Resection of the primary tumor when there are metastases can also potentially offer symptomatic and survival benefits.[23–27] One SEER database study demonstrated that surgery significantly improved survival in contrast to no surgery (114 months vs 35 months). The improvement in survival was identified in patients with localized, regional, and metastatic disease.[23] It is therefore generally recommended that patients be evaluated by an experienced surgeon regardless of tumor stage. Surgery is recommended for all functional localized PNETs to alleviate symptoms and improve quality of life. For nonfunctional PNETs, tumor size may impact surgical decision making. Surgery is recommended for tumor sizes greater than 2 cm because these tumors demonstrate greater risk of malignancy and metastatic potential.[5,18,21,22] Oncologic pancreatic resection is considered for those tumors greater than 2 cm in size whereby pancreatic duct involvement or proximity is a concern, intermediate- or high-grade tumors, or with regional lymph node involvement.[18,22] Preoperative imaging with cross-sectional imaging, such as CT scan or MRI as well as EUS, can play an important role in defining the tumor relationship to critical anatomic structures. Intraoperative ultrasound and intraoperative evaluation for local and distant metastases may impact the tumor stage and determine resectability. Generally, enucleation that is performed for curative intent is reserved for localized, well-circumscribed, well-differentiated tumors, with no involvement of the pancreatic duct, and no evidence of regional lymph node or distant metastases.[5,18,22]

Small Nonfunctional Pancreatic Neuroendocrine Tumors

The management of nonfunctional tumors less than 2 cm in size is controversial. Given their indolent and benign nature, tumors less than 2 cm in size that are low grade can be considered for observation with serial cross-sectional imaging according to various guidelines.[5,18,21,22] However, some studies have also demonstrated that PNET less than 2 cm in size may have lymph node metastases in nearly 30% of patients, and it is unclear how this impacts long-term survival.[18,28,29] One study showed no survival benefit to performing lymphadenectomy for tumors less than 2 cm in size.[30] At this time, guidelines accept nonoperative management for small PNETs as long as frequent surveillance is maintained and the tumors are low grade on biopsy.[22]

Primary Tumor Resection with Unresectable Distant Metastases

Management of the primary tumor in the setting of unresectable stage IV disease is also a topic of controversy. Several large database studies have demonstrated a survival benefit for primary tumor resection in functional and nonfunctional PNETS when there is unresectable distant metastatic disease.[23–27] However, these studies are retrospective and therefore are likely to be affected by selection bias. In addition, there may additional indications for primary tumor resection in order to alleviate symptoms of obstruction, bleeding, or extrinsic compression on nearby structures.

Postoperative Surveillance

Regardless of the type of surgery performed, close surveillance is recommended to evaluate for tumor recurrence. Surveillance should be performed using serial cross-sectional imaging every 3 to 12 months. This interval may be increased if there is no sign of recurrence or progression of disease over time.[22] There is no consensus regarding the frequency of surveillance imaging at this time. Cross-sectional imaging with CT scan or MRI is recommended, whereas the use of [68]Gallium-DOTATATE PET CT may be beneficial for cases where the findings are unclear on CT or MRI or to assess for metastatic disease.[21,22] In addition, if serum tumor markers are elevated before surgery, they should be followed postoperatively to monitor for recurrence.[18,20,31,32]

Patient selection is an important consideration for surgical decision making. Patients must undergo appropriate preoperative evaluation for pancreatic surgery and be educated on the potential morbidities of the operation. The benefit of pancreas-preserving enucleation procedures must be weighed against the higher risk of pancreatic fistula formation. Oncologic resection has the benefit of removal of regional lymph nodes; however, there is still a significant risk of pancreatic fistula and pancreatic insufficiency.[33] Moreover, a recent study suggests that resection margins may not influence survival in patients with PNETs, indicating that parenchymal-sparing pancreatic procedures, such as enucleations, may be appropriate when feasible.[34]

RESECTION OF REGIONAL LYMPH NODES

PNETs are diagnosed with regional lymph node metastases in greater than 20% of patients and predict for worse survival compared with disease confined to the pancreas.[23] Both the AJCC and the European Neuroendocrine Tumor Society (ENETS) staging systems include lymph node status.[10,18,22,23] Guidelines advocate surgical resection and regional lymphadenectomy in patients with PNETs greater than 2 cm in size with or without lymph node metastases evident on preoperative imaging; however, the role of routine lymph node dissection has not been prospectively established.

The utility of lymphadenectomy in PNETs less than 2 cm in size is less clear. These tumors have historically demonstrated a more indolent course, and either enucleation or frequent surveillance has been suggested according to current guidelines. Studies have found conflicting data as to the behavior of these smaller tumors. One study identified the presence of lymph node metastases in nearly 30% of tumors less than 2 cm in size, but lymphadenectomy did not change overall survival.[30]

SURGICAL MANAGEMENT OF LIVER METASTASES

Hepatic metastases are a key determinant of overall survival of patients with PNETs because the liver is the most common site of distant metastases, and most patients with metastatic PNETs die of their liver disease.[24,35] A multidisciplinary approach is key to the management of hepatic metastases and should include surgeons, oncologists, and interventional radiologists with experience in neuroendocrine tumors. Numerous surgical and nonsurgical therapeutic approaches exist for the management of neuroendocrine liver metastases. These approaches include surgical debulking comprising lobar, segmental, or nonanatomic resections and/or tumor ablations (microwave or radiofrequency ablation) or liver-directed therapies, such transarterial embolization with or without chemotherapy and selective intraarterial radiation therapy.[35,36] Systemic approaches to treat liver metastases include somatostatin analogues, PRRT, and chemotherapy; however, none of these systemic approaches consistently decreases hepatic tumor burden.[35]

There is significant variability in the behavior of PNET hepatic metastases, from indolent to rapidly progressive disease. Because of the rare nature of this disease, the wide spectrum of biological behavior of liver metastases, and multiple liver-directed and systemic treatment options, there is a lack of evidence-based guidelines for the management of hepatic metastases. It is likely however that surgery impacts survival.[36,37] Complete resection of both the primary and the hepatic metastases should be considered with curative intent for surgical candidates according to the most recent National Comprehensive Cancer Network guidelines.[38] Whether to stage these procedures or perform the pancreas resection and the liver resection at the same time depends on the hepatic disease burden, the complexity of the liver resection, and whether a pancreaticoduodenectomy will be performed (**Fig. 1**). For patients who are not candidates for complete resection, surgical debulking of liver tumor burden has shown significant survival benefit in large retrospective studies and remains an effective tool for symptomatic relief in functional tumors that are resistant to octreotide therapy.[5,18,22,36–39] Therefore, hepatic cytoreduction or debulking surgery represents an important therapeutic tool for PNETs with hepatic metastases.

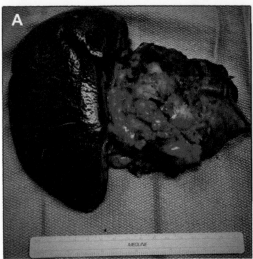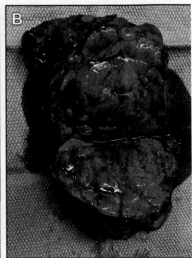

Fig. 1. Surgical specimens of a synchronous resection of a pancreatic tail tumor (with spleen) (*A*) and a single liver metastasis in segment VI (*B*).

Studies in small bowel NETs demonstrated no survival difference when comparing R0/R1 hepatic resection to R2 resections, and patients with R0 hepatic resections still developed disease recurrence.[18,39] These findings also hold true for liver metastases from PNETs, although the time to disease recurrence or liver progression after debulking is shorter than in patients with small bowel NETs.[40] Despite this and because of the limited efficacy of systemic therapies in reducing liver tumor burden, hepatic cytoreduction remains an important component for patients with metastatic PNETs to the liver.[41–43]

The threshold for hepatic debulking for PNETs has been studied by several groups. A recent study compared outcomes in patients undergoing liver cytoreduction of 100%, 90%, or 70% of their hepatic tumor burden. Overall survival was 81% at 5 years across the 3 groups. There was no significant difference in overall survival or liver progression-free survival with different levels of cytoreduction. The only significant factor correlating with survival was liver tumor size greater than 5 cm. An expanded threshold for surgical debulking in PNETs to greater than 70% would allow more patients to undergo surgery with the potential for a survival benefit.[40] Whether to cytoreduce patients with extrahepatic metastases remains controversial, but there are retrospective data suggesting a survival benefit in this setting as well compared with no resection.[24]

Liver transplant is a potential but rarely used treatment option for neuroendocrine hepatic metastases for those with unresectable liver-only disease.[44] Approximately 0.2% to 0.3% of liver transplantations are performed for NET hepatic disease.[45] There is an overall survival at 5 years after transplant that ranges from 36% to 90%, but tumor recurrence is frequently unavoidable. Given the limited data available for liver transplant in NETs and PNETs specifically, the selection criteria recommendations have not been clearly established at this time. Contraindications to liver transplantation are grade 3 neuroendocrine tumors, nonportal systemic tumor drainage, extrahepatic metastases, and active tumor progression on medical therapy.[46]

The optimal surgical treatment of liver metastases may require a sequential combination of liver-directed therapies and systemic therapies, aiming to reduce and control tumor burden even if a cure cannot be obtained long term. As with resection of primary tumors, patients who undergo hepatic surgery also need close surveillance to evaluate for tumor recurrence or progression of disease. Surveillance with serial tumor markers of hormones elevated preoperatively with imaging at intervals ranging anywhere from 3 to 12 months is recommended.

PROGNOSIS

Prognosis varies widely with PNETs depending on their functionality, stage, grade, and biological behavior.[5] Understanding of the patient's prognosis may direct management decisions, ranging from nonoperative surveillance, curative resection, or multimodal treatment strategies. Many prognostication systems exist by using variations of predictive factors, such as tumor grade, presence of metastases, tumor size, age, Ki-67 index, and others. The most commonly used prognostication systems include the WHO criteria, which include both mitoses and Ki-67 index. Both TNM staging systems, the ENETS and AJCC 7th edition prognostication criteria, include tumor size and invasion, lymph nodes, and distant metastases.[47–49] In the last 2 decades there have also been many modifications of these criteria as well as novel criteria that are institution specific. Upon review of these systems, most included age, tumor size, lymph nodes, distant metastases, Ki-67 index, and number of mitoses. The WHO 2010 criteria, ENETS, and AJCC prognostication systems were the most commonly used; however, no international consensus currently exists.[50] Despite the high numbers of patients presenting with stage IV disease, the prognosis of patients with PNETs is favorable compared with other malignancies of the pancreas of similar stage. Among GEP-NETs, one study demonstrated an increase in 5-year overall survival in all GEP-NETs; particularly, stage IV PNETs saw the biggest improvements, possibly reflecting an improvement in treatment modalities.[3] As the understanding of tumor biology continues to expand, the development of prognostication systems will continue to evolve, and surgeons will be better equipped to counsel patients on their individual prognosis and direct their care.

DISCLOSURE

The authors have no relationship with a commercial company that has a direct financial interest in subject matter or materials discussed in this article or with a company making a competing product.

REFERENCES

1. Ehehalt F, Saeger HD, Schmidt CM, et al. Neuroendocrine tumors of the pancreas. Oncologist 2009;14:456–67.
2. Halfdanarson T, Rabe K, Rubin J, et al. Pancreatic neuroendocrine tumors (PNETs): incidence, prognosis and recent trend toward improved survival. Ann Oncol 2008;19:1727–33.
3. Dasari A, Shen C, Halperin D, et al. Trends in the incidence, prevalence, and survival outcomes in patients with neuroendocrine tumors in the United States. JAMA Oncol 2017;10:1335–42.
4. Hallet J, Law CH, Cukier M, et al. Exploring the rising incidence of neuroendocrine tumors: a population-based analysis of epidemiology, metastatic presentation, and outcomes. Cancer 2015;121:589–97.
5. Kulke MH, Anthony LB, Bushnell DL, et al. NANETS treatment guidelines: well-differentiated neuroendocrine tumors of the stomach and pancreas. Pancreas 2010;39:735–52.
6. Lawrence B, Gustafsson BI, Chan A, et al. The epidemiology of gastroenteropancreatic neuroendocrine tumors. Endocrinol Metab Clin North Am 2011; 40:1–18.
7. Zhang J, Francois R, Iyer R, et al. Current understanding of the molecular biology of pancreatic neuroendocrine tumors. J Natl Cancer Inst 2013;105:1005–17.
8. Scott AT, Howe JR. Evaluation and management of neuroendocrine tumors of the pancreas. Surg Clin North Am 2019;99:793–814.
9. Keutgen XM, Hammel P, Choyke PL, et al. Evaluation and management of pancreatic lesions in patients with von Hippel-Lindau disease. Nat Rev Clin Oncol 2016;13(9):537–49.
10. Amin MB, Edge S, Greene F, et al, editors. AJCC Cancer Staging Manual. (8th edition). Springer International Publishing: American Joint Commission on Cancer; 2017.
11. Bosman FT, Carneiro F, Hruban RH, et al. WHO classification of tumours of the digestive system. 4th edition. Geneva (Switzerland): World Health Organization; 2010.
12. Lloyd RV, Osamura R, Kloppel G, et al. 4th edition. WHO classification of tumours of endocrine organs, vol. 10. Lyon (France): IARC Press; 2017.

13. Kloppel G, Couvelard A, Hruban RH, et al. Introduction. In: Lloyd RV, Osamura R, Kloppel G, et al, editors. WHO classification of tumours of endocrine organs. Lyon (France): IARC; 2017.

14. Inzani F, Petrone G, Rindi G. The New World Health Organization classification for pancreatic neuroendocrine neoplasia. Endocrinol Metab Clin North Am 2018;47: 463–70.

15. Vinik AI. Advances in diagnosis and treatment of pancreatic neuroendocrine tumor. Endocr Pract 2014;20:1222–30.

16. van Adrichem RCS, Kamp K, Vandamme T, et al. Serum neuron-specific enolase level is an independent predictor of overall survival in patients with gastroenteropancreatic neuroendocrine tumors. Ann Oncol 2016;27(4):746–7.

17. O'Dorisio TM, Krutzik SR, Woltering EA, et al. Development of a highly sensitive and specific carboxy-terminal human pancreastatin assay to monitor neuroendocrine tumor behavior. Pancreas 2010;39:611–6.

18. Howe JR, Cardona K, Fraker DL, et al. The surgical management of small bowel neuroendocrine tumors: consensus guidelines of the North American Neuroendocrine Tumor Society. Pancreas 2017;46:715–31.

19. Tierney JF, Kosche C, Schadde E, et al. [68]Gallium-DOTATATE positron emission tomography-computed tomography (PET CT) changes management in a majority of patients with neuroendocrine tumors. Surgery 2019;165:178–85.

20. Metz DC, Jensen RT. Gastrointestinal neuroendocrine tumors: pancreatic endocrine tumors. Gastroenterology 2008;135:1469–92.

21. Kunz PL, Reidy-Lagunes D, Anthony LB, et al. Consensus guidelines for the management and treatment of neuroendocrine tumors. Pancreas 2013;42:557–77.

22. Falconi M, Eriksson B, Kaltsas G, et al. ENETS consensus guidelines update for the management of patients with functional pancreatic neuroendocrine tumors and non-functional pancreatic neuroendocrine tumors. Neuroendocrinology 2016;103:153–71.

23. Hill JS, McPhee JT, McDade TP, et al. Pancreatic neuroendocrine tumors: the impact of surgical resection on survival. Cancer 2009;115:741–51.

24. Tierney JF, Poirier J, Chivukula S, et al. Primary tumor site affects survival in patients with gastroenteropancreatic and neuroendocrine liver metastases. Int J Endocrinol 2019;2019:9871319.

25. Tierney JF, Chivukula SV, Wang X, et al. Resection of primary tumor may prolong survival in metastatic gastroenteropancreatic neuroendocrine tumors. Surgery 2019;165:644–51.

26. Keutgen XM, Nilubol N, Kebebew E. Malignant-functioning neuroendocrine tumors of the pancreas: a survival analysis. Surgery 2016;159:1382–9.

27. Keutgen XM, Nilubol N, Glanville J, et al. Resection of primary tumor site is associated with prolonged survival in metastatic nonfunctioning pancreatic neuroendocrine tumors. Surgery 2016;159:311–8.

28. Lee LC, Grant CS, Salomao DR, et al. Small, nonfunctioning, asymptomatic pancreatic neuroendocrine tumors (PNETs): role for nonoperative management. Surgery 2012;152:965–74.

29. Finkelstein P, Sharma R, Picado O, et al. Pancreatic neuroendocrine tumors (panNETs): analysis of overall survival of nonsurgical management versus surgical resection. J Gastrointest Surg 2017;21:855–66.

30. Pura J, Dinan M, Roman S, et al. Impact of extent of surgery on survival in patients with small nonfunctional pancreatic neuroendocrine tumors in the United States. Ann Surg Oncol 2014;21:3515–21.

31. Modlin IM, Gustafsson BI, Moss SF, et al. Chromogranin A—biological function and clinical utility in neuro endocrine tumor disease. Ann Surg Oncol 2010;17:2427.

32. Campana D, Nori F, Piscitelli L, et al. Chromogranin A: is it a useful marker of neuroendocrine tumors? J Clin Oncol 2007;25:1967–73.

33. Jilesen APJ, van Eijck CHJ, Busch ORC, et al. Postoperative outcomes of enucleation and standard resections in patients with a pancreatic neuroendocrine tumor. World J Surg 2016;40:715–28.

34. Zhang XF, Wu Z, Cloyd J, et al. Margin status and long-term prognosis of primary pancreatic neuroendocrine tumor after curative resection: results from the US Neuroendocrine Tumor Study Group. Surgery 2019;165:548–56.

35. Keutgen XM, Schadde E, Pommier RF, et al. Metastatic neuroendocrine tumors of the gastrointestinal tract and pancreas: a surgeon's plea to centering attention on the liver. Semin Oncol 2018;45:232–5.

36. Chamberlain R, Canes D, Brown K, et al. Hepatic neuroendocrine metastases: does intervention alter outcomes? J Am Coll Surg 2000;190:432–45.

37. Scott AT, Breheny PJ, Keck KJ, et al. Effective cytoreduction can be achieved in patients with numerous neuroendocrine tumor liver metastases (NETLMs). Surgery 2019;165:166–75.

38. Neuroendocrine tumors of the pancreas. National Comprehensive Cancer Network Guidelines; 2019. Version 1.2019. Available at: https://www.nccn.org/professionals/physician_gls/pdf/neuroendocrine.pdf.

39. Mayo SC, de Jong MC, Pulitano C, et al. Surgical management of hepatic neuroendocrine tumor metastasis: results from an international multi-institutional analysis. Ann Surg Oncol 2010;17:3129–36.

40. Morgan RE, Pommier SJ, Pommier RF. Expanded criteria for debulking of liver metastasis also apply to pancreatic neuroendocrine tumors. Surgery 2018;163(1):218–25.

41. Caplin ME, Pavel M, Ruszniewski P. Lanreotide in metastatic enteropancreatic neuroendocrine tumors. N Engl J Med 2014;371:1556–7.

42. Yao JC, Shah MH, Ito T, et al. Everolimus for advanced pancreatic neuroendocrine tumors. N Engl J Med 2011;364:514–23.

43. Raymond E, Dahan L, Raoul JL, et al. Sunitinib malate for the treatment of pancreatic neuroendocrine tumors. N Engl J Med 2011;364:501–13.

44. Shimata K, Sugawara Y, Hibi T. Liver transplantation for unresectable pancreatic neuroendocrine tumors with liver metastases in an era of transplant oncology. Gland Surg 2018;7:42–6.

45. Gedaly R, Daily MF, Davenport D, et al. Liver transplantation for the treatment of liver metastases from neuroendocrine tumors: an analysis of the UNOS database. Arch Surg 2011;146:953–8.

46. Frilling A, Modlin I, Kidd M, et al. Recommendations for management of patients with neuroendocrine liver metastases. Lancet Oncol 2014;15:8–21.

47. Rindi G, Kloppel G, Couvelard A, et al. TNM staging of midgut and hindgut (neuro) endocrine tumors: a consensus proposal including a grading system. Virchows Arch 2007;451:757–62.

48. Edge BD, Compton CC, Fritz AG, et al. AJCC cancer staging manual. 7th edition. New York: Springer; 2010.

49. Ferrone CR, Tang LH, Tomlinson J, et al. Determining prognosis in patients with pancreatic endocrine neoplasms: can the WHO classification system be simplified? J Clin Oncol 2007;25:5609–15.

50. Teo RYA, Teo TZ, Tai DWM, et al. Systematic review of current prognostication systems for pancreatic neuroendocrine neoplasms. Surgery 2019;165:672–85.

Management of Other Gastric and Duodenal Neuroendocrine Tumors

Amanda M. Laird, MD*, Steven K. Libutti, MD

KEYWORDS

- Neuroendocrine • Gastric neuroendocrine tumor • Duodenal neuroendocrine tumor
- Zollinger-Ellison syndrome • Carcinoid tumor

KEY POINTS

- Gastric and duodenal neuroendocrine tumors are increasing in frequency likely because of increased use of endoscopy and cross-sectional imaging.
- Treatment is influenced by tumor type because each have different etiologies.
- Type I gastric neuroendocrine tumors have a good prognosis, managed most often with local endoscopic resection and surveillance.
- Type II gastric neuroendocrine tumors develop in the setting of a gastrinoma, for which resection is recommended.
- Most type III gastric neuroendocrine tumors and duodenal neuroendocrine tumors are managed surgically with anatomic resection and regional lymphadenectomy.

INTRODUCTION

Gastric and duodenal neuroendocrine tumors (NETs) are tumors that arise from the neuroendocrine cells within their respective locations. NETs can occur in many locations throughout the body including the gastrointestinal (GI) tract and pancreas and in the lung and respiratory tract. Gastric NETs and duodenal NETs are found much less frequently than those found in other portions of the aerodigestive tract, with gastric NETs making up about 9% of all GI NETs and duodenal NETs occurring approximately 3% of the time.[1,2] Overall the incidence of NETs of all types is increasing including gastric and duodenal NETs, which is thought to be caused by incidental discovery or better recognition of the tumor type on cytology.[3] Both types may occur with multiple endocrine neoplasia type 1 (MEN1), or they may be sporadic. Gastric NETS are

Section of Endocrine Surgery, Rutgers Cancer Institute of New Jersey, Rutgers Robert Wood Johnson Medical School, 195 Little Albany Street, New Brunswick, NJ 08903, USA
* Corresponding author.
E-mail address: amanda.laird@cinj.rutgers.edu

Surg Oncol Clin N Am 29 (2020) 253–266
https://doi.org/10.1016/j.soc.2019.11.009
1055-3207/20/© 2019 Elsevier Inc. All rights reserved.

further classified according to their suspected cause and are typed either I, II, or III, and the clinical course of gastric NETs is influenced by the specific type of the tumor identified. Each may be nonfunctional, or less commonly, gastrin-producing in the case of duodenal NETs.

INCIDENCE

Although NETs of any type occur less often than many malignancies, the incidence overall and within specific types is increasing. An analysis of the Surveillance, Epidemiology, and End Results database from 1973 to 2004 revealed that the incidence of gastric NETs was 0.3/100,000 population and duodenal NETs was 0.19/100,000. In that same group, gastric NETs were more common in women, whereas duodenal NETs occurred more often in men.[2] Gastric NETs have been reported to make up a greater proportion of GI NETs comprising 23% of a prospectively studied Austrian group.[4] Prevalence varies across other countries ranging from 5.2% to 11%.[5] Duodenal NETs comprise 5% to 8% of GI NETs.[6]

LOCATION AND CLINICAL FEATURES
Type I Gastric Neuroendocrine Tumors

Type I gastric NETs are the most common of the three types making up 70% to 80% of all gastric NETs. They occur secondarily as a result of conditions that increase gastrin secretion. Associated conditions include chronic atrophic gastritis (CAG) and intrinsic factor deficiency (IFD). In the setting of CAG or IFD, tumors develop via enterochromaffin cell hyperplasia. Enterochromaffin-like cells (ECL) become hyperplastic as a result of stimulation from gastrin. Gastrin production is increased in CAG and IFD because of achlorhydria that develops as a result of either condition. That, in turn, stimulates gastrin production, and a hallmark in patients with type I gastric NETs is elevated gastrin levels but a normal pH. Proton pump inhibitors are believed to contribute to the formation of gastric NETs but there are conflicting data on this. The tumors themselves are asymptomatic, but patients may present with symptoms related to the presence of CAG and may have dyspepsia. These tumors are typically small, found throughout the stomach, are in the mucosa or submucosal, and are found more commonly in women.[7] Although they are typically benign and well-differentiated (grade 1), there is a possibility of malignant transformation, because metastases are found in 2% to 5% of patients.[8] Treatment of the primary cause can lead to regression of the tumors; however, surgery may play a role in some cases. Use of somatostatin analogues (SSA) has also been investigated as either a primary or adjunctive treatment of type I gastric NETs. SSA have an antiproliferative effect and they are used to limit ECL cell growth. Their routine use is debated, and outcomes are not clear.[8] Netazepide is an oral agent investigated as a potential treatment of type I gastric NETs. It is an antagonist of the gastrin/cholecystokinin-2 receptor. In one trial, treatment with netazepide led to resolution or reduction in number of tumors,[9] but the treatment must be continuous otherwise gastric NETs recur. Characteristics are summarized in **Table 1**.

Type II Gastric Neuroendocrine Tumors

Type II NETs also occur in the setting of hypergastrinemia, but in this case, the cause of hypergastrinemia differs. Tumors form through the same mechanism of ECL cellular hypertrophy, but hypergastrinemia occurs as a result of a gastrinoma, which produces excess gastrin, termed Zollinger-Ellison syndrome (ZES). Like type I gastric NETs, the type II gastric NETs themselves are asymptomatic, but patients may have symptoms

Table 1
Characteristics of gastric NETs

	Type I	Type II	Type III
% of gastric NETs	70–80	5	14–25
Size, cm	<1–2	<1–2	>2
Gender	F > M	F = M	M > F
Multiplicity	+	+	-
Cause	CAG, IFD	ZES, ZES in MEN1	None
Serum gastrin levels	Elevated	Elevated	Normal
Gastric pH	Elevated	Low	Normal
Metastases present, %	2–5	10–30	50–100

Abbreviation: ZES, Zollinger-Ellison syndrome.
Data from Delle Fave G, Kwekkeboom DJ, Van Cutsem E, et al. ENETS Consensus Guidelines for the management of patients with gastroduodenal neoplasms. Neuroendocrinology. 2012;95(2):74-87; and Sato Y, Hashimoto S, Mizuno K, et al. Management of gastric and duodenal neuroendocrine tumors. World J Gastroenterol. 2016;22(30):6817-6828; with permission.

of peptic ulcer disease, which occurs as a result of excess gastrin and resulting increased gastric acid production. For reasons that are unclear, they occur more often in patients with MEN1 and ZES rather than in patients with a sporadic gastrinoma.[10] Tumors are typically small and multiple and occur least commonly of each of the three types at 5% to 8%. Compared with type I gastric NETs, they have a greater malignant potential with metastases identified 10% to 30% of the time.[8] Distribution is similar between men and women (see **Table 1**).

Type III Gastric Neuroendocrine Tumors

Type III gastric NETs occur sporadically and not as a result of another condition. Patients may be asymptomatic, or they develop symptoms related to tumor progression including pain and bleeding. They are solitary rather than multiple and behave more aggressively with metastases 50% to 100% of the time. They are larger than types I and II, ranging from 2 to 5 cm. They comprise up to 20% of gastric NETs and occur more often in men.[11] Because they are a primary tumor, gastrin and gastric pH levels are normal (see **Table 1**).

Duodenal Neuroendocrine Tumors

Most duodenal NETs are found in the first and second portion of the duodenum. Most are nonfunctional; functional tumors produce gastrin and are thus termed gastrinomas and result in ZES. Nonfunctional tumors tend to be solitary, whereas gastrinomas that occur in the setting of MEN1 may be multiple. They tend to be mucosal-based or submucosal and size ranges from a few millimeters up to 2 cm. Metastases to regional lymph nodes are common and found in 40% to 60% of patients, although patients are less likely to have liver metastases, which occur in 10%.

DIAGNOSIS AND STAGING
Endoscopy

Esophagogastroduodenoscopy (EGD) plays a critical role in the diagnosis of gastric and duodenal NETs for obtaining tissue for diagnosis and, in some cases, surveillance. In many cases, EGD is the initial diagnostic study because many gastric and duodenal NETs are found incidentally. EGD allows for biopsy of the primary tumor and of the surrounding gastric or duodenal mucosa, if needed. Endoscopic ultrasound allows for T-staging to assess depth of invasion of the primary tumor and to assess for any adjacent malignant-appearing lymphadenopathy.[12] EGD is used in follow-up of gastric and duodenal NETs; however, the frequency at which it should be performed is not clearly outlined. Guidelines from the European Neuroendocrine Tumor Society (ENETS) recommend endoscopy at least every 2 years and at a shorter interval if clinically indicated.[13]

Other Imaging

Depending on the type of gastric NET identified, cross-sectional imaging including computed tomography (CT) or MRI may add little value unless there is a greater likelihood of metastatic disease. For type I gastric NETs, CT and MRI are not as valuable as EGD in follow-up because of the indolent nature of the disease. For types II and III gastric NETs and duodenal NETs, CT and MRI may aid in the detection of metastatic disease.[13] **Fig. 1** demonstrates the utility of CT in evaluation for nodal metastases with enlarged lymph nodes adjacent to the head of the pancreas. Other types of NETs are imaged with SSA including octreotide somatostatin receptor scintigraphy (SRS) and ^{68}Ga-SSA PET. Data on the use of ^{68}Ga-SSA PET are limited for gastric NETs, although in small case series it demonstrated superior results compared with SRS and identified the primary tumor.[14] SRS is proven to be more sensitive than MRI and CT in the detection of gastrinoma including the primary tumor and lymph node

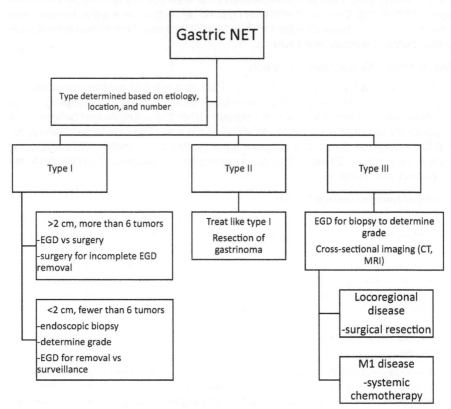

Fig. 1. Treatment algorithm for gastric neuroendocrine tumors.

metastases but did not perform better than intraoperative inspection.[15] SRS may also detect gastric carcinoids,[16] but it may not be more useful than endoscopic surveillance or other cross-sectional imaging. Both types of functional imaging could play a role in planning nonsurgical therapy in the case of metastatic disease because they would determine if an SSA could be used as part of treatment.

Staging

Gastric and duodenal NETs are classified by either pathologic stage or grade. The traditional American Joint Committee on Cancer staging uses tumor size, nodal status, and presence of metastases (TNM) staging to understand extent of anatomic involvement and predict clinical course. In addition, they may be categorized according to tumor grade based on the World Health Organization 2010 classification system.[17] Of the two, grade is the better overall predictor of clinical course and is incorporated into staging outlined by the ENETS.[13] Grade is determined by a combination of mitotic rate and the percentage of cells that immunostain for Ki-67 antigen, a marker of cellular proliferation known as Ki-67 index. Grade 1 (low grade) tumors have a mitotic index of less than 2 per high-power field and a Ki-67 index less than or equal to 3%, whereas grade 2 (intermediate grade) tumors have a mitotic index of 2 to 20 per high-power field and Ki-67 of 3% to 20%. Grade 3 (high grade) tumors are classified as such when the mitotic index is greater than 20 or Ki-67 is greater than 20% (**Table 2**). Grade is determined by the higher of the two between mitotic rate and Ki-67 index. In a group of Spanish patients with NETs of any type, Ki-67 index was shown to be an independent predictor of survival.[18] Along with ENETS, the North American Neuroendocrine Tumor Society incorporates tumor grade into management recommendations, highlighting its clinical relevance.[19]

Other Tests

In conjunction with endoscopy with or without cross-sectional imaging, certain serum biomarkers can support diagnosis and aid in follow-up. Guidelines recommend routine testing of gastrin levels and gastric pH because gastric pH differentiates types I and II gastric NETS and distinguishes functional from nonfunctional duodenal NETs. Chromogranin A and 5-hydroxyindoleacetic acid may be useful adjuncts to aid in follow-up.[19] Chromogranin A is a glycoprotein found within ECL cells, and is also useful in follow-up of NETs that arise from other tissues. Chromogranin A may be falsely elevated with proton pump inhibitor use and this should be taken into consideration when interpreting results.[20]

Table 2 Classification of NETs based on histology		
Mitotic Index (per HPF)	**Ki-67 Index (%)**	**Classification**
<2	≤2	ENETS G1, WHO G1
2–20	3–20	ENETS G2, WHO G2
>20	>20	ENETS G3, WHO G3

Abbreviations: HPF, high-powered field; WHO, World Health Organization.
Data from Delle Fave G, O'Toole D, Sundin A, et al. ENETS Consensus Guidelines Update for Gastroduodenal Neuroendocrine Neoplasms. Neuroendocrinology. 2016;103(2):119-124 and Bosman FT, Carneiro F, Hruban RH, Theise ND, eds. WHO Classification of Tumours of the Digestive System. 4th ed. Lyon, France: IARC Press; 2010.

Testing for the *MEN1* gene should be considered in patients found to have a gastrinoma because patients with gastrinomas are found to have MEN1 approximately 30% of the time. Therefore, genetic testing should be considered in patients with gastrinoma or type II gastric NETs. Development of sporadic gastrinoma may also have a genetic influence. Data suggest an association between the *MEN1* gene and apparently sporadic gastrinoma. In a small series of patients, the gene was found to be mutated in one-third suggesting that alterations in the gene, especially loss of heterozygosity, lead to tumorigenesis.[21] Mutations in the *MEN1* gene have also been identified in type I gastric NETs, and type III gastric NETs have an association with mutations in p53.[22]

RESECTION OF PRIMARY TUMOR

EGD plays a key role in diagnosis of gastric and duodenal NETs and may also be used in treatment depending on tumor type. Endoscopic resection is possible for gastric NETs types I and II and for duodenal NETs depending on their specific presentation and tumor characteristics. Endoscopic resection is not appropriate for type III gastric NETs, which are managed surgically.

Recommendations for management vary between published guidelines slightly but all are in favor of endoscopic management when possible for type I gastric NETs. Tumor size and number determine appropriateness for endoscopic resection. Tumors less than 1 cm may be followed with EGD for surveillance or removed endoscopically. Tumors measuring 1 to 2 cm and when six or fewer are present may be either surveilled with EGD every 3 years or removed endoscopically. Tumors greater than 2 cm when six or fewer are present may be either managed with endoscopic resection if technically feasible versus surgical resection. Tumors greater than 2 cm and when more than six are present should be removed surgically.[13,19] Surgical resection with partial gastrectomy may be considered for incompletely resected lesions. Another surgical approach in management is antrectomy, which is performed to remove all gastrin-producing tissue, which in turn downregulates stimulation of ECL cells and involution of tumors. In a series of 52 patients, antrectomy reduced the need for EGD surveillance and lowered the risk of recurrence compared with polypectomy alone.[23] In another series of patients, 5.5% of those with type I gastric NETs developed gastric adenocarcinoma, suggesting that even in the setting of surgical intervention, life-long surveillance is recommended.[24]

Management of type II gastric NETs is largely dictated by the presence of a gastrin-producing tumor. That should be managed as described in the duodenal NET section to follow. The gastric-based NETs are managed similarly to type I gastric NETs based on size.[19] Data show that removal of the gastrin-producing tumor leads to resolution of the gastric NETs.[25] If the gastrinoma is not resectable, acid hypersecretion is managed with proton pump inhibitors.

Endoscopic management is not recommended for type III gastric NETs, because they are more aggressive and have greater potential for metastasis. Therefore, surgical resection is recommended to limit potential metastatic spread and control tumor-related symptoms, such as bleeding and pain.[13,19] The operation of choice depends on size and location of the tumor and includes partial and subtotal gastrectomy with nodal dissection based on the clinical situation. Patients should undergo preoperative staging with either CT or MRI to assess for locoregional involvement or distant metastases. Treatment is summarized in **Fig. 2**.

Duodenal NETs are managed based on size, location, grade, stage, and whether they are functional, and occur in the setting of MEN1. Because duodenal NETs

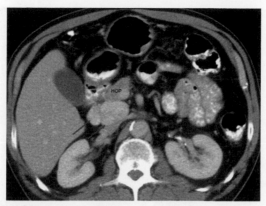

Fig. 2. Computed tomography in a patient with a sporadic gastrinoma. Metastatic lymph nodes (*arrows*) adjacent to head of pancreas (HOP).

have greater malignant potential, all patients should have cross-sectional imaging because the presence of regional or distant metastases would change management making endoscopic resection inappropriate. Proximity to the ampulla of Vater influences management and all periampullary tumors should undergo surgical resection. Tumors less than 1 cm are appropriate for endoscopic resection as in **Fig. 3**. All patients with tumors greater than 2 cm should undergo surgical resection, and there is debate about the best management of tumors between 1 and 2 cm.[13] In patients with gastrinoma, surgery is preferred and may be curative because it limits the potential for metastases.[26] **Fig. 4** demonstrates the typical appearance of a gastrinoma and the technique of bimanual palpation to evaluate for additional lesions. Surgical resection should also be considered for grade 2 and 3 tumors, because grade is an independent risk factor for recurrence.[27]

RESECTION OF REGIONAL NODAL METASTASES

Regional lymph node metastases are less common in type I and II gastric NETs but occur in nearly all cases of type III gastric NETs. They are also common in duodenal NETs, especially in gastrinomas. There are little data specific to the management of nodal metastases in gastric NETs, but en bloc removal is recommended.[28] Lymph node removal allows for better tumor staging and can yield information used to determine clinical course. In small bowel NETs, overall survival and disease-free survival are improved with regional lymph node dissection.[29] Lymphadenectomy should be included at the time of gastrectomy and include all perigastric nodes and those along the left gastric artery. No additional benefit has been shown by more extensive lymphadenectomy as would be performed for gastric adenocarcinoma.

Resection of lymph node metastases and prophylactic lymphadenectomy may have different implications for duodenal NETs, particularly if the tumor is gastrin-producing. Lymphadenectomy appropriately stages the tumor and aids in better understanding the expected clinical course. Gastrin-producing NETs or gastrinomas are unique in that lymph node involvement influences clinical course and may be responsible for persistent hypergastrinemia. In a population of ZES patients who underwent removal of the primary tumor and adjacent lymph nodes, 38% had persistent hypergastrinemia. Of those with an initial biochemical cure, one-third recurred because of nodal disease with a median time to recurrence of 4.2 years.[30] Disease-free survival is reduced

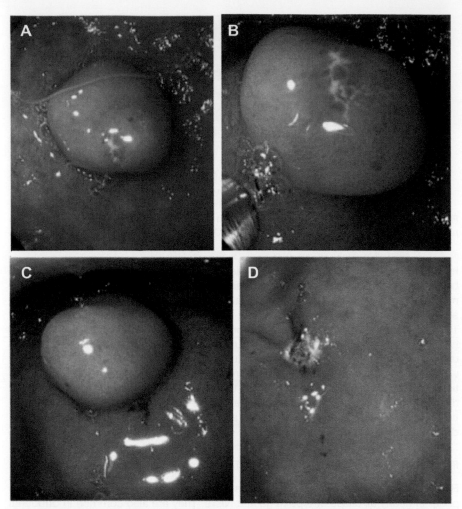

Fig. 3. Endoscopic removal of a duodenal NET. (*A*) Duodenal NET in first portion of duo-denum. (*B*) Lifting the duodenal NET. (*C*) Submucosa lifted in preparation for removal. (*D*) Lesion excision site postremoval. (*Courtesy of* H Shahid, M.D., New Brunswick, NJ.)

in patients with duodenal NETs and nodal metastases suggesting that regional lym-phadenectomy may influence outcomes.[31] Periduodenal lymph nodes may also be the primary location of a gastrinoma, therefore lymph node resection should be included in operations for ZES.[32] Guidelines recommend lymphadenectomy for duodenal NETs that are managed with surgery to be done at the time of the initial operation.[8]

MANAGEMENT OF LIVER METASTASES

Liver metastases may be managed surgically, with systemic therapy, with locoregional therapies, or a combination of the three. The approach to management should be tailored to the individual clinical situation because there are no clinical trials comparing options to each other alone or in combination. Patients treated with any or a

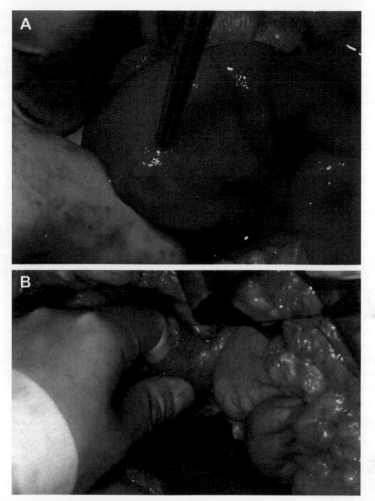

Fig. 4. Intraoperative pictures of resection of a gastrinoma. (*A*) Primary tumor as indicated by forceps. (*B*) Bimanual palpation via duodenotomy to evaluate for additional lesions. (*Courtesy of* A Laird, MD, FACS, New Brunswick, NJ.)

combination of the three approaches have a survival advantage and a longer progression-free survival. In the setting of gastrinoma, treatment may also be used to ameliorate symptoms of hormone excess (ie, ulcer disease) if symptoms are refractory to medical therapy.

Surgical Therapy

Surgical candidacy in management of NET metastases to the liver is determined by resectability of the primary tumor and whether the volume and location of liver metastases makes surgery feasible. Both anatomic liver resection and parenchyma-sparing techniques, such as wedge resection or enucleation, may be used. Gastric and duodenal NETs occur significantly less often than pancreatic and small bowel NETs, but recommendations for management can be extrapolated from data based on the management of more commonly occurring NETs. Surgery should be considered in patients with metastases except when lesions are diffuse and multifocal or when there is extrahepatic disease,[33] although the latter is a matter of debate. Surgical resection of metastases is recommended for grade 1 and 2 NETs of any origin, whereas surgery in the setting of metastases from grade 3 NETs is not recommended unless the lesions are isolated and resectable with low morbidity.[33] In a series of 108 patients with small bowel and pancreas NETs and liver metastases, patients who had at least 70% of liver parenchyma debulked had improved progression-free survival and overall survival.[34] This approach has been demonstrated to be successful with improved progression-free and overall survival by other groups.[35] Guidelines recommend resection of liver metastases for grade 1 and 2 NETs when possible.[8]

Local Ablative and Locoregional Therapy

Local and locoregional therapies for liver metastases include radiofrequency ablation, microwave ablation, transarterial embolization, transarterial chemoembolization, or radioembolization. Much like surgical data, experience with these therapies is primarily from treatment of pancreas and small bowel NETs but use may be considered in patients with low- and intermediate-grade gastric and duodenal NETs.[8] Radiofrequency ablation and microwave ablation may be used either alone or in combination with surgical resection.[36] Outcomes data are limited but a small series of NET patients reported a median survival of 3.9 years from the time of initial ablation.[37] Transarterial embolization, transarterial chemoembolization, and radioembolization are typically reserved for patients who are not surgical candidates, and no data have shown that either approach is superior to the other.[33] They are contraindicated in portal vein thrombosis and in patients with severe liver dysfunction. Transarterial embolization and transarterial chemoembolization achieve radiographic response in 32% to 82% of patients with a progression-free survival of 18 to 24 months.[38]

Systemic Therapy

Recommendations for systemic therapy in gastric and duodenal NETs are based on grade where high-grade tumors differ because they are treated more like adenocarcinomas and receive cytotoxic chemotherapy. Systemic therapy is reserved for those patients who are not surgical candidates either by way of extent of disease or having a high-grade NET.

Options for management of grades 1 and 2 tumors include SSA, certain mTOR inhibitors (everolimus), and peptide-receptor radiotherapy.[8] Commonly used SSAs include long-acting (LAR) octreotide and lanreotide. Octreotide LAR (PROMID trial) and lanreotide (CLARINET trial) have been shown to improve progression-free survival in clinical trials.[39,40] Everolimus (RADIANT-3 trial) may be used as an alternative or in patients with progressive disease and also improves progression-free survival.[41] Neither is recommended in patients with grade 3 NETs. Peptide-receptor radiotherapy is the newest option for management of liver metastases and its efficacy was demonstrated in the NETTER1 clinical trial.[42] Peptide-receptor radiotherapy is used in patients with isolated liver metastases caused by NETs that have progressed on treatment with SSAs. To be eligible for treatment, tumors must demonstrate somatostatin-avidity by functional imaging. Patients are administered treatment with [177]Lutetium-dotatate over three to four cycles. When compared with octreotide-LAR, progression-free survival at 20 months was improved at 65.2% compared with 10.8%.[42]

High-grade tumors are managed more like adenocarcinomas with cytotoxic chemotherapy. Combination therapy with cisplatin and etoposide is recommended provided patient performance status is adequate.[43] Other options studied include 5-fluorouracil or capecitabine with oxaliplatin or irinotecan.[33]

PROGNOSIS

Outcomes for gastric and duodenal NETs are determined by tumor type, grade, TNM stage, and the clinical setting in which they occur. Types I and II gastric NETs tend to be low grade and therefore outcomes are better than in those with type III gastric NETs. Outcomes of duodenal NETs are also influenced by grade, but occurring in the setting of MEN1 increases complexity.

An analysis of Surveillance, Epidemiology, and End Results data from 2000 to 2012 demonstrated better overall survival in low-grade gastric NETs without regional or distant metastatic disease.[3] The 5-year survival of all gastric NETs is approximately 49% but this is lowered by inclusion of more aggressive grade 3 tumors.[11] Single-institutional data demonstrated a disease-specific survival of 100% for type I gastric NETs and 75% for type III gastric NETs at 30.7 months of follow-up.[44] Prognosis for type II gastric NETs is good with a less than 10% mortality.[22]

Outcomes of duodenal NETs are generally good because most are grade 1 or 2. In a single-institutional series of patients with duodenal NETs managed with resection of any type (endoscopic or surgical), 2- and 5-year recurrence-free survival were 84% and 81%, respectively.[27] The prognosis for duodenal NETs is thought to be similar to all GI NETs with 5-year survival of 80% to 95% with localized disease, 65% to 75% with locoregional disease, and 20% to 40% in the setting of distant metastatic disease.[8]

SUMMARY

Gastric and duodenal NETs are being more frequently identified, most likely caused by the increased use of endoscopy and cross-sectional imaging. Tumor location and concomitant medical conditions aid in understanding tumor etiology. Biopsy of the tumor is critical because grade influences decision-making in treatment and outcomes. Options for intervention include either endoscopic or surgical resection with systemic therapies available in the setting of advanced disease. Recognition of gastric and duodenal NETs as distinct neoplasms should allow for appropriate treatment planning.

DISCLOSURE

The authors have nothing to disclose.

REFERENCES

1. Modlin IM, Lye KD, Kidd M. A 5-decade analysis of 13,715 carcinoid tumors. Cancer 2003;97(4):934–59.
2. Yao JC, Hassan M, Phan A, et al. One hundred years after "carcinoid": epidemiology of and prognostic factors for neuroendocrine tumors in 35,825 cases in the United States. J Clin Oncol 2008;26(18):3063–72.
3. Dasari A, Shen C, Halperin D, et al. Trends in the incidence, prevalence, and survival outcomes in patients with neuroendocrine tumors in the United States. JAMA Oncol 2017;3(10):1335–42.
4. Niederle MB, Hackl M, Kaserer K, et al. Gastroenteropancreatic neuroendocrine tumours: the current incidence and staging based on the WHO and European

Neuroendocrine Tumour Society classification: an analysis based on prospectively collected parameters. Endocr Relat Cancer 2010;17(4):909–18.

5. Boyce M, Thomsen L. Gastric neuroendocrine tumors: prevalence in Europe, USA, and Japan, and rationale for treatment with a gastrin/CCK2 receptor antagonist. Scand J Gastroenterol 2015;50(5):550–9.

6. Sato Y, Hashimoto S, Mizuno K, et al. Management of gastric and duodenal neuroendocrine tumors. World J Gastroenterol 2016;22(30):6817–28.

7. Borch K, Ahren B, Ahlman H, et al. Gastric carcinoids: biologic behavior and prognosis after differentiated treatment in relation to type. Ann Surg 2005; 242(1):64–73.

8. Delle Fave G, Kwekkeboom DJ, Van Cutsem E, et al. ENETS Consensus Guidelines for the management of patients with gastroduodenal neoplasms. Neuroendocrinology 2012;95(2):74–87.

9. Boyce M, Moore AR, Sagatun L, et al. Netazepide, a gastrin/cholecystokinin-2 receptor antagonist, can eradicate gastric neuroendocrine tumours in patients with autoimmune chronic atrophic gastritis. Br J Clin Pharmacol 2017;83(3):466–75.

10. Norton JA, Melcher ML, Gibril F, et al. Gastric carcinoid tumors in multiple endocrine neoplasia-1 patients with Zollinger-Ellison syndrome can be symptomatic, demonstrate aggressive growth, and require surgical treatment. Surgery 2004; 136(6):1267–74.

11. Modlin IM, Lye KD, Kidd M. Carcinoid tumors of the stomach. Surg Oncol 2003; 12(2):153–72.

12. Dalenback J, Havel G. Local endoscopic removal of duodenal carcinoid tumors. Endoscopy 2004;36(7):651–5.

13. Delle Fave G, O'Toole D, Sundin A, et al. ENETS consensus guidelines update for gastroduodenal neuroendocrine neoplasms. Neuroendocrinology 2016;103(2): 119–24.

14. Cavallaro A, Zanghi A, Cavallaro M, et al. The role of 68-Ga-DOTATOC CT-PET in surgical tactic for gastric neuroendocrine tumors treatment: our experience: a case report. Int J Surg 2014;12(Suppl 1):S225–31.

15. Alexander HR, Fraker DL, Norton JA, et al. Prospective study of somatostatin receptor scintigraphy and its effect on operative outcome in patients with Zollinger-Ellison syndrome. Ann Surg 1998;228(2):228–38.

16. Gibril F, Reynolds JC, Lubensky IA, et al. Ability of somatostatin receptor scintigraphy to identify patients with gastric carcinoids: a prospective study. J Nucl Med 2000;41(10):1646–56.

17. Kim BS, Park YS, Yook JH, et al. Comparison of the prognostic values of the 2010 WHO classification, AJCC 7th edition, and ENETS classification of gastric neuroendocrine tumors. Medicine (Baltimore) 2016;95(30):e3977.

18. Garcia-Carbonero R, Capdevila J, Crespo-Herrero G, et al. Incidence, patterns of care and prognostic factors for outcome of gastroenteropancreatic neuroendocrine tumors (GEP-NETs): results from the National Cancer Registry of Spain (RGETNE). Ann Oncol 2010;21(9):1794–803.

19. Kunz PL, Reidy-Lagunes D, Anthony LB, et al. Consensus guidelines for the management and treatment of neuroendocrine tumors. Pancreas 2013;42(4):557–77.

20. Verbeek WH, Korse CM, Tesselaar ME. GEP-NETs UPDATE: secreting gastroenteropancreatic neuroendocrine tumours and biomarkers. Eur J Endocrinol 2016;174(1):R1–7.

21. Zhuang Z, Vortmeyer AO, Pack S, et al. Somatic mutations of the MEN1 tumor suppressor gene in sporadic gastrinomas and insulinomas. Cancer Res 1997; 57(21):4682–6.

22. Corey B, Chen H. Neuroendocrine tumors of the stomach. Surg Clin North Am 2017;97(2):333–43.
23. Jenny HE, Ogando PA, Fujitani K, et al. Laparoscopic antrectomy: a safe and definitive treatment in managing type 1 gastric carcinoids. Am J Surg 2016; 211(4):778–82.
24. Chen WC, Warner RR, Ward SC, et al. Management and disease outcome of type I gastric neuroendocrine tumors: the Mount Sinai experience. Dig Dis Sci 2015; 60(4):996–1003.
25. Richards ML, Gauger P, Thompson NW, et al. Regression of type II gastric carcinoids in multiple endocrine neoplasia type 1 patients with Zollinger-Ellison syndrome after surgical excision of all gastrinomas. World J Surg 2004;28(7):652–8.
26. Fraker DL, Norton JA, Alexander HR, et al. Surgery in Zollinger-Ellison syndrome alters the natural history of gastrinoma. Ann Surg 1994;220(3):320–8 [discussion: 328–30].
27. Untch BR, Bonner KP, Roggin KK, et al. Pathologic grade and tumor size are associated with recurrence-free survival in patients with duodenal neuroendocrine tumors. J Gastrointest Surg 2014;18(3):457–62 [discussion: 462–3].
28. Xie SD, Wang LB, Song XY, et al. Minute gastric carcinoid tumor with regional lymph node metastasis: a case report and review of literature. World J Gastroenterol 2004;10(16):2461–3.
29. Howe JR, Cardona K, Fraker DL, et al. The surgical management of small bowel neuroendocrine tumors: consensus guidelines of the North American Neuroendocrine Tumor Society. Pancreas 2017;46(6):715–31.
30. Arnold WS, Fraker DL, Alexander HR, et al. Apparent lymph node primary gastrinoma. Surgery 1994;116(6):1123–9 [discussion: 1129–30].
31. Zogakis TG, Gibril F, Libutti SK, et al. Management and outcome of patients with sporadic gastrinoma arising in the duodenum. Ann Surg 2003;238(1):42–8.
32. Norton JA, Alexander HR, Fraker DL, et al. Possible primary lymph node gastrinoma: occurrence, natural history, and predictive factors: a prospective study. Ann Surg 2003;237(5):650–7 [discussion 657–9].
33. Pavel M, Baudin E, Couvelard A, et al. ENETS Consensus Guidelines for the management of patients with liver and other distant metastases from neuroendocrine neoplasms of foregut, midgut, hindgut, and unknown primary. Neuroendocrinology 2012;95(2):157–76.
34. Maxwell JE, Sherman SK, O'Dorisio TM, et al. Liver-directed surgery of neuroendocrine metastases: what is the optimal strategy? Surgery 2016;159(1):320–33.
35. Farley HA, Pommier RF. Treatment of neuroendocrine liver metastases. Surg Oncol Clin N Am 2016;25(1):217–25.
36. Pawlik TM, Izzo F, Cohen DS, et al. Combined resection and radiofrequency ablation for advanced hepatic malignancies: results in 172 patients. Ann Surg Oncol 2003;10(9):1059–69.
37. Mazzaglia PJ, Berber E, Milas M, et al. Laparoscopic radiofrequency ablation of neuroendocrine liver metastases: a 10-year experience evaluating predictors of survival. Surgery 2007;142(1):10–9.
38. Vogl TJ, Naguib NN, Zangos S, et al. Liver metastases of neuroendocrine carcinomas: interventional treatment via transarterial embolization, chemoembolization and thermal ablation. Eur J Radiol 2009;72(3):517–28.
39. Rinke A, Muller HH, Schade-Brittinger C, et al. Placebo-controlled, double-blind, prospective, randomized study on the effect of octreotide LAR in the control of tumor growth in patients with metastatic neuroendocrine midgut tumors: a report from the PROMID Study Group. J Clin Oncol 2009;27(28):4656–63.

40. Caplin ME, Pavel M, Cwikla JB, et al. Lanreotide in metastatic enteropancreatic neuroendocrine tumors. N Engl J Med 2014;371(3):224–33.
41. Yao JC, Shah MH, Ito T, et al. Everolimus for advanced pancreatic neuroendocrine tumors. N Engl J Med 2011;364(6):514–23.
42. Strosberg J, El-Haddad G, Wolin E, et al. Phase 3 trial of (177)Lu-Dotatate for midgut neuroendocrine tumors. N Engl J Med 2017;376(2):125–35.
43. Moertel CG, Kvols LK, O'Connell MJ, et al. Treatment of neuroendocrine carcinomas with combined etoposide and cisplatin. Evidence of major therapeutic activity in the anaplastic variants of these neoplasms. Cancer 1991;68(2):227–32.
44. Postlewait LM, Baptiste GG, Ethun CG, et al. A 15-year experience with gastric neuroendocrine tumors: does type make a difference? J Surg Oncol 2016; 114(5):576–80.

Neuroendocrine Tumors of the Appendix, Colon, and Rectum

Jennifer Hrabe, MD

KEYWORDS

- Neuroendocrine tumor • Carcinoid • Neuroendocrine carcinoma
- Hindgut neuroendocrine neoplasm • Appendiceal neuroendocrine neoplasm
- Colorectal neuroendocrine neoplasm

KEY POINTS

- Appropriate pathologic evaluation with assessment of size, location, grade, differentiation, and lymphovascular invasion is critical to guiding staging and surgical treatment.
- Appendectomy in tumors less than 2 cm is generally appropriate unless there are high-risk features.
- Colonic tumors tend to be more aggressive and are best treated with segmental colectomy and regional lymphadenectomy.
- Rectal tumors less than 2 cm can be managed by local resections unless there are high-risk features; tumors equal to or greater than 2 cm or with high-risk features should prompt total mesorectal excision.

INTRODUCTION

Neuroendocrine tumors (NETs) encompass a range of pathologies and behaviors, ranging from indolent tumors often discovered incidentally, to poorly differentiated and aggressive carcinomas whose presence is detected late in the disease. Their nomenclature adds to the complexity, with the term "neuroendocrine tumor" and "carcinoid" variably being reserved for low- and intermediate-grade neoplasms and "neuroendocrine carcinoma" referring to poorly differentiated, high-grade neoplasms. This article adheres to those conventions and focuses on NETs in the appendix, colon, and rectum.

INCIDENCE
Appendix

NETs are the most common neoplasm affecting the appendix, with estimates that NETs account for 60% to 88% of all appendiceal tumors.[1–4] The appendix is the

Colorectal Surgery, University of Iowa Hospitals and Clinics, 200 Hawkins Drive, Iowa City, IA 52242, USA
E-mail address: Jennifer-hrabe@uiowa.edu

Surg Oncol Clin N Am 29 (2020) 267–279
https://doi.org/10.1016/j.soc.2019.11.010
1055-3207/20/Published by Elsevier Inc.

surgonc.theclinics.com

most common site for gastrointestinal NETs.[1] In Western series, slightly more women than men are affected, although in other reports the overall incidence of appendiceal NETs was similar between women and men.[2,3,5] The age at diagnosis has been reported to range from 33 to 51 years, although some investigators posit that the mean age is likely lower as many small tumors found incidentally are deemed benign and thus are not reported.[2,3,5] Appendiceal NETs do occur in pediatric patients, in ages as young as 4.5 years.[2]

Most of the appendiceal NETs are diagnosed incidentally on pathologic review of the appendix removed for appendicitis. In one series of 2724 emergency appendectomies, less than 1% of specimens demonstrated NET on histopathology; in another series of 14,850 patients having appendectomies over a 14-year period, 1.45% had histologically confirmed NETs.[1,3] Other series echo this frequency and estimate that NETs are discovered at a rate of 3 to 5/1000 appendectomies.[2]

Colon

Approximately 7.5% of NETs are of colonic origin. NETs of the colon and rectum are often discovered incidentally during screening colonoscopies. Perhaps related to improved colon cancer screening, the incidence of colon NETs has increased 10-fold in the United States over the last 3 decades.[6] The median age at diagnosis for cecal NEN is 68 years and for the colon overall is 65 years.[5,6] In the United States, cecal NETs affect women and men equally and are more common in individuals of black race as compared with white and Asian races.[7]

Rectum

Rectal NETs may present with symptoms such as bleeding or change in bowel habits, but nearly half of patients are asymptomatic and are diagnosed on screening colonoscopy.[4] These tumors now represent 18% of all NETs and 27% of gastrointestinal NETs and have surpassed small intestine NENs in frequency.[4,6,8] Similar to colonic NETs, their incidence has increased in the United States.[6] The median age at diagnosis for rectal NETs is 56 years, and men are slightly more affected than women, with a male-to-female ratio of 1.1.[4] In the United States, racial discrepancies exist, with the ratio of NETs in blacks versus whites being 2.30 and in Asians versus non-Asians 4.99.[4]

DIAGNOSIS AND STAGING
Pathology

The nomenclature as related to tumor grade is summarized in **Table 1**. In general, well-differentiated tumors are low or intermediate grade, although they are also well-differentiated high-grade NETs. These are rare yet demonstrate improved prognosis compared with the poorly differentiated high-grade neuroendocrine carcinomas, which typically have large-cell and small-cell morphology.[9–11] The terms NET versus neuroendocrine carcinoma are typically reserved for well versus poorly differentiated tumors, respectively. However, as the terms have been used interchangeably in some publications, they must be qualified by details of grade and differentiation to convey meaningful pathology data.[5] Pathologic staging is via the TNM staging system.[12,13]

Elements critical to the pathology report are tumor size and depth of invasion, margin involvement, tumor grade, differentiation, presence of lymphovascular or mesoappendix invasion, and lymph node involvement. For appendiceal neoplasms, tumor location—whether the tumor is at the appendiceal base—should be reported, as well.

Table 1
Nomenclature and tumor grading system

Nomenclature	Differentiation	Grade	Ki-67 Index	Mitotic Rate, Mitoses/High Power Fields (HPF)
Neuroendocrine tumor	Well differentiated	Low grade (G1)	≤2%	<2/10 HPF
Neuroendocrine tumor	Well differentiated	Intermediate grade (G2)	3%–20%	2–20/10 HPF
Neuroendocrine carcinoma	Poorly differentiated	High grade (G3)	>20%	>20/10 HPF

Data from Refs.[4,5,16,39]

These factors influence tumor staging and whether a formal oncologic segmental resection is needed.

Biochemical Evaluation

For small, early stage, well-differentiated appendiceal NETs confined to the appendix and with negative margins on pathologic review, no further biochemical studies are needed. However, for all other appendiceal NETs, laboratory studies should be considered. Serum chromogranin A (CgA) testing is recommended by the North American Neuroendocrine Tumor Society (NANETS) and European Neuroendocrine Society (ENETS) for advanced metastatic disease, although its role in diagnosis and surveillance has yet to be determined, and is a disputed recommendation in National Comprehensive Cancer Network (NCCN) guidelines.[2,13,14] Both NANETS and NCCN guidelines recommend obtaining 24-hour urine 5′-hydroxyindoleacetic acid.[13,14] These tests can be falsely elevated by medications and diet, thus, prior cessation of proton pump inhibitors as well as medications and foods that elevate serotonin is necessary. For tumors in the colon and rectum, NANETS and ENETS recommend serum CgA testing and consideration of obtaining urine 5-HIAA, although both note that tumors of the colon and rectum rarely secrete serotonin.[14]

Imaging

Cross-sectional imaging for staging NENs depends on the extent of the disease. For R0 resections of early stage appendiceal NENs harboring no high-risk features, postoperative cross-sectional imaging is not indicated.[13,14] For completely resected, well-differentiated tumors between 1 and 2 cm, ENETS recommends cross-sectional imaging with either computed tomography (CT) or MRI of the abdomen and pelvis to evaluate for lymph node or distant metastasis.[2] For tumors greater than 2 cm, those with invasion beyond 3 mm into the mesoappendix, or with positive margins, cross-sectional imaging combined with somatostatin receptor imaging (SSTR-PET) should be obtained.[2,5,15]

Rectal neoplasms greater than 1 cm in size or with high-risk features should prompt pelvic MRI and/or endorectal ultrasound (EUS) to determine depth of invasion and lymph node status. For colon and rectal NENs larger than 2 cm, with invasion deeper than the submucosa, or with positive lymph nodes, NANETS, ENETS, and NCCN guidelines recommend CT or MRI of the abdomen and pelvis.[4,13,14,16] If not already done, full colonoscopy to evaluate the colon and rectum should be performed.

Advances in imaging techniques have improved disease detection for staging and surveillance. One such advance is in somatostatin receptor imaging. Somatostatin receptors (SSTR) are overexpressed in most NETs. Imaging with radiolabeled somatostatin analogues allows improved identification of disease. The newest agents use labeled gallium and include DOTATATE (Food and Drug Administration approved) and DOTATOC. Together, these are referred to SSTR-PET and replace ^{111}In-Pentetreotide scintigraphy (OctreoScan). SSTR-PET should be performed with intravenous contrast and should be combined with either CT or MRI cross-sectional imaging. PET/MRI is better for imaging of liver metastasis, whereas PET/CT offers improved visualization of mesenteric, bone, and pulmonary disease.[13,15] Except in very low–risk disease (eg, <2 cm low-grade appendiceal NET with negative margins or <1 cm low-grade rectal NET), SSTR-PET should be considered for staging. If a patient did not undergo SSTR-PET before surgical resection, consider obtaining this postoperatively to complete the staging.[15]

LOCATION

Appendiceal NETs can occur anywhere along the appendix, with 60% to 75% at the tip, 5% to 20% occurring in the midportion, and less than 10% occurring at the base of the appendix.[1,2,6] Those at the base may be more prone to an incomplete resection with appendectomy.

In 2 large series of NETs identified incidentally on appendectomy, tumors tended to be small and most were early stage. The series reported by Amr and colleagues[1] demonstrated the median tumor size to be 5 mm, with two-thirds measuring less than 1 cm. In a series reported by Pawa and colleagues[3] of 14,850 patients undergoing appendectomies at 3 European referral centers, of which 215 patients were identified to have NETs, the mean tumor size was 9.8 mm (1–50 mm); 24.2% of patients had tumors 1 to 2 cm and 29.3% had tumors greater than 2 cm. Mesoappendiceal lymph node metastases were present in 7.9% of specimens and 12 of the 49 patients who underwent subsequent right hemicolectomy had positive lymph nodes. Two of 215 patients presented with synchronous liver metastases.

NETs of the appendix are usually low or intermediate grade. Pape and colleagues[2] reported that 93% of NENs in their series were Grade 1, and all patients with Grade 2 or 3 tumors had positive locoregional lymph nodes. Although appendiceal NENs are rarely symptomatic, locally advanced tumors or those with distant metastases may be accompanied by abdominal pain or signs of bowel obstruction. Carcinoid syndrome is extremely rare and is consistent with metastatic disease.

In the pediatric population, the rate of NETs in appendectomy specimens seems to be slightly lower than in adults, with an incidence of 0.2% to 0.9%.[17,18] In 2 large series of pediatric appendectomies, the mean age of patients with NETs was 12.5 to 13.8 years; tumor size in these series resembled that of adults, with median sizes reported as 6.5 to 7 mm.[17,18] Neither series reported any recurrence of disease and noted a paucity of data to support surveillance following diagnosis.

NETs occur throughout the colon. Well-differentiated tumors in the cecum behave similarly to terminal ileal NETs. Unfortunately, colonic NETs tend to be more aggressive, poorly differentiated, and up to 40% are high-grade.[4,8] In a recent review of 1208 high-grade neuroendocrine carcinomas of the colon and rectum in the National Cancer Database (NCDB), 62.5% of these aggressive tumors occurred in the colon.[19] Unlike appendiceal neoplasms, there is a roughly even presentation across stages. Many more (approximately 30%–40%) of these tumors have metastases at diagnosis, perhaps because of late detection due to absence of symptoms with early disease.

Metastases are to the liver, lymph nodes, the mesentery, and peritoneum.[16] Symptoms that can occur with colon NETs are similar to colon adenocarcinomas, and include diarrhea, abdominal pain, weight loss, gastrointestinal bleeding and anemia, bowel obstruction, and a palpable mass.

Most rectal NETs are located in the midrectum, roughly 5 to 10 cm from the anal verge.[4]

Approximately 40% of rectal NETs are found incidentally on lower endoscopy, appearing as yellow-tinged sessile or submucosal polyps that can have a central depression or ulceration.[8,10] Patient symptoms, when present, include hematochezia, anorectal pain, tenesmus, altered bowel habits, and weight loss. Carcinoid syndrome is rare because tumors do not tend to produce serotonin.[10] The median size of these lesions is 0.6 cm and the majority (75%–85%) of rectal NETs are localized at diagnosis, with distant metastases at diagnosis in 2% to 8%.[4,16]

In rectal NETs, tumor size and depth of invasion have been linked to the likelihood of metastases. Historical data suggest a 2% incidence of metastases with rectal NENs less than 1.0 cm, versus 10% to 15% in tumors 1 to 2 cm and 60% to 80% in tumors greater than 2.0 cm.[20] Invasion of the muscularis propria significantly increases the risk of metastasis.[4,16] Other factors associated with metastatic behavior include high grade, poor differentiation, and lymphovascular and perineural invasion.[16]

RESECTION OF THE PRIMARY TUMOR AND REGIONAL LYMPH NODES
Appendix

The recommended surgical treatment of appendiceal NENs is fairly straightforward for tumors under 1 cm (appendectomy) or greater than 2 cm (segmental colectomy with regional lymphadenectomy). For tumors between 1 and 2 cm, the extent of resection necessary is less defined and weighing risks of incomplete resection with morbidity of segmental colectomy is required (**Fig. 1**).

For appendiceal NENs less than 1 cm, simple appendectomy is appropriate for most tumors. NANETS guidelines recommend appendectomy for tumors less than 1 cm while indicating the controversial role for right hemicolectomy in tumors with mesenteric invasion, higher grade, and involvement of the appendiceal base.[14] ENETS guidelines recommend appendectomy for tumors less than 1 cm except in the rare occurrence of tumor at the base of the appendix or mesoappendix invasion of greater than 3 mm on pathologic assessment. In either situation, a right hemicolectomy "seems advisable," but the investigators note a lack of evidence for improvement of prognosis.[2] ENETS incorporates mesoappendix invasion into their TNM staging system and reports that invasion greater than 3 mm may reflect a more aggressive neoplasm. Tumors of any size with mixed histology including goblet cell carcinoid or adenocarcinoid should be treated in the same manner as adenocarcinoma.[5] Right hemicolectomy should follow oncologic principles including adequate resection of the mesenteric lymph nodes.

Tumors 1 to 2 cm in overall dimension require more complex decision-making. Factors that portend increased risk of nodal or distant metastases or of disease recurrence are not clearly defined. The NCCN guidelines note the risk of lymph node metastases even in tumors less than 2 cm and support consideration of right hemicolectomy when poor prognostic features are present, such as mesoappendix infiltration or lymphovascular invasion.[13] NANETS guidelines recommend a formal right hemicolectomy in the setting of high-risk features including mesenteric invasion, tumor location at the appendiceal base, intermediate and high grades, lymphovascular invasion, obvious mesenteric lymph node involvement, and positive margins.[5] ENETS

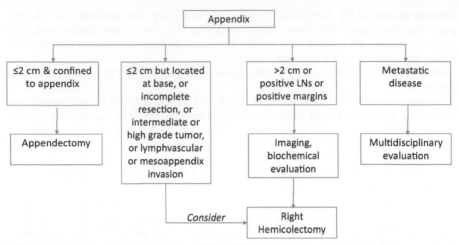

Fig. 1. Surgical management of appendiceal NETs.

guidelines offer similar recommendations, noting the risk of metastases particularly in tumors greater than 1.5 cm, whereas acknowledging lack of data supporting improved survival with more extensive resection.[2]

As noted earlier, the challenge for these intermediate-sized tumors is in predicting which will metastasize or recur. A review of 916 patients in the NCDB with 1 to 2 cm NENs compared survival for patients undergoing primary resection versus right hemicolectomy with lymphadenectomy. The investigators found no difference in survival between the 2 treatments, although there was insufficient stage and grade data for the investigators to include these in the hazards model.[21] Another review from the SEER database from 1988 to 2003 examined 89 patients with NENs with complete pathologic data and found that 47% of patients with tumors 1 to 2 cm had positive lymph nodes.[22] Factors associated with metastases with smaller tumors include small vessel invasion as well as invasion into or through the muscularis propria, independent of tumor size.[23,24]

Colon

If not already performed at time of diagnosis of a colonic NET, full colonoscopy for synchronous lesions or adenomatous lesions should be completed. Often found incidentally on colonoscopy, NETs that have been biopsied will require subsequent segmental colectomy for definitive treatment. To ensure an appropriate resection is performed, the NET location should be tattooed unless it is in an unambiguous location (cecum, ileocecal valve); this is critical because endoscopic identification of colonic location is not always accurate (**Fig. 2**).

Colonic NETs often present late and tend to behave more aggressively. For low- and intermediate-grade colonic NENs with size less than 2 cm, ENETS guidelines support endoscopic excision.[16] In comparison, NANETS guidelines recommend a right hemicolectomy for cecal NETs.[14] For distal colonic NETs, the 2013 NANETS guidelines are somewhat ambiguous in that the investigators lump distal colonic tumors with rectal tumors and suggest small NETs may be suitable for endoscopic resection. On closer review of the 2013 and 2010 NANETS guidelines, however, it seems that the recommendations for endoscopic resection are really only for rectal lesions.[4,14] Given the reported aggressive biology of colonic NETs, segmental colectomy performed in an

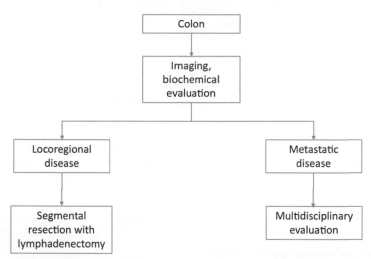

Fig. 2. Surgical management of colonic NETs.

oncologically sound fashion is likely most appropriate. Occasionally, patients with metastatic disease present with symptoms from the primary tumor; in these cases, one should consider resecting or diverting for palliation.

Rectum

The surgical management of rectal NETs mimics that of appendiceal neoplasms, with more discrete guidelines for tumors less than 1 cm or greater than 2 cm but less rigid recommendations for 1 to 2 cm lesions. This reflects a lack of data on the risks of metastases and recurrence with intermediate-sized rectal NETs (**Fig. 3**).

For rectal NETs less than 1 cm, local resection is recommended by both NANETS and ENETS guidelines.[4,14,16] The method of local resection can be either endoscopic or transanal surgery. Endoscopic techniques include traditional polypectomy, endoscopic mucosal resection (EMR), EMR band ligation, and endoscopic submucosal dissection.[8] Transanal excision approaches include traditional instrumentation as well as minimally invasive approaches such as transanal minimally invasive surgery and transanal endoscopic microsurgery. The advantages of each of these techniques are beyond the scope of this article.

For NETs 1 to 2 cm, EUS and/or MRI of the pelvis should be obtained to evaluate for invasion into the muscularis propria and evidence of regional lymph node metastases. Barring the presence of either of these, 1 to 2 cm rectal NETs can be removed by the aforementioned local resection methods, although techniques that facilitate en bloc resection with negative margins such as ESD or transanal surgical approaches should be considered, particularly for larger lesions.[4,16] Patients whose tumors are incompletely removed with polypectomy may be considered for repeat excision via transanal resection, although emerging data indicate that R1 resections (<1 mm resection margins) often do not recur within 5 years, so whether patients should simply be monitored versus reresected remains to be seen.[10,14] Locoregional positive lymph nodes or invasion of the muscularis propria should prompt discussion of radical mesorectal excision with either low anterior resection (LAR) or abdominoperineal resection (APR).[14]

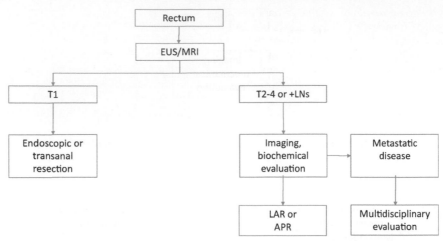

Fig. 3. Surgical management of rectal NETs.

In addition to size greater than 2 cm, factors favoring aggressive behavior in rectal NETs include high grade, poor differentiation, invasion of the muscularis propria, and lymphovascular invasion.[16] Because of these additional factors and the possibility of aggressive behavior in intermediate-sized lesions, there is debate over the optimal resection technique for 1 to 2 cm lesions. A recent evaluation of 321 patients in the NCDB from 2004 to 2013 who underwent excision of nonmetastatic 1 to 2 cm rectal NETs examined outcomes by resection type. In this study, 274 patients underwent local excision, whereas 47 underwent radical resection (LAR, APR, Hartmann proced-ure). Those undergoing radical resection had more advanced tumors, with 35.3% be-ing stage 3 versus none in the local resection group. Of those having local resection, 8.2% of patients had positive margins. This retrospective study was limited by its lack of information on depth of invasion. After adjusting for resection type, age, sex, comor-bidities, margin status, and lymph node status, there was no difference in outcomes between the 2 groups.[25] This finding was echoed by another review of 1794 patients in the NCDB from 1998 to 2012 with tumor size less than 2.0 cm; 89% of the patients in this subset underwent local excision. On Kaplan-Meier survival estimates, no differ-ence in survival was observed between those undergoing local resection versus radical surgery.[26] Although these are not the definitive answer to management of 1 to 2 cm rectal neoplasms, they point to the importance of discussing with patients the risks of incomplete resection along with the morbidities of radical resection. For tumors greater than 2 cm, patients should undergo mesorectal excision with LAR or APR.[14,16]

High-Grade Neuroendocrine Carcinoma

Patients with poorly differentiated, high-grade neuroendocrine carcinomas present a treatment dilemma. To date, there is mixed evidence as to the survival benefit conferred by surgical resection. Data from 1367 patients with high-grade NEC from the SEER database from 2000 to 2011 indicate that resection of localized non–small cell NEC offered survival benefit (median 21 months with surgery vs 6 months without, $P<.0001$), but there was no significant survival benefit seen with resection of small- cell NEC.[27] A series of 126 patients with high-grade colorectal NECs treated at Memorial Sloan Kettering between 1991 and 2010 demonstrated no improvement for patients undergoing resection of the primary, regardless of whether they had metastatic disease.[28] A review of 1208 patients in the NCDB with high-grade NEC observed a median survival of 10.5 months for those who underwent surgical resection versus 6.9 months for those who did not ($P<.001$). The investigators also reported that on multivariate analysis surgical resection was associated with improved overall survival (hazard ratio 0.54, confidence interval 0.44–0.66) and this association held even with patients with metastatic disease.[19]

Surgery in the Setting of Functional Neuroendocrine Tumors and Advanced Disease

Patients with functional neuroendocrine neoplasms should receive octreotide preoperatively to prevent carcinoid crisis. This should be administered intravenously before induction of anesthesia in a bolus of 250 to 500 ug, with additional doses administered as necessary throughout the surgery. It can be discontinued on postoperative day one if there are no issues.[13,14] In patients with advanced disease who are likely to receive long-term octreotide or lanreotide postoperatively, it is recommended that cholecystectomy be performed at the time of their surgical resection. With long-term octreotide administration, these patients are at risk for developing cholelithiasis and biliary symptoms.[13]

Management of Liver Metastases

Patients with NETs frequently die from liver failure due to hepatic metastases. Treating liver metastases should focus on improving symptoms and quality of life and extending survival.[5] The treatment modalities available for NETs with liver metastases are varied and depend on the individual patient's disease as well as local expertise. In addition, many of the recommendations for treatment are based on expert opinion only. Because of this, appropriate treatment of these patients demands discussion and review of imaging and pathology of each patient in a multidisciplinary tumor board at an institution experienced in NETs. Decisions on how and whether to treat liver metastases depend on the patient's symptomatology, burden of disease, and fitness to undergo various interventions.[29]

Pathologic diagnosis of liver metastasis via fine-needle aspirate, core needle, or surgical specimen is recommended to evaluate tumor differentiation and grade.[30] SSTR-PET CT or MRI should be obtained to assist in operative planning if tumor debulking is considered.[15] Options for controlling liver disease include systemic chemotherapy and peptide receptor–targeted radiotherapy, which are covered elsewhere. Locoregional and ablative therapies include transarterial embolization, transarterial chemoembolization, selective internal radiation therapy, radiofrequency ablation, and microwave ablation. There is a lack of data to suggest one locoregional therapy over another, although most are associated with tumor shrinkage and improvement in symptoms in more than 50% of patients.[29,30]

In well-selected patients, surgical debulking should be considered for palliation of symptoms associated with tumor bulk or hormone production. Patients with liver-predominant and hormonally active disease benefit from improved symptom control even if less than 90% of the disease burden can be removed.[29] Resection for improving survival has historically been advocated only if at least 90% of the tumor can be resected or ablated.[4] However, recent series are demonstrating clinically relevant improved survival when the threshold for liver debulking is 70%.[31–33] In a systematic review of liver resection for neuroendocrine metastases, Lesurtel and colleagues[34] did not find any evidence that surgical resection offered improved overall or progression-free survival when compared with other liver-directed therapies. In super-selected patients, including those in whom extrahepatic disease has been excluded and whose symptoms are refractory to medical management, liver transplantation may be considered.[29]

PROGNOSIS

Most patients with appendiceal NETs present at lower stage and therefore enjoy extremely good outcomes. With localized disease only, the 5-year overall survival is estimated between 95% and 100%.[2,3,35] Although size is associated with survival, one study reported no difference in 5-year overall survival for tumors less than 1 cm as compared with tumors 1 to 2 cm in size.[35] Tumors 2 cm or larger have a 5-year survival of 70.5%.[6] Five-year survival estimates for patients with regional disease range from 78% to 100%.[2,6,22,36] Unfortunately, patients presenting with distant metastases are faced with relatively poor 5-year survival of less than 25% and a median survival of 31 months.[2,7,36]

Colon NETs are, as noted earlier, more aggressive and have worse survival compared with small bowel, appendiceal, and rectal NETs. Across all stages, the average 5-year survival is estimated between 40% and 70%.[16] Based on a large multi-decade analysis of NETs, the 5-year survival for localized, regional, and metastatic colon NETs is 76%, 72%, and 30%, respectively.[36] In a review of SEER data on NETs from 1998 to 2004, the median survival for cecal NETs was 135, 107, and 55 months for localized, regional, and metastatic disease, respectively. The median survival for colon NETs excluding cecum is 52 months for regional disease and 7 months for metastatic disease.[7]

Compared with NETs of the lung, small intestine, stomach, colon, and pancreas, rectal NETs demonstrate the best overall and cancer specific survival.[37] Five-year overall survival for rectal NETs is estimated at 76% to 88% with a median survival across all stages of 240 months.[7,16,36] Median survival for localized, regional, and metastatic disease is 290, 90, and 26 months, respectively.[7] Five-year survival ranges from 15% to 32% if distant metastases are present.[4,38] In a recent evaluation of 687 patients in the NCDB who underwent radical resection for NET, the investigators found that patients with 1 to 4 positive lymph nodes had a 57.8% 5-year overall survival versus 32.6% overall survival in patients with 5 or more positive lymph nodes, suggesting opportunities for refining prognostication by lymph node stage.[38]

High-grade neuroendocrine cancers portend a poor prognosis. The median survival of all stages of colorectal neuroendocrine carcinoma in the SEER database from 2000 to 2011 was 8.1 months and in the NCDB from 2004 to 2015 was 9.0 months.[19,27] In a series from Memorial Sloan Kettering, Smith and colleagues[28] identified 126 patients with high-grade colorectal NECs where the median survival was 13.2 months.

SUMMARY

NENs of the appendix, colon, and rectum are rare and are increasing in incidence. Appropriate treatment depends in part on thorough histopathologic assessment. For intermediate-sized appendiceal and rectal tumors, guidelines are less rigid in their recommendations for extent of resection. Weighing risks of metastatic and recurrent disease with the morbidities accompanying more extensive resection are critical. Patients with advanced or metastatic disease are best served by centers with dedicated multidisciplinary tumor boards and practitioners experienced in NETs. Poorly differentiated, high-grade neuroendocrine carcinomas continue to demonstrate aggressive and lethal behavior.

REFERENCES

1. Amr B, Froghi F, Edmond M, et al. Management and outcomes of appendicular neuroendocrine tumours: Retrospective review with 5-year follow-up. Eur J Surg Oncol 2015;41(9):1243–6.
2. Pape UF, Niederle B, Costa F, et al. ENETS consensus guidelines for neuroendocrine neoplasms of the appendix (excluding goblet cell carcinomas). Neuroendocrinology 2016;103(2):144–52.
3. Pawa N, Clift AK, Osmani H, et al. Surgical management of patients with neuroendocrine neoplasms of the appendix: appendectomy or more. Neuroendocrinology 2018;106(3):242–51.
4. Anthony LB, Strosberg JR, Klimstra DS, et al. The NANETS consensus guidelines for the diagnosis and management of gastrointestinal neuroendocrine tumors (NETs): well-differentiated nets of the distal colon and rectum. Pancreas 2010; 39(6):767–74.
5. Boudreaux JP, Klimstra DS, Hassan MM, et al. The NANETS consensus guideline for the diagnosis and management of neuroendocrine tumors: well-differentiated neuroendocrine tumors of the Jejunum, Ileum, Appendix, and Cecum. Pancreas 2010;39(6):753–66.
6. Byrne RM, Pommier RF. Small bowel and colorectal carcinoids. Clin Colon Rectal Surg 2018;31(5):301–8.
7. Yao JC, Hassan M, Phan A, et al. One hundred years after "carcinoid": epidemiology of and prognostic factors for neuroendocrine tumors in 35,825 cases in the United States. J Clin Oncol 2008;26(18):3063–72.
8. Ramage JK, De Herder WW, Delle Fave G, et al. ENETS consensus guidelines update for colorectal neuroendocrine neoplasms. Neuroendocrinology 2016; 103(2):139–43.
9. Klimstra DS, Modlin IR, Coppola D, et al. The pathologic classification of neuroendocrine tumors: a review of nomenclature, grading, and staging systems. Pancreas 2010;39(6):707–12.
10. Ramage JK, Valle JW, Nieveen van Dijkum EJM, et al. Colorectal neuroendocrine neoplasms: areas of unmet need. Neuroendocrinology 2019;108(1):45–53.
11. Garcia-Carbonero R, Sorbye H, Baudin E, et al. ENETS consensus guidelines for high-grade gastroenteropancreatic neuroendocrine tumors and neuroendocrine carcinomas. Neuroendocrinology 2016;103(2):186–94.
12. Amin MB, Edge SB, Greene FL, et al, editors. AJCC Cancer Staging Manual. 8th ed. New York: Springer; 2017.
13. National Comprehensive Cancer Network. Neuroendocrine and adrenal tumors (Version 1.2019). 2019. Available at: https://www.nccn.org/professionals/physician_gls/pdf/neuroendocrine.pdf.
14. Kunz PL, Reidy-Lagunes D, Anthony LB, et al. Consensus guidelines for the management and treatment of neuroendocrine tumors. Pancreas 2013;42(4):557–77.
15. Hope TA, Bergsland EK, Bozkurt MF, et al. Appropriate use criteria for somatostatin receptor PET imaging in neuroendocrine tumors. J Nucl Med 2018;59(1): 66–74.
16. Caplin M, Sundin A, Nillson O, et al. ENETS Consensus Guidelines for the management of patients with digestive neuroendocrine neoplasms: colorectal neuroendocrine neoplasms. Neuroendocrinology 2012;95(2):88–97.
17. Vandevelde A, Gera P. Carcinoid tumours of the appendix in children having appendicectomies at Princess Margaret Hospital since 1995. J Pediatr Surg 2015; 50(9):1595–9.

18. Fallon SC, Hicks MJ, Carpenter JL, et al. Management of appendiceal carcinoid tumors in children. J Surg Res 2015;198(2):384–7.
19. Fields AC, Lu P, Vierra BM, et al. Survival in patients with high-grade colorectal neuroendocrine carcinomas: the role of surgery and chemotherapy. Ann Surg Oncol 2019;26(4):1127–33.
20. Mani S, Modlin IM, Ballantyne G, et al. Carcinoids of the rectum. J Am Coll Surg 1994;179(2):231–48.
21. Nussbaum DP, Speicher PJ, Gulack BC, et al. Management of 1- to 2-cm Carcinoid tumors of the appendix: using the national cancer data base to address controversies in general surgery. J Am Coll Surg 2015;220(5):894–903.
22. Mullen JT, Savarese DM. Carcinoid tumors of the appendix: a population-based study. J Surg Oncol 2011;104(1):41–4.
23. Kleiman DA, Finnerty B, Beninato T, et al. Features associated with metastases among well-differentiated neuroendocrine (Carcinoid) tumors of the appendix: the significance of small vessel invasion in addition to size. Dis Colon Rectum 2015;58(12):1137–43.
24. Mosquera C, Fitzgerald TL, Vora H, et al. Novel nomogram combining depth of invasion and size can accurately predict the risk for regional nodal metastases for appendiceal neuroendocrine tumors (A-NET). J Surg Oncol 2017;116(6):651–7.
25. Fields AC, Saadat LV, Scully RE, et al. Local excision versus radical resection for 1- to 2-cm neuroendocrine tumors of the rectum: a national cancer database analysis. Dis Colon Rectum 2019;62(4):417–21.
26. Ezekian B, Adam MA, Turner MC, et al. Local excision results in comparable survival to radical resection for early-stage rectal carcinoid. J Surg Res 2018;230:28–33.
27. Shafqat H, Ali S, Salhab M, et al. Survival of patients with neuroendocrine carcinoma of the colon and rectum: a population-based analysis. Dis Colon Rectum 2015;58(3):294–303.
28. Smith JD, Reidy DL, Goodman KA, et al. A retrospective review of 126 high-grade neuroendocrine carcinomas of the colon and rectum. Ann Surg Oncol 2014;21(9):2956–62.
29. Pavel M, O'Toole D, Costa F, et al. ENETS consensus guidelines update for the management of distant metastatic disease of intestinal, pancreatic, bronchial Neuroendocrine Neoplasms (NEN) and NEN of unknown primary site. Neuroendocrinology 2016;103(2):172–85.
30. Strosberg JR, Halfdanarson TR, Bellizzi AM, et al. The North American Neuroendocrine Tumor Society Consensus guidelines for surveillance and medical management of Midgut neuroendocrine tumors. Pancreas 2017;46(6):707–14.
31. Maxwell JE, Sherman SK, O'Dorisio TM, et al. Liver-directed surgery of neuroendocrine metastases: What is the optimal strategy? Surgery 2016;159(1):320–33.
32. Scott AT, Breheny PJ, Keck KJ, et al. Effective cytoreduction can be achieved in patients with numerous neuroendocrine tumor liver metastases (NETLMs). Surgery 2019;165(1):166–75.
33. Graff-Baker AN, Sauer DA, Pommier SJ, et al. Expanded criteria for carcinoid liver debulking: Maintaining survival and increasing the number of eligible patients. Surgery 2014;156(6):1369–76 [discussion: 76–7].
34. Lesurtel M, Nagorney DM, Mazzaferro V, et al. When should a liver resection be performed in patients with liver metastases from neuroendocrine tumours? A systematic review with practice recommendations. HPB (Oxford) 2015;17(1):17–22.

35. Landry CS, Woodall C, Scoggins CR, et al. Analysis of 900 appendiceal carcinoid tumors for a proposed predictive staging system. Arch Surg 2008;143(7):664–70 [discussion: 70].
36. Modlin IM, Lye KD, Kidd M. A 5-decade analysis of 13,715 carcinoid tumors. Cancer 2003;97(4):934–59.
37. Man D, Wu J, Shen Z, et al. Prognosis of patients with neuroendocrine tumor: a SEER database analysis. Cancer Manag Res 2018;10:5629–38.
38. Fields AC, McCarty JC, Ma-Pak L, et al. New lymph node staging for rectal neuroendocrine tumors. J Surg Oncol 2019;119(1):156–62.
39. Rindi G, Arnold R, Bosman FT, et al. Nomenclature and classification of neuroendocrine neoplasms of the digestive system. In: Bosman FT, Carneiro F, Hruban RH, et al, editors. WHO classification of tumours of the digestive system. 4th edition. Lyon (France): IARC; 2010. p. 13–4.

Management of Metastatic GEPNETs

Kristen E. Limbach, MD[a,1], Rodney F. Pommier, MD[b],*

KEYWORDS

• GEPNETS • NETS • Metastases

KEY POINTS

• The chief causes of death of patients with GEPNETs are liver failure from hepatic replacement by tumor in the majority and bowel obstruction in the remainder.

• Many patient with liver metastases are actually eligible for hepatic cytoreductive operations, even if numerous bilobar metastases are present, provided 70% of the tumor volume can be removed.

• Patients with higher liver tumor burden can have liver metastases treated with intra-arterial therapies, such as embolization or chemoembolization.

• Cytoreductive operations including peritoneal stripping and bowel resections are recommend for patients with peritoneal carcinomatosis.

• Expert consensus recommends bisphosphonate therapy for bone metastases, reserving surgical treatment for patients with mechanical issues and/or potential spinal cord compression.

INCIDENCE

Neuroendocrine tumors (NETs) were originally described as benign, but it has become clear in the modern era that these tumors exhibit malignant behavior far more often than previously thought.[1] The largest series to date, by Modlin and colleagues[1] in 2003, reports that the current rates of metastasis, arranged by primary tumor site, are stomach, 6.5%; pancreas, 59.4%; small intestine, 22.4%; cecum, 41.0%; appendix, 9.9%; sigmoid colon, 6.6%; rectum and rectosigmoid junction, 2.0%; and anus, anal canal, and anorectum, 11.1%. However, some series have reported frequencies of distant metastasis as high as 60% to 80% depending on primary tumor location and type of institution.[2,3]

Frequent metastatic sites include the liver, peritoneum, bone, and lung.[4–6] The most commonly observed location is the liver, which is involved in more than 44% of NETs.[1]

a Department of Surgery, Oregon Health & Science University, Portland, OR, 97239, USA; b Division of Surgical Oncology, Department of Surgery, Mail Code L619, Oregon Health & Science University, Portland, OR 97239, USA
1 Present address: 1530 North Blandena Street, Portland, OR 97217.
* Corresponding author.
E-mail address: pommierr@ohsu.edu

Surg Oncol Clin N Am 29 (2020) 281–292
https://doi.org/10.1016/j.soc.2019.11.001
1055-3207/20/© 2019 Elsevier Inc. All rights reserved.

By contrast, peritoneal metastases were historically considered to be rare,[4] but recent studies have indicated an incidence of 4% to 11% for all gastroenteropancreatic neuroendocrine tumors (GEPNETs).[7,8] The frequency of peritoneal metastases by location of the primary tumor is highest for those with small intestinal and colon NETs (13% for each), 5% for those with occult gastrointestinal NETs, and less than 5% for those with appendiceal, pancreas, and esophageal/stomach NETs.[8] Similarly, bone metastases were also considered to be uncommon, but the modern series by Van Loon and colleagues[9] observed rates of 8.8% for gastrointestinal NETs and 7.8% for pancreatic neuroendocrine tumors (PNETs). Autopsy studies show rates as high as 42%, underscoring the difficulty in diagnosis of neuroendocrine bone metastases.[10] However, the increasing use of [68]gallium-DOTATATE PET-computed tomography (CT) has revealed metastatic disease in sites that had previously eluded other means of clinical detection,[11] which may increase the detection of bone metastases in the future. Most bone metastases originate from foregut and hindgut primaries, with midgut primaries being a less frequent source.[12]

HEPATIC METASTASES

Management of hepatic metastases is of critical importance because liver failure is the major cause of mortality in this population.[13] Consequently, several treatment modalities have been explored in the literature in recent years, including surgical cytoreduction by both formal resection and parenchyma-sparing debulking procedures, radiofrequency or microwave ablation, intraarterial therapies (IAT), liver transplantation, peptide receptor radionuclide therapy (PRRT), and medical management, of which PRRT and medical management are discussed in other articles. Although the uncommon nature of GEPNETs has made level 1 evidence comparing these modalities scarce, it should be noted that the data that are available have shown clear differences in outcomes.

Surgical Cytoreduction

Surgical cytoreduction is the preferred option for management of hepatic metastases, and surgery with clinical curative intent should be at least considered for all low- and intermediate-grade GEPNET patients.[4] Unfortunately, misunderstanding of operative criteria has led to a vast underutilization of surgical cytoreduction for these patients, with many never benefiting from a surgical evaluation.[13,14] Thus, current recommendations emphasize accurate imaging and pathology review in a multidisciplinary tumor board that includes a surgical opinion.[4] Furthermore, consultation of an experienced neuroendocrine surgeon should be considered in every case, even if the patient has been previously deemed unresectable.[14] One high-volume center noted that 67% of patients with advanced GEPNETs for whom they were able to perform surgical cytoreduction had been previously explored and deemed unresectable by another surgeon,[15] demonstrating the necessity of GEPNET-specific experience in determining resectability.

Options for surgical cytoreduction include formal anatomic hepatic resection as well as parenchyma-sparing procedures, which include enucleation and wedge resection.[16] Surgical treatment of metastatic GEPNETs is unique in that many patients present with diffuse, bilobar disease that would render their metastases unresectable in other types of cancer. However, an R0 resection is not required to achieve comparable oncologic outcomes,[13,17] and negative margins are not required.[13,18] Lesions are often peripheral and can be removed by enucleation without major hepatic resection and with low blood loss.[13] Thus, use of parenchyma-sparing procedures with or without ablation can facilitate resection in most patients to the currently accepted debulking threshold of 70%,[3] even when numerous metastases are present.[19] There are no randomized data available at this time to support a specific debulking threshold, but the accumulated retrospective evidence from multiple studies over the past several decades has led to the establishment of progressively lower debulking thresholds as studies reveal comparable oncologic outcomes.

Consistent with the principles used in treatment of other types of cancer, early studies required complete resection of all hepatic disease. In 1990, McEntee and colleagues[20] proposed a 90% debulking threshold for symptom control. Although they were not able to evaluate oncologic outcomes at that time, the proposal was followed by the landmark retrospective series by Sarmiento and colleagues[21] in 2003, which retrospectively examined 170 patients, of whom 95 underwent debulking with a 90% threshold for symptom control and the remainder underwent complete excision. The 2 groups exhibited no significant difference in survival, with a median overall survival (MOS) of 81 months and a 5-year survival rate of 61% for the 2 groups combined. Further studies have more recently indicated that lowering the debulking threshold even further, to 70%, is sufficient to achieve comparable oncologic outcomes. Graff-Baker and colleagues[18] in 2014 demonstrated that in gastrointestinal NETs, a debulking threshold of 70% resulted in comparable hepatic progression-free survival (PFS) and disease-specific survival to the previously proposed threshold of 90%, and additional examination of outcomes after surgical resection of PNET hepatic metastases by Morgan and colleagues[22] also found no difference in overall survival between these groups. These findings were replicated by Maxwell and colleagues,[16] who examined a larger range of debulking percentages (<50% to ≥90%) and found that the 70% threshold was associated with improved overall and hepatic PFS in PNETs as well as improved hepatic PFS in small bowel NETs (SBNETs) when compared with debulking of less than 70%. There was no difference in overall survival between the debulking thresholds of 70% and greater. Thus, current recommendations have established 70% as the threshold for surgical cytoreduction.[3,16,18,19,22]

Overall, multiple retrospective series have shown surgical cytoreduction methods to be safe, with a mortality of less than 5% and an acceptable surgical morbidity.[21,23,24] Benefits of surgical cytoreduction include relief of symptoms from carcinoid syndrome and functional NETs, without requiring continued long-acting somatostatin analogue injections.[21,23] Sarmiento and colleagues[21] demonstrated that this relief is fairly durable, with a 96% symptom response rate and median time to recurrence of 45.5 months. The 5-year recurrence rate was 59%, but recurrent symptoms were notably less severe and typically easily controlled with octreotide.

More importantly, surgical cytoreduction appears to confer a survival advantage over medical therapy alone, although there are currently no randomized controlled trials to conclusively prove this. Retrospective series by Que and colleagues,[23] Sarmiento and colleagues,[21] and Maxwell and colleagues[16] have determined an MOS ranging from 81 to 126 months with 5-year survival rates of 61% to 76.1%. Although difficult to compare directly, these outcomes represent vast improvements over historical data that showed an MOS of 2 to 4 years and a 30% to 40% 5-year survival rate with medical therapy alone.[25] It should be noted, however, that surgical cytoreduction has a significant rate of recurrence, which has been reported to be as high as 84% at 5 years and 94% at 10 years with a median time to recurrence of 21 months.[21] The site of recurrence is most commonly in the liver (82% of cases), but recurrences have also been noted in the bone and lung.[21] In the case of hepatic recurrence, a second liver debulking operation has also been shown to be safe,[18,22,24] and patients should be evaluated for additional cytoreduction procedures.

Ablation Procedures

Radiofrequency ablation (RFA) has also been shown to be a useful modality in the treatment of hepatic neuroendocrine metastases, both on its own and as an adjunct to surgical debulking. RFA works by converting radiofrequency energy into heat; a probe is inserted into the lesion to be ablated and raises the temperature of the surrounding area to approximately 85°C. The diameter of the resulting necrosis can be up to around 4 cm, depending on the probe and technique used, but lesions amenable to RFA are typically less than 2 cm.[26,27] The probe insertion can be done percutaneously, either by an ultrasound or CT-guided approach or by an intraoperative ultrasound-guided approach.[28] Microwave ablation has been replacing RFA in many centers because it is less susceptible to the heat sink effect of nearby blood vessels, giving more complete ablations, but this also makes it more likely to damage nearby adjacent ducts. It is also faster, allowing for many lesions to be ablated in a relatively short period of time, which may be up to 5 cm in size.[19]

One of the most frequently noted benefits of ablation is that it can reach lesions that would be difficult to resect surgically, either because of position within the liver or because of bilobar disease burden. Thus, disease that would have previously been unresectable may still be cytoreduced.[26] Using this combined approach, it has been shown that a 70% debulking threshold can be achieved in most cases,[16] even when there are numerous (>10) metastases present.[19] However, data directly comparing outcomes of a combined approach with those of a purely surgical or ablative approach are lacking. Ablation has been demonstrated to have acceptable morbidity and low mortality,[19,28] and combined procedures, in which ablation is used as an adjunct to surgical cytoreduction, have also been shown to be safe.[16]

Ablation can be performed both for symptom relief and to improve survival. A meta-analysis by Mohan and colleagues[28] in 2015 found that 92% of patients with symptoms experienced either partial or complete symptom relief. Median duration of symptom relief ranged from 14 to 27 months, although there was significant variation in symptom assessment between the included studies. Survival outcomes after laparoscopic RFA of neuroendocrine metastases were also examined by Akyildiz and colleagues,[29] who found that median disease-free survival was 15 months and MOS was 6 years. Combined surgical cytoreduction and ablation survival outcomes have been reported as a median PFS of 23 months to 3.2 years and an MOS of 89 months.[16,19] Thus, ablation appears to be a safe and effective adjunct to surgical cytoreduction to improve survival and relieve symptoms in patients with neuroendocrine liver metastases.

Intraarterial Therapies

Despite the recently expanded criteria and multiple tools available to achieve surgical cytoreduction in patients with metastatic NETs, not all patients are candidates for surgical debulking. One option for these patients is IAT, of which there are several modalities available. These modalities include transarterial bland embolization (TAE), conventional transarterial chemoembolization (cTACE), transarterial chemoembolization using drug-eluting beads (DEB-TACE), and transarterial radioembolization (TARE). TAE functions by inducing selective ischemia in metastatic tumors, which are predominantly supplied by branches of the hepatic arteries. Swärd and colleagues[30] in 2009 found that MOS after treatment with TAE was 56 months, with symptomatic relief in 71% of patients. The procedure carried an associated mortality of 1.9%. TAE is more frequently associated with pain after the procedure than with other, similar procedures, such as cTACE or TARE.[31] However, a small pilot study for a prospective clinical trial comparing TAE with TARE showed that TAE was associated with superior oncologic outcomes (increased response rate at 3 and 6 months after the procedure).[32]

cTACE has been performed for more than 20 years[33] and has been well established to be generally well tolerated.[34] Several studies have examined outcomes with a variety of chemotherapeutic agents, with MOS ranging from 33.8 to 86.1 months[35,36] and 5-year survival rate ranging from 40.8% to 65%. Symptom relief was noted in 47% to 57% of patients with carcinoid syndrome.[35,37] Prospective data comparing cTACE to other IAT modalities are currently limited, but Do Minh and colleagues[36] retrospectively compared cTACE relative to DEB-TACE and TARE. The investigators found a median hepatic PFS of 21.6 months and an MOS of 33.8 months for cTACE, with significantly superior survival outcomes with cTACE than with DEB-TACE (MOS 21.7 months) or TARE (MOS 23.6 months). Retrospective comparison of cTACE with TAE found no difference in outcomes.[37]

DEB-TACE and TARE with yttrium-90 microspheres are 2 additional modalities that initially showed promise in the treatment of neuroendocrine hepatic metastases. However, retrospective comparisons have failed to show a survival benefit over cTACE,[36] and there is concern that there is a significantly higher rate of biochemical toxicity with TARE than with cTACE or TAE.[31] Thus, the role of these modalities remains to be elucidated.[31,36] Consequently, the prospective RETNET trial has been designed to determine differences in outcomes between these modalities and is currently accruing.

Liver Transplantation

Another option for treatment of diffuse liver metastases that are not amenable to surgical cytoreduction or RFA is liver transplantation. However, transplantation remains highly controversial, because prospective data are lacking, particularly data comparing transplant to other treatment modalities. A 2017 metaanalysis of 64 retrospective studies examining outcomes after liver transplantation found 5-year survival rates ranging from 49.2% to 70.7% with recurrence rates of 31.3% to 56.8%.[38] However, a retrospective review of the European Liver Transplant Registry, which included 213 cases of metastatic NET to the liver between 1982 and 2009, found a 3-month postoperative mortality of 10%, mostly related to surgical complications, including severe hemorrhage, thrombosis, and primary graft nonfunction. Retransplantation was required in 11% of patients, and a total of 17% of patients died of either early or late complications of the liver transplant without evidence of recurrent disease. Outcomes for the overall patient population included an MOS of 67 months with a 5-year survival rate of 52% and disease-free survival rate of 17%.[39] Thus, liver transplantation may confer a survival benefit among patients with diffuse neuroendocrine metastases to the liver who are not candidates for surgical cytoreduction, but many concerns remain given the high mortality, high complication rate, high recurrence rate, scarcity of available grafts, and lack of level 1 evidence comparing it to other treatment modalities. Furthermore, there are no strategies available for treatment of hepatic recurrence after transplant.[40]

Summary of Treatment Options for Grade 1 or 2 Hepatic Neuroendocrine Metastases

Surgical cytoreduction and ablative therapies are the preferred treatment of grade 1 or 2 hepatic neuroendocrine metastases,[4] and use of combined surgical and ablative modalities may facilitate resection of hepatic metastases to the currently accepted threshold of 70% debulking in most patients,[16] even when numerous metastases are present.[19] In cases of unresectable metastases, IAT may provide benefit. Liver transplantation is not recommended except in highly select cases.[4]

PERITONEAL METASTASIS

There are no generally agreed on medical or surgical treatment algorithms for peritoneal metastasis. However, patients treated with surgical debulking may achieve long-term survival,[3] and operation is often indicated for prevention and/or treatment of either external or internal bowel obstruction; intestinal hemorrhage; avoidance of complications related to fibrosis, such as accordion pleating of the bowel, mesenteric retraction, or vascular compromise; and treatment of segmental portal hypertension (in PNETs). Thus, the 2010 European Neuroendocrine Tumor Society (ENETS) treatment guidelines emphasize histopathologic confirmation of peritoneal metastasis, staging, and subsequent consideration of surgical treatment, based on expert consensus and retrospective data.[5]

Staging

There are multiple staging classifications for peritoneal metastasis, all of which were originally developed for other cancer types. For staging of GEPNETs, ENETS guidelines specifically recommend the peritoneal carcinomatosis index (PCI) and Gilly's classification.[5] The PCI quantifies the peritoneal burden of disease by region of the abdomen and pelvis and is reported as a composite score between 1 and 39.[41] A simpler and potentially more reproducible classification scheme is Gilly's classification, which is also known as the Lyon prognostic index (LPI) (**Table 1**).[42]

The LPI investigators concede that one of the shortcomings of this staging system is that it does not reflect the resectability of the lesions.[42] However, it has shown promise as a prognostic indicator in GEPNETs.[43]

Management

Candidacy for operation should generally be considered on a case-by-case basis, but surgical cytoreduction may be indicated for any of several reasons, as stated above.[5] The preferred techniques for cytoreductive operations for peritoneal metastasis are determined by the disease burden. Limited areas of peritoneal metastasis may be treated with regional peritoneal excision, whereas more extensive disease may require peritoneal stripping or resection in the areas of the implants, such as diaphragmatic, small bowel, or sigmoid resection. Small bowel and mesenteric implants can be individually excised. Additional tools available include use of electrocautery or argon beam to burn small lesions.[3] Use of hyperthermic intraperitoneal chemotherapy (HIPEC) has also been proposed, although data are lacking regarding its efficacy in NETs.[5] Elias and colleagues[44] combined cytoreductive surgery with HIPEC for treatment of peritoneal metastasis, but the investigators thought that the complications of

Table 1 Lyon prognostic index	
Stage	**Description**
0	No macroscopic disease
1	Lesions <0.5 cm in diameter, localized to 1 part of abdomen
2	Lesions <0.5 cm in diameter, diffuse
3	Lesions >0.5 cm and <2 cm in diameter, localized or diffuse
4	Lesions >2 cm in diameter, localized or diffuse

Data from Glehen O, Mohamed F, Gilly FN. Peritoneal carcinomatosis from digestive tract cancer: new management by cytoreductive surgery and intraperitoneal chemohyperthermia. The Lancet. Oncology. Apr 2004;5(4):219-228.

HIPEC outweighed any potential benefit and stopped using it by the final one-third of the patients in the study. Consequently, society guidelines state that there is no evidence for the use of HIPEC for treatment of peritoneal metastases in GEPNETs.[3,5]

Regardless of the specific operative approach, many of the studies available agree that aggressive surgical resection may yield both symptom relief and survival benefit. One retrospective study of 82 patients, of whom 47.6% had extensive small bowel and mesenteric/peritoneal involvement, found that aggressive surgical debulking led to significant symptom improvement in 91.5% of cases. Of those with partial or complete intestinal obstruction, 92% experienced relief of their obstruction, and all patients with intractable abdominal pain had significant improvement (20 out of 27 weaned off chronic opioid pain medications). Thirty-day mortality was 0%; median actuarial survival was 51.2 months.[15] Elias and colleagues[44] also compared those who underwent cytoreductive operation and intraperitoneal chemotherapy with those who were not operative candidates and found a significantly improved 5-year survival rate in the operative group (66.2% vs 40.9%, $P = .007$). Cause of death in the nonoperative group was liver failure in 60% of patients and bowel obstruction from peritoneal metastasis in the remainder of the patients, leading the investigators to conclude that if untreated, peritoneal metastasis would be a direct cause of death in up to 40% of patients. Moreover, Norlen and colleagues[43] showed that the postoperative burden of disease may have profound implications for patient prognosis. The investigators used the LPI to retrospectively compare outcomes for 672 consecutive patients with SBNETs, of whom 73 had peritoneal carcinomatosis at initial celiotomy. The investigators found that postoperative LPI was an independent predictor of prognosis; MOS for those with postoperative stage 0 was 11.5 years, stage 1 8.5 years, stage 2 6.3 years, stage 3 5.6 years, and stage 4 4.0 years ($P = .007$). It should be noted that outcomes were not statistically different when compared by preoperative LPI ($P = .322$). Thus, these studies as well as additional institutional experiences have led to a consensus expert view that favors meticulous resection of peritoneal metastasis in specialized centers when surgical risk is acceptable,[5] although clinical trials will be necessary to determine the optimal strategy.

The potential benefits of cytoreductive operation in peritoneal metastasis may be somewhat offset by the high rates of morbidity associated with the procedure. Elias and colleagues[45] have reported that combined hepatic and extrahepatic resections constitute major abdominal procedures, with operations lasting longer than 5 hours in 83% of patients. Furthermore, the series by Boudreaux and colleagues[15] and Elias and colleagues[44] reported high rates of morbidity, ranging from 39% to 47%, although in the latter series these may have been adversely affected by the addition of HIPEC. Thus, determination of surgical candidacy should be made on a case-by-case basis, although in many cases operative cytoreduction is reasonable given the worse prognosis and potential complications associated with untreated peritoneal metastasis.[43,46]

Summary of Treatment Options for Grade 1 or 2 Peritoneal Neuroendocrine Metastasis

Although there are no well-established surgical or medical treatment options for peritoneal metastasis, surgical resection is associated with improved outcomes,[3,5] and the greatest volume possible should be removed because a lower postoperative Lyon stage appears to confer survival benefit.[43] Operative peritoneal cytoreduction may be combined with hepatic debulking operations. However, this typically constitutes a major abdominal operation and may be associated with a relatively high morbidity. There is no evidence for improved results by including HIPEC in GEPNET patients with peritoneal metastasis.

BONE METASTASIS

Like peritoneal metastasis, bone metastasis in low- and intermediate-grade GEPNETs has long been considered to be rare, and only recently has the literature begun to acknowledge that bone metastases may be prevalent enough to have a significant negative impact on the quality of life and prognosis of patients with GEPNETs.[9] Thus, there is a paucity of prospective data to guide management.

Symptom Management

Symptomatic patients should be considered for treatment to address their symptoms.[6] Bone pain may be managed with analgesia, including nonsteroidal anti-inflammatory drugs[47] and consideration of radiation therapy.[6] Radiation has been well studied for palliation of bone pain from metastases in other types of cancer, and it appears to be generally safe and provide a reproducible pain response. One retrospective study of 44 NET patients treated with radiation between 1950 and 1986 found that for the 8 included patients with bone metastases, complete or partial response was achieved in 88% of radiation therapy courses, and 78% of patients remained free from in-field tumor progression (no median follow-up provided).[48] Accordingly, ENETS guidelines recommend radiation therapy for palliation of bone pain as well as prophylactically to avoid fractures.[6]

Guidelines additionally suggest treatment with bisphosphonates for all patients with bone metastases, although they have not been validated specifically in GEPNETs.[6] The additional antiresorptive agent denosumab, which is a monoclonal antibody that inhibits osteoclasts, has also been approved for treatment of bone metastases and is another option.[9] Some limited evidence has shown that patients with adrenocortical carcinoma metastatic to the bone may derive benefit from treatment with denosumab, although it has not been studied in GEPNETs.[49] Patients with hypercalcemia may also benefit from adequate hydration.[6]

Treatment Options

There is a paucity of evidence to determine which patients with bone metastases would benefit from surgical intervention. Early reports extrapolated the surgical excision data from studies not aimed to evaluate treatment of bone metastases specifically; these suggested that surgical excision was a reasonable approach because otherwise GEPNETs are generally well treated with surgery.[48] However, the overall lack of evidence has led the 2010 ENETS guidelines for management of GEPNET bone metastases to state that surgery is only recommended for individual lesions or for mechanical reasons, such as instability of the axial skeleton.

For patients with more than a solitary lesion, options for treatment with clinical curative intent generally include only PRRT in somatostatin receptor-positive cases and ^{131}I- metaiodobenzylguanidine in somatostatin receptor-negative cases,[6] although evidence is limited and outcomes have so far not been impressive. Ezziddin and colleagues[50] found that treatment with ^{177}Lu-DOTA octreotate PRRT resulted in complete response in 5% of patients, partial response in 33%, a minor response in 12%, stable disease in 38%, and progressive disease in 12%. Those that had regression of their bone metastases trended toward improved outcomes, because they had not yet reached MOS after 53 months of follow-up (MOS for nonregression group 39 months, $P = .076$). Symptoms of bone metastases completely resolved in 55% of those with bone pain and partially improved in 45%.

Spinal Cord Compression

Patients who present with symptoms concerning spinal cord compression, including numbness, paresthesias, and weakness, should be further evaluated with appropriate imaging. It is generally accepted that those with spinal cord compression should be considered for operative intervention.[47] Evidence is lacking regarding optimal management, but case reports describe symptom relief and improvement in neurologic status with operative spinal cord decompression combined with postoperative radiation therapy.[51]

Summary of Treatment Options for Grade 1 or 2 Bone Neuroendocrine Metastasis

Evidence is lacking to guide treatment of GEPNET bone metastases. Guidelines based on expert consensus recommend bisphosphonates for all patients with bone metastases. Surgery should be reserved for patients with solitary lesions, mechanical issues that would be amenable to surgical intervention, or potentially spinal cord compression.[6] However, PRRT is an emerging option that may have a role in the treatment of bone metastases. Bone pain may be palliated with analgesia and consideration of radiation therapy.

DISCLOSURE

Rodney F. Pommier, MD is a consultant to Novartis Oncology Pharmaceuticals, Ipsen Pharmaceuticals, Lexicon Pharmaceuticals, and Advanced Accelerator Applications.

REFERENCES

1. Modlin IM, Lye KD, Kidd M. A 5-decade analysis of 13,715 carcinoid tumors. Cancer 2003;97(4):934–59.
2. Boudreaux JP, Klimstra DS, Hassan MM, et al. The NANETS consensus guideline for the diagnosis and management of neuroendocrine tumors: well-differentiated neuroendocrine tumors of the jejunum, ileum, appendix, and cecum. Pancreas 2010;39(6):753–66.
3. Howe JR, Cardona K, Fraker DL, et al. The surgical management of small bowel neuroendocrine tumors: consensus guidelines of the North American Neuroendocrine Tumor Society. Pancreas 2017;46(6):715–31.
4. Pavel M, O'Toole D, Costa F, et al. ENETS consensus guidelines update for the management of distant metastatic disease of intestinal, pancreatic, bronchial neuroendocrine neoplasms (NEN) and NEN of unknown primary site. Neuroendocrinology 2016;103(2):172–85.
5. Kianmanesh R, Ruszniewski P, Rindi G, et al. ENETS consensus guidelines for the management of peritoneal carcinomatosis from neuroendocrine tumors. Neuroendocrinology 2010;91(4):333–40.
6. Kos-Kudla B, O'Toole D, Falconi M, et al. ENETS consensus guidelines for the management of bone and lung metastases from neuroendocrine tumors. Neuroendocrinology 2010;91(4):341–50.
7. Garcia-Carbonero R, Capdevila J, Crespo-Herrero G, et al. Incidence, patterns of care and prognostic factors for outcome of gastroenteropancreatic neuroendocrine tumors (GEP-NETs): results from the National Cancer Registry of Spain (RGETNE). Ann Oncol 2010;21(9):1794–803.
8. Madani A, Thomassen I, van Gestel Y, et al. Peritoneal metastases from gastroenteropancreatic neuroendocrine tumors: incidence, risk factors and prognosis. Ann Surg Oncol 2017;24(8):2199–205.

9. Van Loon K, Zhang L, Keiser J, et al. Bone metastases and skeletal-related events from neuroendocrine tumors. Endocr Connect 2015;4(1):9–17.

10. Ross EM, Roberts WC. The carcinoid syndrome: comparison of 21 necropsy subjects with carcinoid heart disease to 15 necropsy subjects without carcinoid heart disease. Am J Med 1985;79(3):339–54.

11. Tierney JF, Kosche C, Schadde E, et al. (68)Gallium-DOTATATE positron emission tomography-computed tomography (PET CT) changes management in a majority of patients with neuroendocrine tumors. Surgery 2019;165(1):178–85.

12. Meijer WG, van der Veer E, Jager PL, et al. Bone metastases in carcinoid tumors: clinical features, imaging characteristics, and markers of bone metabolism. J Nucl Med 2003;44(2):184–91.

13. Farley HA, Pommier RF. Treatment of neuroendocrine liver metastases. Surg Oncol Clin N Am 2016;25(1):217–25.

14. Kelz RR, Fraker DL. Metastatic carcinoid: don't forget the surgical consultation. Surgery 2014;156(6):1367–8.

15. Boudreaux JP, Putty B, Frey DJ, et al. Surgical treatment of advanced-stage carcinoid tumors: lessons learned. Ann Surg 2005;241(6):839–45 [discussion: 845–6].

16. Maxwell JE, Sherman SK, O'Dorisio TM, et al. Liver-directed surgery of neuroendocrine metastases: what is the optimal strategy? Surgery 2016;159(1):320–33.

17. Glazer ES, Tseng JF, Al-Refaie W, et al. Long-term survival after surgical management of neuroendocrine hepatic metastases. HPB (Oxford) 2010;12(6):427–33.

18. Graff-Baker AN, Sauer DA, Pommier SJ, et al. Expanded criteria for carcinoid liver debulking: maintaining survival and increasing the number of eligible patients. Surgery 2014;156(6):1369–76 [discussion: 1376–7].

19. Scott AT, Breheny PJ, Keck KJ, et al. Effective cytoreduction can be achieved in patients with numerous neuroendocrine tumor liver metastases (NETLMs). Surgery 2019;165(1):166–75.

20. McEntee GP, Nagorney DM, Kvols LK, et al. Cytoreductive hepatic surgery for neuroendocrine tumors. Surgery 1990;108(6):1091–6.

21. Sarmiento JM, Heywood G, Rubin J, et al. Surgical treatment of neuroendocrine metastases to the liver: a plea for resection to increase survival. J Am Coll Surg 2003;197(1):29–37.

22. Morgan RE, Pommier SJ, Pommier RF. Expanded criteria for debulking of liver metastasis also apply to pancreatic neuroendocrine tumors. Surgery 2018;163(1):218–25.

23. Que FG, Nagorney DM, Batts KP, et al. Hepatic resection for metastatic neuroendocrine carcinomas. Am J Surg 1995;169(1):36–42 [discussion: 42–3].

24. Soreide JA, van Heerden JA, Thompson GB, et al. Gastrointestinal carcinoid tumors: long-term prognosis for surgically treated patients. World J Surg 2000;24(11):1431–6.

25. Chen H, Hardacre JM, Uzar A, et al. Isolated liver metastases from neuroendocrine tumors: does resection prolong survival? J Am Coll Surg 1998;187(1):88–92 [discussion: 92–3].

26. Elias D, Debaere T, Muttillo I, et al. Intraoperative use of radiofrequency treatment allows an increase in the rate of curative liver resection. J Surg Oncol 1998;67(3):190–1.

27. Goldberg SN, Gazelle GS, Dawson SL, et al. Tissue ablation with radiofrequency: effect of probe size, gauge, duration, and temperature on lesion volume. Acad Radiol 1995;2(5):399–404.

28. Mohan H, Nicholson P, Winter DC, et al. Radiofrequency ablation for neuroendocrine liver metastases: a systematic review. J Vasc Interv Radiol 2015;26(7): 935–42.e1.

29. Akyildiz HY, Mitchell J, Milas M, et al. Laparoscopic radiofrequency thermal ablation of neuroendocrine hepatic metastases: long-term follow-up. Surgery 2010; 148(6):1288–93 [discussion: 1293].

30. Swärd C, Johanson V, Nieveen van Dijkum E, et al. Prolonged survival after hepatic artery embolization in patients with midgut carcinoid syndrome. Br J Surg 2009;96(5):517–21.

31. Chen JX, Rose S, White SB, et al. Embolotherapy for neuroendocrine tumor liver metastases: prognostic factors for hepatic progression-free survival and overall survival. Cardiovasc Intervent Radiol 2017;40(1):69–80.

32. Elf AK, Andersson M, Henrikson O, et al. Radioembolization versus bland embolization for hepatic metastases from small intestinal neuroendocrine tumors: short-term results of a randomized clinical trial. World J Surg 2018;42(2):506–13.

33. Carrasco CH, Charnsangavej C, Ajani J, et al. The carcinoid syndrome: palliation by hepatic artery embolization. AJR Am J Roentgenol 1986;147(1):149–54.

34. Hur S, Chung JW, Kim HC, et al. Survival outcomes and prognostic factors of transcatheter arterial chemoembolization for hepatic neuroendocrine metastases. J Vasc Interv Radiol 2013;24(7):947–56 [quiz: 957].

35. Dhir M, Shrestha R, Steel JL, et al. Initial treatment of unresectable neuroendocrine tumor liver metastases with transarterial chemoembolization using streptozotocin: a 20-year experience. Ann Surg Oncol 2017;24(2):450–9.

36. Do Minh D, Chapiro J, Gorodetski B, et al. Intra-arterial therapy of neuroendocrine tumour liver metastases: comparing conventional TACE, drug-eluting beads TACE and yttrium-90 radioembolisation as treatment options using a propensity score analysis model. Eur Radiol 2017;27(12):4995–5005.

37. Pericleous M, Caplin ME, Tsochatzis E, et al. Hepatic artery embolization in advanced neuroendocrine tumors: efficacy and long-term outcomes. Asia Pac J Clin Oncol 2016;12(1):61–9.

38. Moris D, Tsilimigras DI, Ntanasis-Stathopoulos I, et al. Liver transplantation in patients with liver metastases from neuroendocrine tumors: a systematic review. Surgery 2017;162(3):525–36.

39. Le Treut YP, Gregoire E, Klempnauer J, et al. Liver transplantation for neuroendocrine tumors in Europe–results and trends in patient selection: a 213-case European Liver Transplant Registry study. Ann Surg 2013;257(5):807–15.

40. Rossi RE, Burroughs AK, Caplin ME. Liver transplantation for unresectable neuroendocrine tumor liver metastases. Ann Surg Oncol 2014;21(7):2398–405.

41. Jacquet P, Sugarbaker PH. Clinical research methodologies in diagnosis and staging of patients with peritoneal carcinomatosis. Cancer Treat Res 1996;82: 359–74.

42. Glehen O, Mohamed F, Gilly FN. Peritoneal carcinomatosis from digestive tract cancer: new management by cytoreductive surgery and intraperitoneal chemohyperthermia. Lancet Oncol 2004;5(4):219–28.

43. Norlen O, Edfeldt K, Akerstrom G, et al. Peritoneal carcinomatosis from small intestinal neuroendocrine tumors: clinical course and genetic profiling. Surgery 2014;156(6):1512–21 [discussion: 1521–2].

44. Elias D, Sideris L, Liberale G, et al. Surgical treatment of peritoneal carcinomatosis from well-differentiated digestive endocrine carcinomas. Surgery 2005; 137(4):411–6.

45. Elias D, Lasser P, Ducreux M, et al. Liver resection (and associated extrahepatic resections) for metastatic well-differentiated endocrine tumors: a 15-year single center prospective study. Surgery 2003;133(4):375–82.

46. de Mestier L, Lardiere-Deguelte S, Brixi H, et al. Updating the surgical management of peritoneal carcinomatosis in patients with neuroendocrine tumors. Neuroendocrinology 2015;101(2):105–11.

47. Zamborsky R, Svec A, Kokavec M, et al. Bone metastases in neuroendocrine tumors. Bratisl Lek Listy 2017;118(9):529–34.

48. Schupak KD, Wallner KE. The role of radiation therapy in the treatment of locally unresectable or metastatic carcinoid tumors. Int J Radiat Oncol Biol Phys 1991; 20(3):489–95.

49. Berruti A, Libe R, Lagana M, et al. Morbidity and mortality of bone metastases in advanced adrenocortical carcinoma: a multicenter retrospective study. Eur J Endocrinol 2019;180(5):311–20.

50. Ezziddin S, Sabet A, Heinemann F, et al. Response and long-term control of bone metastases after peptide receptor radionuclide therapy with (177)Lu-octreotate. J Nucl Med 2011;52(8):1197–203.

51. Arnold PM, Floyd HE, Anderson KK, et al. Surgical management of carcinoid tumors metastatic to the spine: report of three cases. Clin Neurol Neurosurg 2010; 112(5):443–5.

Medical Management of Gastroenteropancreatic Neuroendocrine Tumors

Chandrikha Chandrasekharan, MBBS

KEYWORDS

- GEPNETs • Chemotherapy • Somatostatin analogues • Sunitinib • Everolimus
- CAPTEM

KEY POINTS

- Octreotide LAR (long-acting repeatable) and lanreotide both have shown antiproliferative properties in somatostatin expressing in advanced well-differentiated gastroenteropancreatic neuroendocrine tumors (NETs) in addition to their well-established role in the control of symptoms associated with functional NETs.
- Sunitinib is the only US Food and Drug Administration (FDA)–approved tyrosine kinase inhibitor in advanced well-differentiated pancreatic NET.
- Everolimus, a mammalian target of rapamycin complex inhibitor, gained FDA approval for use in well-differentiated NET of lung, gastrointestinal, or pancreatic origin after progression on octreotide analogue therapy.
- Chemotherapy has limited therapeutic efficacy in small bowel NETs; however, its role in pancreatic NETs is well established.
- The question of appropriate sequencing of therapies, the safety and efficacy of combinations, as well as novel drug targets remain to be explored.

INTRODUCTION

Neuroendocrine tumors (NETs) have increased in incidence over time. A recent Surveillance, Epidemiology, and End Results (SEER) database analysis showed that the age-adjusted incidence of NETs has increased nearly 6.4-fold from 1.09 per 100,000 persons in 1973 to 6.98 per 100,000 in 2012.[1] The increasing incidence was noted across all sites, grades, and stages of NETs. The median overall survival (OS) for all patients was 9.3 years. Localized NETs had better median OS (>30 years) compared with regional NETs (10.2 years) and distant NETs (12 months). On evaluation of survival trends over 3 time periods (2000–2004, 2005–2008, and 2009–2012), the improvement in survival was more pronounced in the subgroup with distant gastrointestinal (GI) NETs (hazard ratio [HR], 0.76; 95% confidence interval [CI],

Division of Medical Oncology, University of Iowa, 200 Hawkins Drive, C GH 32, Iowa City, Iowa 52242, USA
E-mail address: Chandrikha-chandrasekharan@uiowa.edu

Surg Oncol Clin N Am 29 (2020) 293–316
https://doi.org/10.1016/j.soc.2019.11.004
1055-3207/20/Published by Elsevier Inc.

surgonc.theclinics.com

0.67–0.86 for 2005–2008 and HR, 0.71; 95% CI, 0.63–0.82 for 2009–2012 compared with 2000–2004). In addition to factors such as increased detection rates and awareness, the improvement in survival is also likely caused by the addition of treatment options for NETs in this time period. This article discusses the systemic therapy options for the management of well-differentiated gastroenteropancreatic NETs (GEPNETs). The management of high-grade or poorly differentiated neuroendocrine carcinomas (NECs) is also discussed briefly.

Treatment of all patients with GEPNETs should be individualized and approached in a multidisciplinary manner. Some important tumor-related factors to consider include the site of origin (small intestine vs pancreas), grade of the tumor, presence or absence of symptoms attributable to the disease, hormonal hypersecretion, and sites and burden of metastases. Some of the patient-related factors that are pertinent in decision making include age, medical comorbidities, and patient preferences. In patients with hepatic metastases only, especially small bowel grade 1 or 2 NETs, surgical debulking should be considered if optimal cytoreduction can be achieved. In asymptomatic patients with low-volume disease, surveillance with periodic clinical and radiographic assessment is also an appropriate first step of management. Upfront systemic therapy should be considered in patients who are symptomatic from tumor bulk or from hormone hypersecretion, especially if significant extrahepatic disease is noted and not appropriate for surgical resection. In such patients, a combination of therapies can also be considered for rapid relief of symptoms.

While pancreatic NETs (pNETs) are more responsive to cytotoxic chemotherapy, small bowel NETs (SBNETs) are relatively refractory to chemotherapy. Everolimus, a mammalian target of rapamycin complex (mTORC) inhibitor, is approved for pancreatic, lung, and SBNETs, whereas sunitinib, a multi–tyrosine kinase inhibitor, is approved for use in pNETs only at this time.[2,3] Peptide receptor radionucleotide therapy (PRRT) may be an option for all low or intermediate GEPNETs that express somatostatin receptors (SSTRs). Although many therapeutic options have been added to the treatment armamentarium for GEPNETs, very little is known about the optimal sequence of these therapies.

SOMATOSTATIN ANALOGUES

For patients with symptoms of hormone secretion from GEPNETs, treatment with a somatostatin analogue (SSA) is often the first step. Somatostatin, a hypothalamic peptide that inhibits growth hormone secretion, was first discovered in 1973.[4] Thereafter, its role in the regulation of multiple other hormones, neuropeptides, as well as secretion of pancreatic enzymes was elucidated. Most well-differentiated GEPNETs express SSTRs on their cell surface. There are 5 subtypes of SSTRs (numbered 1–5), of which the SSTR2 subtype is most commonly overexpressed by GEPNETs. Almost 80% to 100% of cases of well-differentiated grade 1 and 2 GEPNETs express SSTRs.[5] The presence of these receptors is usually confirmed by an octreotide scan or the more sensitive ^{68}Ga-DOTATATE PET. SSTRs are G protein–coupled receptors whose antisecretory function is modulated by inhibition of adenyl cyclase and regulation of calcium and potassium channels. However, they also have potent antiproliferative effects through multiple direct and indirect mechanisms.[6] The direct mechanisms include blocking cell division by blockade of mitogenic growth factor signals through interaction with the mitogen-activated protein kinase/extracellular signal-regulated kinase (MAPK/ERK) pathway or inducing apoptosis. SSAs also exert many indirect antitumor actions through inhibition of secretion of growth factors, antiangiogenic effects, and immunomodulatory effects.

There are currently 2 US Food and Drug Administration (FDA)–approved long-acting SSAs for the management of metastatic or advanced GEPNETs: octreotide LAR (long-acting repeatable) depot and lanreotide. Octreotide, an 8-amino-acid peptide analogue, with more specific and longer duration of activity compared with native somatostatin, was first introduced into clinical practice for the management of carcinoid syndrome in 1986.[7] In this landmark study of 25 patients with symptomatic carcinoid syndrome and increased urinary 5-hydroxyindoleacetic acid (5-HIAA) levels, administration of subcutaneous octreotide led to palliation of symptoms in nearly all the patients and reduction in urinary 5-HIAA levels. The long-acting depot formulation octreotide LAR, administered intramuscularly once every 28 days, was then compared with short-acting subcutaneous octreotide in a randomized trial of 93 patients and showed similar efficacy.[8] Subsequently, multiple studies of octreotide, either alone or in conjunction with other therapies such as interferon, established the role of octreotide LAR in the management of carcinoid syndrome, leading to its FDA approval in 1995. **Table 1** lists some of the important studies with SSAs.

Although octreotide's role in the control of hormone hypersecretion is well established, its role as an antiproliferative agent remained in question. PROMID was the first randomized, double-blind, placebo-controlled prospective study that examined the effect of octreotide LAR on tumor control.[20] Treatment-naive patients with functional or nonfunctional, locally inoperable or metastatic well-differentiated SBNETs received either placebo or long-acting octreotide LAR at a dosage of 30 mg every 28 days. The median time to tumor progression in the octreotide LAR and placebo groups were 14.3 and 6 months respectively (HR = 0.34; 95% CI, 0.20–0.59; P = .000072). At 6 months, stable disease was noted in 66.7% in the octreotide LAR arm versus 37.2% of patients in the placebo arm. Although the long-term median OS was only slightly different between the 2 patients groups (84.7 months and 83.7 months respectively), crossover of most of the patients on the placebo arm (38 out of 43) to the octreotide LAR arm may have confounded this.[21] Only 1 partial response (PR) was noted in either group and no complete responses were noted. The health-related quality of life deteriorated more often and earlier in the placebo group as opposed to the patients who received octreotide LAR.[22]

The PROMID study was limited to SBNETs. The antiproliferative action of SSAs in pNET as well as NET of unknown origin was established by the subsequent CLARINET study.[23] CLARINET was a randomized, double-blind, placebo-controlled study of lanreotide 120 mg administered deep subcutaneously every 4 weeks compared with placebo in patients with well-differentiated or moderately differentiated nonfunctional NETs of pancreas, small bowel, or unknown origin. Median progression-free survival (PFS) was not reached in the lanreotide arm versus 18 months for the placebo arm (HR for progression or death, 0.47; 95% CI, 0.30–0.73; P<.001). This pivotal study led to the approval of lanreotide for the treatment of metastatic or unresectable well-differentiated to moderately differentiated GEPNETs by the FDA in 2014. The safety and efficacy of lanreotide as well as its antitumor activity was further confirmed in the open-label extension study.[24] Lanreotide's role in the control of carcinoid syndrome is also well established through multiple studies.[11,25,26]

Higher doses of octreotide LAR or lanreotide are often used in practice for refractory symptoms or disease progression. Although well tolerated, it is hard to draw conclusions regarding their impact on PFS, OS, or symptomatic improvement.[27,28] Ongoing trials such as CLARINET FORTE (National Clinical Trial [NCT] 02651987) may provide an answer to these questions. The role of lanreotide following disease progression on octreotide LAR or vice versa is also not known. In a single-institution retrospective study of 16 patients, treatment with lanreotide following disease progression or

Table 1
Somatostatin analog trials

Trial	Treatment Arm	Number of Patients	Results
Phase 3 randomized prospective Arnold et al,[9] 2005	Octreotide vs Octreotide + IFNα	109	Median OS 32 mo vs 54 mo. Not significant Partial tumor response, 5.7% and 15% in both arms
Phase 3 randomized prospective Faiss et al,[10] 2003	Lanreotide (L) vs IFNα (I) vs Lanreotide + IFNα (L + I)	83	Partial tumor regression in 1 (L), 1 (I) and 2 (L + I)
Phase 3 randomized, double blind, placebo controlled ELECT Vinik et al,[11] 2016	Lanreotide depot vs Placebo	115	Percentage of days with rescue octreotide use 33.7% vs 48.5%
Phase 2 single arm Kvols et al,[7] 1986	Octreotide subcutaneous Different doses	25	72% biochemical response
Phase 2 single arm in pancreatic islet cell Kvols et al,[12] 1987	Octreotide subcutaneous	22	63% biochemical response
Phase 2 single arm Saltz et al,[13] 1993	Octreotide subcutaneous	34	No objective response 50% stable disease 71% biochemical or symptom response
Phase 2 single arm, prospective Arnold et al,[14] 1996	Octreotide subcutaneous	103	No objective tumor regression 36.5% stable disease 64% improvement in carcinoid syndrome
Phase 2 single arm, prospective di Bartolomeo et al,[15] 1996	Octreotide subcutaneous in 2 dosing schedules	58	3% PR 73% symptomatic control 77% biochemical response
Phase 2 single arm, pilot Eriksson et al,[16] 1997	Lanreotide daily subcutaneous	19	5% tumor regression 70% stable disease 58% biochemical response
Phase 2 single arm, prospective Wymenga et al,[17] 1999	Lanreotide depot	56	47% biochemical response 6% tumor regression 81% stable disease
Phase 2 single arm Ducreux et al,[18] 2000	Lanreotide every 14 d or lanreotide 30 mg every 10 d	46	5% objective response rate 70% stable disease
Phase 2/3 dose titration study Ruszniewski et al,[19] 2004	Lanreotide depot titrated from 90 mg to 120 mg	71	38% overall symptom response 81% flushing improvement 75% diarrhea improvement

Abbreviations: IFN, interferon; PR, partial response.

poor tolerance was reported to be favorable; however, many of these patients also received additional disease-directed therapies.[29]

Pasireotide, an SSA with avid binding affinity to SSTRs 1, 2, 3, and 5, has been evaluated in multiple trials.[30,31] However, higher rates of higher rates of grade 3 or 4 hyperglycemia without a benefit in PFS limited its usage and approval in NETs. Novel oral octreotide and subcutaneous depot formulations of octreotide are in early clinical trials and may add more therapy options in the future. **Table 2** lists some ongoing clinical trials of octreotide or lanreotide.

In summary, multiple studies have unequivocally established the role of SSAs in the management of both functional and nonfunctional metastatic GEPNETs, making it a category 1 recommendation in National Comprehensive Cancer Network (NCCN) guidelines as well as in European Neuroendocrine Tumor Society (ENETS) and North American Neuroendocrine Tumor Society (NANETS) guidelines.[32–34] The most frequent side effects are related to steatorrhea, flatulence, hyperglycemia, and gallstones. Drug discontinuation because of side effects is infrequent. Most neuroendocrine experts consider either of the drugs appropriate for the management of carcinoid syndrome and for tumor control.

HISTORICAL RESULTS WITH CHEMOTHERAPY

Before the discovery of agents targeting specific molecular pathways in NETs, most clinical trials examined the role of chemotherapeutic agents in the management of GEPNETs. Many of these early trials used end points such as decrease in the size of hepatomegaly, reduction in urinary 5-HIAA level, or other biomarkers to assess response, as opposed to the more modern and accepted response criteria such as radiographic Response Evaluation Criteria in Solid Tumors (RECIST) criteria. Thus, the response rates reported by these trials are likely an overestimation of the actual benefit from chemotherapy. Nevertheless, any discussion regarding systemic therapy options in GEPNETs is incomplete without reviewing some of these pioneering trials. To date, streptozocin (STZ), which was approved in 1982, is the only FDA-approved chemotherapeutic agent for the management of advanced pancreatic islet cell tumors.

CHEMOTHERAPY IN NONPANCREATIC GASTROINTESTINAL CARCINOID TUMORS

Early clinical trials in metastatic carcinoid tumors using the combination of STZ with 5-fluorouracil (5-FU) or cyclophosphamide noted response rates of 44% and 37% respectively in carcinoids of small bowel origin with no difference in survival between the two arms.[35] A subsequent Eastern Cooperative Oncology Group (ECOG) study investigated the combination of a modified schedule of 5-FU + STZ versus doxorubicin in 172 patients, and roughly one-third of the patients had a confirmed NET of small intestine origin. The response rates in the combination 5-FU + STZ arm was lower than in the prior ECOG study at 22%.[36] Dacarbazine as a single agent in metastatic carcinoid showed a response rate of 16% (9 out of 56 patients).[37] Based on these studies, a 3-arm study comparing 5-FU + doxorubicin, 5-FU + STZ, and dacarbazine was conducted using more objective radiographic criteria to assess response.[38] Response rates to all 3 regimens were modest (15.9% vs 16% vs 8.2% respectively). A randomized phase 3 clinical trial in 64 patients with progressive metastatic carcinoids comparing interferon alpha with 5-FU/STZ combination showed no statistically significant difference in PFS and OS between the two arms and very few objective responses (9% and 3% respectively).[39] In an analysis of 2 phase II trials investigating the safety and efficacy of bevacizumab + FOLFOX (5-FU and oxaliplatin)

Table 2
Somatostatin analogue ongoing or recently completed clinical trials

Trial Name Phase	Disease Site	Therapy	Number of Patients	NCT
REMINET Prospective multicenter double-blind randomized	Unresectable duodenopancreatic grade 1, 2	Lanreotide vs placebo as maintenance after chemotherapy	118	NCT02288377
PLANET Phase 1 b/2	GEPENT grade 1/2	Pembrolizumab 200 mg intravenous and lanreotide 90 mg every 3 wk	26	NCT03043664
Phase 2 study of ramucirumab with SSA in advanced carcinoid tumors	Carcinoids Excluding pancreatic	Octreotide or lanreotide plus ramucirumab	43	NCT02795858
METNET-2 Pilot 1-arm open-label prospective study	Advanced GI or lung well-differentiated NETs	Lanreotide and metformin 2550 mg daily	20	NCT02823691
Sandostatin LAR and axitinib vs placebo Phase II/III randomized double blind	G1 G2 NET of nonpancreatic origin	Sandostatin + axitinib vs sandostatin + placebo	148	NCT01744249

or CAPOX (capecitabine and oxaliplatin), response rate in the carcinoid arm was 13.6% (3 out of 22 patients) with a median PFS of 19.3 months, whereas the response rates were higher in pNET at 41.7% (4 out of 12 patients).[40] Phase 2 nonrandomized studies of single-agent capecitabine or in combination with bevacizumab have also shown much lesser response rates than historical data in SBNETs.[41–43] In a retrospective study of 18 patients with GI NETs, 4 of them of small bowel origin, combination capecitabine and temozolomide (CAPTEM) showed 1 complete response, 1 PR, and 1 stable disease.[44] Similarly, temozolomide-based therapy in small bowel carcinoid was associated with no radiographic response and 1 biochemical response, as opposed to response rates of 34% in pNET.[45] In a systematic meta-analysis of chemotherapy in nonpancreatic NETs by Lamarca and colleagues,[46] the investigators concluded that most of the studies were of level C evidence with heterogeneous populations and treatments, limiting any conclusions. There is a lack of evidence showing objective response rates, OS, or PFS benefit with chemotherapy in well-differentiated GI NETs except of pancreatic origin. Thus, their use in small bowel–origin NETs is generally considered only if patients have exhausted other standard therapy options. A summary of some of these trials is presented in **Table 3**.

CHEMOTHERAPY IN PANCREATIC NEUROENDOCRINE TUMORS

Broder and Carter[55] were one of the first groups to report response rates of 37% with STZ in advanced pancreatic islet cell tumors in a single-arm 52-patient study. This work was followed by a randomized ECOG study comparing STZ + 5-FU with STZ alone in advanced islet cell tumors.[56] Patients who received the combination chemotherapy were noted to have double the response rates compared with single-agent STZ (63% vs 36%) but no statistical difference in OS (24 months vs 17 months). Complete response rate of 33% was reported with the combination arm, defined as the disappearance of all clinical or laboratory evidence of malignant disease and not by radiographic assessment. STZ/doxorubicin compared with 5-FU/STZ in a prospective randomized trial of 102 patients with pNETs was noted to be superior, with response rates of 69% versus 45% respectively.[57] Dacarbazine, another alkylating agent like STZ, showed a response rate of 34% in a 50-patient study.[58] Despite the robust response rates noted in pNETs, the widespread use of dacarbazine and STZ is limited because of their toxicity. The advent of temozolomide (TMZ), an oral alkylating agent with a better toxicity prolife and tolerance, has rendered the use of STZ and dacarbazine in pNETs obsolete in modern times.

CAPECITABINE AND TEMOZOLOMIDE FOR PANCREATIC NEUROENDOCRINE TUMORS

Alkylating agents such as STZ work by inhibiting nucleoside incorporation during cell cycle division. The discovery of temozolomide, an oral alkylating agent that is converted to its active agent MTIC [(methyl-triazene-1-yl)-imidazole-4-carboxamide] similar to dacarbazine, gave another treatment option with a more favorable toxicity profile. In a pilot phase 1 study of 30 patients with advanced NETs excluding small cell carcinomas, temozolomide in combination with an antiangiogenic agent, thalidomide, showed an overall response rates of 25% (45% in pNET and 7% in SBNET).[54] Temozolomide, administered in a dose-intense regimen of 150 mg/m^2 days 1 to 7 and days 15 to 21, was then studied in combination with bevacizumab, a monoclonal antibody targeting vascular endothelial growth factor (VEGF), in a 34 patient study.[59] Five out of 15 patients with pNETs had radiographic response, whereas none of the patients with carcinoid tumor had an objective response. Another phase 1/2 study of

Table 3
Chemotherapy in nonpancreatic carcinoids

Type of Study	Regimen	Number of Patients	Response Rates	Median OS
RCT Moertel & Hanley,[35] 1979	STZ + cyclophosphamide Vs STZ+5-FU	89 total	26% vs 33%	12.5 mo vs 11.2 mo
RCT phase 2/3 Engstorm et al,[36] 1984	5-FU + STZ vs Doxorubicin	172 total	22% Vs 21%	64 wk vs 48 wk
RCT phase 2/3 study Sun et al,[38] 2005	5-FU + Doxorubicin Vs 5-FU + STZ Vs Dacarbazine	249 total Including pancreatic	15.9% 16% 8.2%	15.7 mo 24.3 mo 11.9 mo
RCT phase 3 Dahan et al,[39] 2009	5-FU + STZ Vs IFN-α-2a	64 total 36 midgut	1 PR in midgut Vs 2 PR in midgut	PFS 8.5 mo vs 14.1 mo (midgut) PFS and OS difference not significant
Phase 2 single arm Bukowski et al,[37] 1994	Dacarbazine	56 total 28 midgut	16% PR total	20 mo
Phase 2 combined analysis Kunz et al,[40] 2016 Included pNETs	FOLFOX + bevacizumab CAPOX + bevacizumab	22 20	13.6% PR 5% PR	33.1 mo 42.2 mo
BETTER-1 phase 2 nonrandomized trial Mitry et al,[41] 2014	Capecitabine + bevacizumab	49	No complete response 18% PR	Median OS not reached Median PFS 23.4 mo
Phase 2 single arm Berruti et al,[42] 2014	Capecitabine + Bevacizumab + Octreotide LAR	13	11.5% radiographic PR (including lung and unknown primary)	Median PFS 14.3 mo
Phase 2 open label single arm Medley et al,[43] 2011	Capecitabine	20	11% biochemical PR No radiographic PR/CR	36.5 mo
Phase 2 trial Bukowski et al,[47] 1987	5FU + adriamcyin + Cyclophosphamide + STZ	63	31% response rate	10.8 mo

Study	Regimen	n	Response	Survival
2-arm nonrandomized study Van Hazel et al,[48] 1983	Dactinomycin Dacarbazine	17 15	1 PR 2 PRs	28 wk 47 wk
Phase 2 randomized Oberg et al,[49] 1989	5–FU + STZ Vs IFNα	10 10	0 biochemical or radiographic response 50% biochemical response, 20% radiographic response	Not reported
Phase 2 randomized Janson et al,[50] 1992	IFNα Vs IFNα + STZ + doxorubicin	12 11	1 biochemical response 2 radiographic response 0 biochemical or radiographic response	Not reported
Phase 2 single arm Kulke et al,[51] 2004	Docetaxel	21 11 midgut	0% response rate in midgut	Median PFS10 mo Median OS 24 mo
Phase 2 single arm Di Bartolomeo et al,[52] 1995	5–FU + Epirubicin + Dacarbazine	38 total	2 out of 20 carcinoid	Not reported
Retrospective study Kaltsas et al,[53] 2002	5–FU + lomustine	31	21%	48 mo
Phase 2 single arm Kulke et al,[54] 2006	Temozolamide + Thalidomide	29 total 14 carcinoid	25% radiographic response in all 7% radiographic response in carcinoid	Median OS not reached for entire cohort

Abbreviations: CR, complete response; RCT, randomized controlled trial; OS, overall survival.

everolimus in combination with temozolomide in patients with advanced pNETs showed a PR rate of 40% and a median PFS of 15.4 months.[60]

The CAPTEM combination was first reported by Fine and colleagues[61] in 2005. They hypothesized that because most pNETs are wild-type p53, the resistance to cell cycle specific cytotoxic agents is more likely a function of the tumor's low Ki-67 and indolent nature rather than a p53 mutation, a phenomenon called cytokinetic resistance. Thus, the synergistic combination of an alkylating agent that induces apoptosis in a static G0 cell phase and an antimetabolite such as 5-FU has sound scientific rationale. They also noted a synergistic cell kill in BON1 cell line if these agents were delivered in a schedule-dependent manner with 5-FU exposure preceding TMZ. Capecitabine is an oral pro-drug for 5-FU that gets activated in the liver to its active metabolites. Temozolomide mediates most of its cytotoxicity by methylation at the O6 guanine position. Tumors with high levels of the O6-methylguanyl methyltransferase (MGMT) repair enzyme are thus known to be more resistant to the action of temozolomide, such as in glioblastoma and vice versa.[62,63] pNETs in general have been shown to have low or absent levels of O6-MGMT enzyme.[45] Even in pNETs with sufficient O6-MGMT, it is postulated that the initial administration of capecitabine may deplete the thymidine pools by inhibition of thymidylate synthase, leading to decreased O6-MGMT enzyme repair activity and potentiation of temozolomide effect on the tumor. In their initial 10 patient series treated on this combination, they noted 1 complete response and 2 PRs.[64]

Following this, CAPTEM was reported by Strosberg and colleagues[65] in grade 1 and 2 advanced pNETs. In a single-institution retrospective series of 30 patients who received capecitabine at 750 mg/m^2 twice daily on days 1 to 14 and oral temozolomide at 200 mg/m^2 once daily on days 10 to 14, the overall radiographic response rate was 70% (21 patients with PR, 8 patients with stable disease). The combination as well as the dose of temozolomide used was well tolerated, with less nausea and lymphopenia than on the dose-intense schedules used before. In a retrospective review of 18 patients, including both pNETs and SBNETs, most of whom had also received prior chemotherapy (61%), the combination of CAPTEM still showed a response rate of 61% and median PFS of 14 months.[44] A meta-analysis of 15 published studies with pooled data from 384 patients, including some with grade 3 and non pancreatic NETs, treatment with CAPTEM noted disease control rates of 72.89% (95% CI, 64.04% to 81.73%; $P<.01$).[66] ECOG 2211, a 2-arm, randomized, phase II clinical trial comparing single-agent temozolomide versus CAPTEM in low-intermediate grade advanced pNETs was presented at the Annual American Society of Clinical Oncology (ASCO) GI meeting in 2018.[67] At a median follow-up of 29 months, the median PFS for the combination arm of CAPTEM was 22.7 months versus 14.4 months for single-agent temozolomide (HR, 0.58; 95% CI, 0.36–0.93). Median OS was 38 months in the temozolomide arm and had not been reached in the combination arm. An objective response rate of 33% was noted with the combination, similar to what has been noted in prior retrospective studies. This trial is the first and only prospective trial that clearly validates the role of CAPTEM chemotherapy in patients with pNETs and also reported the longest PFS on any therapy in patients with pNETs to date.

Based on the early trials from 1980 to 1990s as well as the collective evidence through recent retrospective case series and the randomized ECOG 2211 trial, cytotoxic chemotherapy is an important treatment option in pNETs. Chemotherapy should be considered as an initial treatment option in patients with advanced pNETs with a significant tumor burden, especially when symptomatic and if a rapid progressive clinical course is noted. With the robust response rates noted with this combination, their use in a neoadjuvant setting for borderline resectable or locally advanced pNETs may also be considered.[68]

ROLE OF INTERFERONS

Interferons were first introduced for the treatment of carcinoid tumors in 1982 by Oberg and colleagues.[69] Nine patients with midgut carcinoid tumors, 6 of them with symptomatic carcinoid syndrome, were treated with daily intramuscular doses of leukocyte interferon at 3×10^6 U/d for 1 month and 6×10^6 U/d for another 2 months. Treatment with interferon resulted in prompt and decreased levels of urinary 5-HIAA in 6 patients with liver metastases with resolution of the carcinoid symptoms. Since then, multiple studies of interferon either as a single agent or in combination with SSAs showed biochemical response rates of about 40% to 50% and tumor response of 10% to 15%.[70] Studies have also assessed the role of interferon beta as well as polyethylene glycol–modified (PEGylated) interferon, a once-weekly long-acting formulation of interferon.[71,72] The antitumor effects of interferons include a direct effect on cell cycle inducing arrest in G1 and G0 phase of synthesis, inhibition of growth factor production, antiangiogenic effects, and an immunomodulatory effect by increasing expression of class 1 antigens on tumor cells. Interferons have also been studied in combination with SSAs and bevacizumab. A list of some important randomized clinical trials using interferons is summarized in **Table 4**. A high incidence of flulike symptoms, severe fatigue, depression, and myelosuppression limit their widespread use in the management of NETs. While NCCN guidelines list the use of interferons in NETs as a category 3 recommendation, the NANETS does not recommend the use of interferon alpha unless no other options are available.[32,33] The ENETS includes interferons as a second-line therapy for refractory carcinoid syndrome and as an antiproliferative agent in midgut carcinoid tumors with limited options.[34]

MOLECULAR TARGETED THERAPIES
Tyrosine Kinase Inhibitors

GEPNETs are highly vascular tumors that have been shown to express high levels of VEGF, VEGF receptor (VEGFR) 2, VEGFR 3, platelet-derived growth factor receptor

Table 4
Randomized clinical trials with interferons

Trial	Treatment Arms	Number of Patients	Results
RCT Kolby et al,[73] 2003	IFNα + octreotide vs Octreotide	68 metastatic SBNETs	No difference in 5-y OS 56.8% vs 36.6% IFNα-treated patients with reduced risk of tumor progression ($P = .008$)
RCT Arnold et al,[9] 2005	IFNα + octreotide vs Octreotide	105 metastatic GEPNETs	Long-term OS similar at 35 mo for monotherapy and 51 mo for combination (HR, 1.19; 95% CI, 0.67–2.13; $P = .55$). PFS similar
RCT Faiss et al,[10] 2003	Lanreotide + IFNα vs Lanreotide vs IFNα	80 therapy naive metastatic GEPNETs	No statistically significant difference in rates of partial remission, stable disease, or tumor progression in all 3 arms
RCT open label Yao et al,[74] 2017	Octreotide + bevacizumab vs Octreotide + IFNα-2b	427 advanced grade 1 and 2 NETs	No difference in PFS 16.6 mo vs 15.4 mo (HR, 0.93; 95% CI, 0.73–1.18; $P = .55$)

(PDGFR) alpha, PDGFR beta, and the stem cell receptor c-kit.[75–77] Further, inhibition of the VEGF pathway in a mouse pancreatic neuroendocrine model provided proof of concept for multiple studies using angiogenesis inhibitors in GEPNETs. The VEGF pathway can be targeted either through tyrosine kinase inhibitors (TKIs), which inhibit multiple other growth factor receptors in addition to VEGF, or through monoclonal antibody against VEGF receptors such as bevacizumab. Although sunitinib is the only drug in this category that has gained FDA approval at this time, several TKIs have been tested or are undergoing clinical trials.

Sunitinib for Pancreatic Neuroendocrine Tumors

Sunitinib is a broad-spectrum TKI that works by inhibition of VEGFR1-2, PDGFR alpha, PDGFR beta, KIT, RET, FMS-like tyrosine kinase-3 (FLT3), and colony-stimulating factor receptor (CSF)-1R. Studies of sunitinib in Rip-Tag2 mouse models of pancreatic islet tumors suggested clinical activity.[78,79] In addition, in a phase 1 clinical trial of sunitinib in multiple advanced solid tumors, antitumor activity was noted in 1 out of 4 patients with NETs.[80] This observation led to an open-label, multicenter, phase 2 study with 109 patients(n = 41 carcinoids, n = 66 pNETs) that showed an overall objective response rate (ORR) of 16.7% in pNETs (11 of 66 patients) and stable disease in 68% (45 of 66 patients).[81] The ORR was less, at 2.4%, in carcinoid tumors. Subsequently, a phase 3, randomized, double-blind, placebo-controlled trial was conducted in 171 patients with advanced and metastatic pNETs with evidence of disease progression before trial enrollment.[82] Patients were randomized to receive a 37.5-mg daily dose of sunitinib or placebo. Because of clear differences in efficacy and the occurrence of more adverse events in the placebo arm, the trial was amended to allow crossover to the treatment arm. Median PFS was 11.4 months in patients treated with sunitinib compared with 5.5 months in the placebo arm (HR for disease progression or death, 0.42; 95% CI, 0.26–0.66; $P<.001$). Including 2 patients with complete response and 6 with PR, the overall response rate on the sunitinib arm was 9.3%. The most common adverse events noted were diarrhea, nausea, asthenia, vomiting, hypertension, hand-foot syndrome, and neutropenia. This landmark study led to the FDA approval of sunitinib for the management of metastatic pNETs in 2011.

Pazopanib

Pazopanib, another oral TKI that targets VEGF receptors, PDGFR alpha and beta, fibroblast growth factor receptors 1 and 3, and cKIT has been evaluated in both pNETs and SBNETs. In a parallel cohort study of patients with grade 1 to 2 carcinoid tumors (n = 20) or pNET (n = 32), 7 of 32 patients with pNETs achieved an objective response.[83] In another nonrandomized, open-label, single-center phase II study in 37 patients with metastatic GEPNETs, an ORR of 18.9% was noted.[84] A more recent study presented at ASCO 2019 showed that VEGF targeting may still be a relevant therapeutic option in advanced nonpancreatic NETs[85]; 171 patients with low-grade or intermediate-grade nonpancreatic GI NETs were randomized to pazopanib versus placebo. Median PFS was 11.6 months in the pazopanib arm versus 8.5 months in the placebo arm (HR, 0.53; $P = .0005$). Although pazopanib was associated with more symptoms such as diarrhea, fatigue, and grade 4 hypertension, the overall quality of life was similar between the treatment arms.

Cabozantinib

In preclinical models of pNETs in RIP-Tag2 transgenic mice, VEGF inhibition by sunitinib was accompanied by strong immunoreactivity for c-met in tumor lymphatics. c-met blockade was shown to significantly reduce metastases to local lymph nodes.[86]

Concurrent c-met and VEGF inhibition showed reduced invasion and metastases.[87] These findings led to a phase II 2-cohort clinical trial to evaluate the efficacy of cabozantinib, a potent kinase inhibitor with activity against AXL; FLT-3; c-met; VEGFRs 1, 2, and 3; and RET in patients with progressive, well-differentiated grade 1 to 2 carcinoid or pNET.[88] Three of 20 patients with pNETs achieved PR (ORR 15%), with a median PFS of 21.8 months (95% CI, 8.5–32 months). An ongoing phase 3, randomized clinical trial is evaluating the role of cabozantinib in advanced or metastatic NET with Ki-67 less than 20% of any origin (NCT03375320).

Other Tyrosine Kinase Inhibitors

Sorafenib showed a PR rate of 10% in carcinoids and pNETs in a phase 2 consortium study of 93 patients with metastatic GEPNETs.[89] Axitinib, approved in the treatment of metastatic renal cell carcinoma, showed a median PFS of 26.7 months (95% CI, 11.4–35.1) in an open-label, single-arm, phase 2 study of 30 patients with metastatic low-grade to intermediate-grade NET.[90] Lenvatinib, another oral TKI, currently approved for use in advanced hepatocellular carcinoma and medullar thyroid cancers, also showed significant antitumor activity in GEPNETs in a single-arm phase 2 study, with an overall response rate of 29%.[91]

Bevacizumab

Bevacizumab is a recombinant humanized monoclonal antibody that blocks angiogenesis by binding and neutralizing VEGF. Bevacizumab has been studied in NETs in many clinical trials in combination with SSAs, TKIs, as well as chemotherapy.[40–42,59,72,74,92] In a systematic review of bevacizumab-based combination therapies in NETs, median PFS was reported in 8 out of 9 studies ranging from 8.2 months to 16.5 months.[93] However, it is hard to draw any conclusions because of the heterogeneity of the patients included and the different drug combinations used.

Everolimus in Pancreatic and Small Bowel Neuroendocrine Tumors

Mammalian target of rapamycin (mTOR) is a serine threonine kinase that plays a key role in the control of cell growth, proliferation, and cell death. It signals downstream of many receptor tyrosine kinases, such as VEGF, IGF, Akt/PKB, and ERK1/2.[94] Patients with genetic cancer syndromes affecting the mTOR pathway genes such as neurofibromatosis (NF1), tuberous sclerosis (TSC1 and TSC2), and von Hippel-Lindau disease have an increased incidence of NETs.[95–98] Further, multiple gene expression profiling studies indicate a role for the (PI3K/AKT/mTOR) pathway in neuroendocrine tumorigenesis.[99–101] Everolimus, a selective mTORC1 oral inhibitor previously known as RAD-001, showed antitumor activity by itself or in combination with octreotide in multiple preclinical studies in NET cell lines.[102,103] Temsirolimus, an intravenous agent that inhibits the mTOR pathway, was first studied in a phase 2 clinical trial in 37 patients with progressive NETs of GI origin. A response rate of 5.6% was noted and the median time to progression was 6 months.[104] In a phase 2 study in advanced low-grade to intermediate-grade NETs, treatment with everolimus at 5 mg or 10 mg daily in combination with octreotide LAR showed promising antitumor activity with a PR rate of 22%.[105] RADIANT-1 (RAD001 in Advanced Neuroendocrine Tumors) was a multinational, open-label, phase II, nonrandomized trial to assess the antitumor activity of everolimus 10 mg in advanced well-differentiated to moderately differentiated pNETs with progressive disease during or after cytotoxic chemotherapy.[106] Patients were stratified to receive either everolimus or everolimus and octreotide LAR. ORR was 9.6% by central radiology review, with a median PFS of 9.7 months in the everolimus arm (95% CI, 8.3–13.3 months).

RADIANT-2 was a randomized, double-blind, placebo-controlled, phase 3 study in 429 patients with low-grade or intermediate-grade advanced NET associated with carcinoid syndrome.[107] Patients with disease progression within the past 12 months before enrollment were assigned to receive everolimus 10 mg daily or placebo in conjunction with octreotide LAR. Treatment with everolimus was associated with a 5.1-month improvement in median PFS; however, the difference did not reach the prespecified threshold for statistical significance (HR, 0.77; $P = .026$). This finding was partly attributed to imbalances in the baseline characteristics of the arms and the crossover design, all favoring the placebo arm.

RADIANT -3 investigated everolimus 10 mg daily versus placebo in advanced low-grade to intermediate-grade pNETs in a prospective, randomized, double-blind, placebo-controlled multicenter study of 410 patients.[108] The median PFS was 11 months in the everolimus group compared with 4.6 months in the placebo group, representing a 65% reduction in the risk of progression or death by central independent assessment (HR for disease progression or death, 0.35; 95% CI, 0.26- 0.44; p< 0.001). The ORR was 5% as assessed by local investigators compared with 2% in placebo arm. This study led to the FDA approval of everolimus for the treatment of advanced pNET in 2011, the same year as the approval of sunitinib, nearly 30 years after the last drug approval for NETs. The RADIANT-4 trial led to the FDA approval of everolimus in well to moderately differentiated nonpancreatic NETs as well in 2016.[109] Everolimus was associated with a 52% reduction in the estimated risk of progression or death (HR, 0.48; 95% CI, 0.35–0.67; P<0.00001). A trend toward improved OS was noted in the interim analysis. Although somatic mutations in the mTOR pathway are less frequently described in nonpancreatic NETs, the antitumor activity was postulated to be caused by other factors, such as inhibition of growth factor signaling, epigenetic modulation, and other undiscovered mechanisms of action of everolimus. The grade 3 or 4 adverse events noted with everolimus across the RADIANT-3 and RADIANT-4 trials include fatigue (2%–4%), stomatitis (7%–9%), diarrhea (7%–10%), infections (2%–7%), anemia (4%–6%), and hyperglycemia (4%–5%). Other pertinent side effects of all grades include rash, asthenia, peripheral edema, pneumonitis, nausea, and weight loss. However, the drug discontinuation rates because of side effects in the RADIANT-3 and RADIANT-4 trials were 13% and 12% respectively.

The RADIANT trials have firmly established everolimus as a therapeutic option for well-differentiated NETs of any GI, lung, or unknown origin. Although RADIANT-3 and RADIANT-4 trials did not allow concurrent SSA therapy and enrolled only nonfunctional NETs, the combination of everolimus and SSAs is known to be safe and well tolerated. Several studies have also alluded to the role of everolimus in the control of functional NETs.[110,111]

Combined mTOR and VEGF Data or Sequencing VEGF/mTOR

While targeting VEGF and mTOR pathway individually has shown success, the combination of these agents has been limited due to increased toxicity noted in multiple clinical trials. In a phase 1 standard dose-escalation study of 12 patients combining everolimus with sorafenib, dose-limiting toxicity was noted within the first cycle of therapy.[112] Another phase 2 study that combined temsirolimus and bevacizumab in well to moderately differentiated pNETs showed response rates of 41%, and median PFS and OS were 13.2 months and 34 months (95% CI, 27.1 months to not reached), respectively.[113] Again, higher rates of grade 3 to 4 adverse events were noted. The combination of everolimus and bevacizumab in the Cancer and Leukemia Group B (CALGB) 80701 study also noted higher rates of toxicity without additional benefits.[93]

Combination of two angiogenesis inhibitors sorafenib and bevacizumab also showed unacceptable toxicity rates.[114]

Fewer studies have investigated sequencing therapies in the management of NETs. Pazopanib was studied in a phase 2 clinical trial in patients with advanced GEPNETs who had shown disease progression on at least 1 antiangiogenic therapy or mTORC inhibitor.[115] Clinical benefit rate, defined as complete response plus PR plus stable disease, was noted in 60% of patients with prior mTOR inhibitor therapy, 73% of patients with prior antiangiogenic therapy, and 25% of patients with both. An ongoing randomized open-label study in advanced pNETs to compare the efficacy and safety of everolimus followed by chemotherapy with STZ/5-FU on progression or the reverse sequence, SEQTOR (NCT02246127), may shed further light on the question of sequencing therapies. There are also multiple trials ongoing to help answer the question of where PRRT fits in the sequence of treatment. The phase III COMPETE trial is a randomized, open-label, multicenter phase II study to evaluate ^{177}Lu-edotreotide PRRT compared twice with everolimus in patients with advanced SSTR-positive GEPNETs (NCT03049189). Another ongoing randomized, open-label, phase II trial will assess the efficacy and safety of ^{177}Lu-octreotate versus sunitinib in well-differentiated pNETs (NCT02230176).

High-Grade Neuroendocrine Carcinoma

High-grade NECs are characterized by a very aggressive clinical course, high Ki-67, and a propensity to metastasize early. The World Health Organization classification of pNETs was updated in 2017 to reflect the heterogeneity of grade 3 neuroendocrine neoplasms.[116] Well-differentiated grade 3 pNETs usually have a better prognosis than poorly differentiated small cell or large cell NECs. In large population-based studies of high-grade NETs of GI origin, a Ki-67 greater than 55% has been shown to be predictive of response to platinum-based therapy.[117] There is a lack of prospective clinical trial data to guide the management of these high-grade extrapulmonary NECs, both in the metastatic and locally advanced settings. Although surgery can be curative in a subset of patients with locally advanced tumors, the high risk of early metastatic dissemination raises the question of neoadjuvant therapy and careful patient selection in a multidisciplinary setting before such surgery is performed. In a SEER database study of 14,732 extrapulmonary NECs, the 5-year survival ranged from 58% to 60% in local-stage NEC of the female genital tract and small intestine to 25% for esophageal-origin NEC.[118] A Nordic multicenter cohort study evaluating the role of surgery in 119 patients with high-grade pNETs that included both well-differentiated and poorly differentiated grade 3 tumors,14 patients underwent surgery in a nonmetastatic setting.[119] All these patients experienced recurrent disease, with a median time to recurrence or metastasis of 7 months (range, 2–14 months). In another single-institution study of 44 poorly differentiated pNECs of all stages, 2-year survival rates were 22.5%.[120]

Based on extrapolated data from small cell lung cancers, chemotherapy with a platinum combination, usually cisplatin/etoposide or carboplatin/etoposide, is often the first line of therapy in metastatic poorly differentiated extrapulmonary NECs. The IMpower 133 study led to the approval of the combination of atezolizumab, a checkpoint inhibitor, and platinum doublet chemotherapy in 2019 as first-line therapy for extensive-stage lung cancer.[121] However, the upfront use of checkpoint inhibitors in extra pulmonary small cell cancers cannot yet be advocated for in the absence of well-designed clinical trials. In a preliminary report of the neuroendocrine tumor cohort of a basket trial of dual immune checkpoint inhibitors using ipilimumab plus nivolumab in rare cancers, objective response rates were seen in 8 out of 19 patients with high grade neuroendocrine tumors in a second-or third-line setting. (ORR 42%).[122] However, 2 other clinical trials using single-agent checkpoint inhibitors in high-grade extrapulmonary NETs only yielded 5% ORRs.[123,124] Thus, there is no clear evidence yet of OS benefit to recommend immunotherapy as a standard line of therapy, and its role continues to be debated. The optimal second-line chemotherapy in the platinum-refractory setting is also not well established. Options include irinotecan-based regimens, topotecan, temozolomide, and taxol. Because of a paucity of data, participation in clinical trials is encouraged.

FUTURE DIRECTIONS

In addition to sequencing existing therapy options, there is ongoing interest in combination therapies as well as novel therapeutic targets.[125] mTORC1/mTORC2 inhibitors have shown encouraging results in early-phase clinical trials.[126] Early-phase spelling- trials with CDK4/CDK6 inhibitors alone (NCT03891784) or in combination with everolimus (NCT03070301) are either underway or have been recently completed.[127,128] Ongoing trials are evaluating the combination of chemotherapy, immunotherapy, or molecular targeted therapy in conjunction with PRRT (NCT02358356, NCT03457948, NCT03629847 respectively). Although reported trials have shown low response rates with single-agent immunotherapy, there are many ongoing studies of immune checkpoint inhibitors alone or in combination with other therapies (NCT03457948, NCT03043664, NCT03095274).[123,129] Novel SSA-DM1 conjugate molecules such as PEN-221, an antibody-drug conjugate containing the tubulin inhibitor mersantine, has shown preliminary evidence of antitumor activity,[130] and expansion cohorts in pNETs and SBNETs are underway (NCT02936323). Phase 1 study of XmAb 18087, a bispecific antibody that engages the immune system against tumors by binding to SSTR 2 and CD3, is ongoing in NETs and GI stromal tumors (NCT03411915).

SUMMARY

The systemic therapy options for the management of NETs have come a long way from the discovery of somatostatin in 1973 to the most recent FDA approval of ^{177}Lu-PRRT in 2018. A better understanding of the underlying molecular biology of NETs has paved the way for the addition of many new therapies within the past 15 years. The significant improvement in OS even in advanced GEPNETs between the 2000 to 2004 period and the 2009 to 2012 period as noted in the recent SEER database study may possibly be caused by the addition of these new therapeutic agents in this time frame.[1] With the addition of many therapeutic agents comes the challenge of appropriate treatment selection and sequencing. Patient-centric and tumor-centric factors remain paramount in the management of NETs, making this the perfect example of how the science and art of cancer therapy come together to improve patient outcomes.

DISCLOSURE

The author is on the Lexicon pharmaceuticals scientific advisory board. The author is supported by SPORE P50 CA174521-01 Grants.

REFERENCES

1. Dasari A, Shen C, Halperin D, et al. Trends in the incidence, prevalence, and survival outcomes in patients with neuroendocrine tumors in the United States. JAMA Oncol 2017;3(10):1335–42.

2. Available at: https://www.fda.gov/drugs/resources-information-approved-drugs/everolimus-afinitor.

3. Blumenthal GM, Cortazar P, Zhang JJ, et al. FDA approval summary: sunitinib for the treatment of progressive well-differentiated locally advanced or metastatic pancreatic neuroendocrine tumors. Oncologist 2012;17(8):1108–13.

4. Ling N, Burgus R, Rivier J, et al. The use of mass spectrometry in deducing the sequence of somatostatin–a hypothalamic polypeptide that inhibits the secretion of growth hormone. Biochem Biophys Res Commun 1973;50(1):127–33.

5. Reubi JC, Waser B. Concomitant expression of several peptide receptors in neuroendocrine tumours: molecular basis for in vivo multireceptor tumour targeting. Eur J Nucl Med Mol Imaging 2003;30(5):781–93.

6. Susini C, Buscail L. Rationale for the use of somatostatin analogs as antitumor agents. Ann Oncol 2006;17(12):1733–42.

7. Kvols LK, Moertel CG, O'Connell MJ, et al. Treatment of the malignant carcinoid syndrome. Evaluation of a long-acting somatostatin analogue. N Engl J Med 1986;315(11):663–6.

8. Rubin J, Ajani J, Schirmer W, et al. Octreotide acetate long-acting formulation versus open-label subcutaneous octreotide acetate in malignant carcinoid syndrome. J Clin Oncol 1999;17(2):600–6.

9. Arnold R, Rinke A, Klose K, et al. Octreotide versus octreotide plus interferon-alpha in endocrine gastroenteropancreatic tumors: a randomized trial. Clin Gastroenterol Hepatol 2005;3(8):761–71.

10. Faiss S, Pape UF, Bohmig M, et al. Prospective, randomized, multicenter trial on the antiproliferative effect of lanreotide, interferon alfa, and their combination for therapy of metastatic neuroendocrine gastroenteropancreatic tumors—the International Lanreotide and Interferon Alfa Study Group. J Clin Oncol 2003;21(14):2689–96.

11. Vinik AI, Wolin EM, Liyanage N, et al. Evaluation of lanreotide depot/autogel efficacy and safety as a carcinoid syndrome treatment (ELECT): a randomized ,double-blind, placebo-controlled trial. Endocr Pract 2016;22(9):1068–80.

12. Kvols LK, Buck M, Moerterl CG, et al. Treatment of metastatic islet cell carcinoma with a somatostatin analogue (SMS 201-995). Ann Intern Med 1987;107:162–8.

13. Saltz L, Trochanowski B, Buckley M, et al. Octreotide as an antineoplastic agent in the treatment of functional and nonfunctional neuroendocrine tumors. Cancer 1993;72:244–8.

14. Arnold R, Trautmann ME, Creutzfeldt W, et al. the German Sandostatin Multicentre Study Group. Somatostatin analogue octreotide and inhibition of tumor growth in metastatic endocrine gastroenteropancreatic tumors. Gut 1996;38:430–8.

15. di Bartolomeo M, Bajetta E, Buzzoni R, et al. Clinical efficacy of octreotide in the treatment of metastatic neuroendocrine tumors. A study by the Italian Trials in Medical Oncology Group. Cancer 1996;77(2):402–8.

16. Eriksson B, Renstrup J, Iman H, et al. High-dose treatment with lanreotide of patients with advanced neuroendocrine gastrointestinal tumor: clinical and biological effects. Ann Oncol 1997;8:1041–4.

17. Wymenga ANM, Eriksson B, Salmela PI, et al. Efficacy and safety of prolonged-release lanreotide in patients with gastrointestinal neuroendocrine tumors and hormone-related symptoms. J Clin Oncol 1999;17(4):1111.

18. Ducreux M, Ruszniewski P, Chayvialle JA, et al. The antitumoral effect of the long-acting somatostatin analog lanreotide in neuroendocrine tumors. Am J Gastroenterol 2000;95(11):3276–81.

19. Ruszniewski P, Ish-Shalom S, Wymenga M, et al. Rapid and sustained relief from the symptoms of carcinoid syndrome: results from an open 6-month study of the 28-day prolonged-release formulation of lanreotide. Neuroendocrinology 2004; 80(4):244–51.

20. Rinke A, Müller HH, Schade-Brittinger C, et al. Placebo-controlled, double-blind, prospective, randomized study on the effect of octreotide LAR in the control of tumor growth in patients with metastatic neuroendocrine midgut tumors: a report from the PROMID Study Group. J Clin Oncol 2009;27(28):4656–63.

21. Rinke A, Wittenberg M, Schade-Brittinger C, et al. Placebo-controlled, double-blind, prospective, randomized study on the effect of octreotide LAR in the control of tumor growth in patients with metastatic neuroendocrine midgut tumors (PROMID): results of long-term survival. Neuroendocrinology 2017;104(1): 26–32.

22. Rinke A, Neary MP, Eriksson J, et al. Health-related quality of life for octreotide long-acting vs. placebo in patients with metastatic midgut neuroendocrine tumors in the phase 3 PROMID trial. Neuroendocrinology 2019;109(2):141–51.

23. Caplin ME1, Pavel M, Ćwikła JB, et al. Lanreotide in metastatic enteropancreatic neuroendocrine tumors. N Engl J Med 2014;371(3):224–33.

24. Caplin ME, Pavel M, Ćwikła JB, et al. Anti-tumor effects of lanreotide for pancreatic and intestinal neuroendocrine tumors: the CLARINET open-label extension study. Endocr Relat Cancer 2016;23(3):191–9.

25. Khan MS, El-Khouly F, Davies P, et al. Long-term results of treatment of malignant carcinoid syndrome with prolonged release Lanreotide (Somatuline Autogel). Aliment Pharmacol Ther 2011;34(2):235–42.

26. O'Toole D, Ducreux M, Bommelaer G, et al. Treatment of carcinoid syndrome: a prospective crossover evaluation of lanreotide versus octreotide in terms of efficacy, patient acceptability, and tolerance. Cancer 2000;88(4):770–6.

27. Broder MS, Beenhouwer D, Strosberg JR, et al. Gastrointestinal neuroendocrine tumors treated with high dose octreotide-LAR: a systematic literature review. World J Gastroenterol 2015;21(6):1945–55.

28. Chan DL, Ferone D, Albertelli M, et al. Escalated-dose somatostatin analogues for antiproliferative effect in GEPNETS: a systematic review. Endocrine 2017; 57(3):366–75.

29. Saif MW, Fu J, Smith MH, et al. Treatment with Lanreotide Depot Following Octreotide Long-Acting Release among Patients with Gastroenteropancreatic Neuroendocrine Tumors. J Pancreat Cancer 2018;4(1):64–71.

30. Wolin EM, Jarzab B, Eriksson B, et al. Phase III study of pasireotide long-acting release in patients with metastatic neuroendocrine tumors and carcinoid symptoms refractory to available somatostatin analogues. Drug Des Devel Ther 2015; 9:5075–86.

31. Kulke MH, Ruszniewski P, Van Cutsem E, et al. A randomized, open-label, phase 2 study of everolimus in combination with pasireotide LAR or everolimus alone in advanced, well-differentiated, progressive pancreatic neuroendocrine tumors: COOPERATE-2 trial. Ann Oncol 2017;28(6):1309–15.

32. Available at: https://www.nccn.org/professionals/physician_gls/pdf/neuroendocrine_blocks.pdf.

33. Strosberg JR1, Halfdanarson TR, Bellizzi AM, et al. The North American Neuro-endocrine Tumor Society Consensus Guidelines for Surveillance and Medical Management of Midgut Neuroendocrine Tumors. Pancreas 2017;46(6):707–14.
34. Pavel M, O'Toole D, Costa F, et al. ENETS Consensus Guidelines update for the Management of Distant Metastatic Disease of Intestinal, Pancreatic, Bronchial Neuroendocrine Neoplasms (NEN) and NEN of Unknown Primary Site. Neuroen-docrinology 2016;103(2):172–85.
35. Moertel CG, Hanley JA. Combination chemotherapy trials in metastatic carci-noid tumor and the malignant carcinoid syndrome. Cancer Clin Trials 1979; 2(4):327–34.
36. Engstrom PF, Lavin PT, Moertel CG, et al. Streptozocin plus fluorouracil versus doxorubicin therapy for metastatic carcinoid tumor. J Clin Oncol 1984;2(11): 1255–9.
37. Bukowski RM, Tangen CM, Peterson RF, et al. Phase II trial of dimethyltriazenoi-midazole carboxamide in patients with metastatic carcinoid. A Southwest Oncology Group study. Cancer 1994;73(5):1505–8.
38. Sun W, Lipsitz S, Catalano P, et al. Phase II/III study of doxorubicin with fluoro-uracil compared with streptozocin with fluorouracil or dacarbazine in the treat-ment of advanced carcinoid tumors: Eastern Cooperative Oncology Group Study E1281. J Clin Oncol 2005;23(22):4897–904.
39. Dahan L, Bonnetain F, Rougier P, et al. Phase III trial of chemotherapy using 5-fluorouracil and streptozotocin compared with interferon alpha for advanced carcinoid tumors: FNCLCC-FFCD 9710. Endocr Relat Cancer 2009;16(4): 1351–61.
40. Kunz PL, Balise RR, Fehrenbacher L, et al. Oxaliplatin-fluoropyrimidine chemo-therapy plus bevacizumab in advanced neuroendocrine tumors: an analysis of 2 phase II trials. Pancreas 2016;45(10):1394–400.
41. Mitry E, Walter T, Baudin E, et al. Bevacizumab plus capecitabine in patients with progressive advanced well-differentiated neuroendocrine tumors of the gastro-intestinal (GI-NETs) tract (BETTER trial)–a phase II non-randomized trial. Eur J Cancer 2014;50(18):3107–15.
42. Berruti A, Fazio N, Ferrero A, et al. Bevacizumab plus octreotide and metro-nomic capecitabine in patients with metastatic well-to-moderately differentiated neuroendocrine tumors: the XELBEVOCT study. BMC Cancer 2014;14:184.
43. Medley L, Morel AN, Farrugia D. Phase II study of single agent capecitabine in the treatment of metastatic non-pancreatic neuroendocrine tumours. Br J Can-cer 2011;104(7):1067–70.
44. Fine RL, Gulati AP, Krantz BA, et al. Capecitabine and temozolomide (CAPTEM) for metastatic, well-differentiated neuroendocrine cancers: the Pancreas Center at Columbia University experience. Cancer Chemother Pharmacol 2013;71(3): 663–70.
45. Kulke MH, Hornick JL, Frauenhoffer C, et al. O6-methylguanine DNA methyl-transferase deficiency and response to temozolomide-based therapy in patients with neuroendocrine tumors. Clin Cancer Res 2009;15(1):338–45.
46. Lamarca A, Elliott E, Barriuso J, et al. Chemotherapy for advanced non-pancreatic well-differentiated neuroendocrine tumours of the gastrointestinal tract, a systematic review and meta-analysis: a lost cause? Cancer Treat Rev 2016;44:26–41.
47. Bukowski RM, Johnson KG, Peterson RF, et al. A phase II trial of combination chemotherapy in patients with metastatic carcinoid tumors. A Southwest Oncology Group Study. Cancer 1987;60(12):2891–5.

48. Van Hazel GA, Rubin J, Moertel CG. Treatment of metastatic carcinoid tumor with dactinomycin or dacarbazine. Cancer Treat Rep 1983;67(6):583–5.
49. Oberg K, Norhein I, Alm G. Treatment of malignant carcinoid tumors: a randomized controlled study of streptozocin plus 5-FU and human leukocyte interferon. Eur J Cancer Clin Oncol 1989;25(10):1475–9.
50. Janson ET, Ronnblom L, Ahlstrom H, et al. Treatment with alpha-interferon versus alpha-interferon in combination with streptozocin and doxorubicin in patients with malignant carcinoid tumors: a randomized trial. Ann Oncol 1992;3(8): 635–8.
51. Kulke MH, Kim H, Stuart K, et al. A phase II study of docetaxel in patients with metastatic carcinoid tumors. Cancer Invest 2004;22(3):353–9.
52. Di Bartolomeo M, Bajetta E, Bochicchio AM, et al. A phase II trial of dacarbazine, fluorouracil and epirubicin in patients with neuroendocrine tumours. A study by the Italian Trials in Medical Oncology (I.T.M.O.) Group. Ann Oncol 1995;6(1):77–9.
53. Kaltsas GA, Mukherjee JJ, Isidori A, et al. Treatment of advanced neuroendocrine tumours using combination chemotherapy with lomustine and 5-fluorouracil. Clin Endocrinol (Oxf) 2002;57(2):169–83.
54. Kulke MH, Stuart K, Enzinger PC, et al. Phase II study of temozolomide and thalidomide in patients with metastatic neuroendocrine tumors. J Clin Oncol 2006;24(3):401–6.
55. Broder LE, Carter SK. Pancreatic islet cell carcinoma. II. Results of therapy with Streptozotocin in 52 patients. Ann Intern Med 1973;79(1):108–18.
56. Moertel CG, Hanley JA, Johnson LA. Streptozocin alone compared with streptozocin plus fluorouracil in the treatment of advanced islet-cell carcinoma. N Engl J Med 1980;303(21):1189–94.
57. Moertel CG, Lefkopoulo M, Lipsitz S, et al. Streptozocin-doxorubicin, streptozocin-fluorouracil or chlorozotocin in the treatment of advanced islet-cell carcinoma. N Engl J Med 1992;326(8):519–23.
58. Ramanathan RK, Cnaan A, Hahn RG, et al. Phase II trial of dacarbazine (DTIC) in advanced pancreatic islet cell carcinoma. Study of the Eastern Cooperative Oncology Group-E6282. Ann Oncol 2001;12(8):1139–43.
59. Chan JA, Stuart K, Earle CC, et al. Prospective study of bevacizumab plus temozolomide in patients with advanced neuroendocrine tumors. J Clin Oncol 2012;30(24):2963–8.
60. Chan JA, Blaszkowsky L, Stuart K, et al. A prospective, phase 1/2 study of everolimus and temozolomide in patients with advanced pancreatic neuroendocrine tumor. Cancer 2013;119(17):3212–8.
61. Fine RL, Fogelman DR, Schreibman SM. Effective treatment of neuroendocrine tumors with temozolomide and capecitabine. J Clin Oncol 2005;23(16S):S4216.
62. Baer JC, Freeman AA, Newlands ES, et al. Depletion of O6-alkylguanine-DNA alkyltransferase correlates with potentiation of temozolomide and CCNU toxicity in human tumour cells. Br J Cancer 1993;67(6):1299–302.
63. Hegi ME, Diserens AC, Gorlia T, et al. MGMT gene silencing and benefit from temozolomide in glioblastoma. N Engl J Med 2005;352:997–1003.
64. Isacoff WH, Moss RA, Pecora AL, et al. Temozolomide/capecitabine therapy for metastatic neuroendocrine tumors of the pancreas. A retrospective review. J Clin Oncol 2006;24(18S):14023.
65. Strosberg JR, Fine RL, Choi J, et al. First-line chemotherapy with capecitabine and temozolomide in patients with metastatic pancreatic endocrine carcinomas. Cancer 2011;117(2):268–75.

66. Lu Y, Zhao Z, Wang J, et al. Safety and efficacy of combining capecitabine and temozolomide (CAPTEM) to treat advanced neuroendocrine neoplasms: a meta-analysis. Medicine (Baltimore) 2018;97(41):e12784.

67. Kunz PL, Catalano PJ, Nimeiri H, et al. A randomized study of temozolomide or temozolomide and capecitabine in patients with advanced pancreatic neuroendocrine tumors: a trial of the ECOG-ACRIN Cancer Research Group (E2211). J Clin Oncol 2018;36(15_suppl):4004.

68. Ambe CM, Nguyen P, Centeno BA, et al. Multimodality management of "borderline resectable" pancreatic neuroendocrine tumors: report of a single-institution experience. Cancer Control 2017;24(5). 1073274817729076.

69. Oberg K, Funa K, Alm G. Effects of leukocyte interferon on clinical symptoms and hormone levels in patients with mid-gut carcinoid tumors and carcinoid syndrome. N Engl J Med 1983;309(3):129–33.

70. Oberg K. Interferon in the management of neuroendocrine GEP-tumors: a review. Digestion 2000;62(Suppl 1):92–7.

71. Pavel M, Hahn EG, Schuppan D, et al. Efficacy and tolerability of pegylated IFN-alpha in patients with neuroendocrine gastroenteropancreatic carcinomas. J Interferon Cytokine Res 2006;26(1):8–13.

72. Yao JC, Phan A, Hoff PM, et al. Targeting vascular endothelial growth factor in advanced carcinoid tumor: a random assignment phase II study of depot octreotide with bevacizumab and pegylated interferon alpha-2b. J Clin Oncol 2008;26(8):1316–23.

73. Kolby L, Persson G, Franzen S, et al. Randomized clinical trial of the effect of interferon alpha on survival in patients with disseminated midgut carcinoid tumours. Br J Surg 2003;90(6):687–93.

74. Yao JC, Guthrie KA, Moran C, et al. Phase III Prospective Randomized Comparison Trial of Depot Octreotide plus Interferon Alfa-2b versus Depot Octreotide Plus Bevacizumab in Patients With Advanced Carcinoid Tumors: SWOG S0518. J Clin Oncol 2017;35(15):1695–703.

75. Terris B, Scoazec JY, Rubbia L, et al. Expression of vascular endothelial growth factor in digestive neuroendocrine tumours. Histopathology 1998;32:133–8.

76. Fjällskog ML, Lejonklou MH, Oberg KE, et al. Expression of Molecular Targets for Tyrosine Kinase Receptor Antagonists in Malignant Endocrine Pancreatic Tumors. Clin Cancer Res 2003;9(4):1469–73.

77. Fjällskog ML, Hessman O, Eriksson B, et al. Upregulated expression of PDGF receptor beta in endocrine pancreatic tumors and metastases compared to normal endocrine pancreas. Acta Oncol 2007;46(6):741–6.

78. Pietras K, Hanahan D. A Multi targeted, metronomic, and Maximum-Tolerated Dose "Chemo-Switch" Regimen is Antiangiogenic, Producing Objective Responses and Survival Benefit in a Mouse Model of Cancer. J Clin Oncol 2005; 23(5):939–52.

79. Yao VJ, Sennino B, Davis RB, et al. Combined anti-VEGFR and anti-PDGFR actions of sunitinib on blood vessels in preclinical tumor models. Eur J Cancer 2006;4(Suppl):27–8. Abstract.

80. Faivre S, Delbaldo C, Vera K. Safety, pharmacokinetic, and antitumor activity of SU11248, a novel oral multitarget tyrosine kinase inhibitor, in patients with cancer. J Clin Oncol 2006;24(1):25–35.

81. Kulke MH, Lenz HJ, Meropol NJ. Activity of sunitinib in patients with advanced neuroendocrine tumors. J Clin Oncol 2008;26(20):3403–10.

82. Raymond E, Dahan L, Raoul JL, et al. Sunitinib malate for the treatment of pancreatic neuroendocrine tumors. N Engl J Med 2011;364(6):501–13.

83. Phan AT, Halperin DM, Chan JA, et al. Pazopanib and depot octreotide in advanced, well-differentiated neuroendocrine tumours: a multicenter, single-group, phase 2 study. Lancet Oncol 2015;16(6):695–703.
84. Ahn HK, Choi JY, Kim KM, et al. Phase II study of pazopanib monotherapy in metastatic gastroenteropancreatic neuroendocrine tumours. Br J Cancer 2013;109(6):1414–9.
85. Bergsland EK, Mahoney MR, Asmis TR, et al. Prospective randomized phase II trial of pazopanib versus placebo in patients with progressive carcinoid tumors (CARC) (Alliance A021202). J Clin Oncol 2019;37(15_suppl):4005.
86. Sennino B, Ishiguro-Oonuma T, Schriver BJ, et al. Inhibition of c-Met reduces lymphatic metastasis in RIP-Tag2 transgenic mice. Cancer Res 2013;73(12):3692–703.
87. Sennino B, Ishiguro-Oonuma T, Wei Y, et al. Suppression of tumor invasion and metastasis by concurrent inhibition of c-Met and VEGF signaling in pancreatic neuroendocrine tumors. Cancer Discov 2012;2(3):270–87.
88. Chan JA, Faris JE, Murphy JE, et al. Phase II trial of cabozantinib in patients with carcinoid and pancreatic neuroendocrine tumors (pNET). J Clin Oncol 2017;35(4_suppl):228.
89. Hobday TJ, Rubin J, Holen K, et al. MC044h, a phase II trial of sorafenib in patients (pts) with metastatic neuroendocrine tumors (NET): a phase II consortium (P2C) study. J Clin Oncol 2007;25(18_suppl):4504.
90. Strosberg JR, Cives M, Hwang J, et al. A phase II study of axitinib in advanced neuroendocrine tumors. Endocr Relat Cancer 2016;23(5):411–8.
91. Capdevila J, Fazio N, Lopez C, et al. Efficacy of lenvatinib in patients with advanced pancreatic (panNETs) and gastrointestinal (giNETs) grade 1/2 (G1/G2) neuroendocrine tumors: results of the international phase II TALENT trial. Ann Oncol 2018;29(suppl_8):viii467–78.
92. Kulke MH, Niedzwiecki D, Foster NR, et al. Randomized phase II study of everolimus versus everolimus plus bevacizumab in patients with locally advanced or metastatic pancreatic neuroendocrine tumors (pNET), CALGB 80701 (Alliance) (abstr). J Clin Oncol 2015;33(15_suppl). 4005–4005.
93. Abdel-Rahman O, Fouad M. Bevacizumab-based combination therapy for advanced gastroenteropancreatic neuroendocrine neoplasms (GEP-NENs): a systematic review of the literature. J Cancer Res Clin Oncol 2015;141(2):295–305.
94. Laplante M, Sabatini DM. mTOR signaling in growth control and disease. Cell 2012;149(2):274–93.
95. Verhoef S, van Diemen-Steenvoorde R, Akkersdijk WL, et al. Malignant pancreatic tumour within the spectrum of tuberous sclerosis complex in childhood. Eur J Pediatr 1999;158(4):284–7.
96. Eledrisi MS, Stuart CA, Alshanti M. Insulinoma in a patient with tuberous sclerosis: is there an association? Endocr Pract 2002;8(2):109–12.
97. Yoshida A, Hatanaka S, Ohi Y, et al. Von Recklinghausen's disease associated with somatostatin-rich duodenal carcinoid (somatostatinoma), medullary thyroid carcinoma and diffuse adrenal medullary hyperplasia. Acta Pathol Jpn 1991;41(11):847–56.
98. Lubensky IA, Pack S, Ault D. Multiple neuroendocrine tumors of the pancreas in von Hippel-Lindau disease patients: histopathological and molecular genetic analysis. Am J Pathol 1998;153(1):223–31.
99. Missiaglia E, Dalai I, Barbi S, et al. Pancreatic endocrine tumors: expression profiling evidences a role for AKT-mTOR pathway. J Clin Oncol 2010;28(2):245–55.

100. Fernandes I, Pacheco TR, Costa A, et al. Prognostic significance of AKT/mTOR signaling in advanced neuroendocrine tumors treated with somatostatin analogs. Onco Targets Ther 2012;5:409–16.

101. Jiao Y, Shi C, Edil BH, et al. DAXX/ATRX, MEN1, and mTOR pathway genes are frequently altered in pancreatic neuroendocrine tumors. Science 2011; 331(6021):1199–203.

102. Moreno A, Akcakanat A, Munsell MF, et al. Antitumor activity of rapamycin and octreotide as single agents or in combination in neuroendocrine tumors. Endocr Relat Cancer 2008;15(1):257–66.

103. Grozinsky-Glasberg S, Franchi G, Teng M, et al. Octreotide and the mTOR inhibitor RAD001 (everolimus) block proliferation and interact with the Akt-mTOR-p70S6K pathway in a neuro-endocrine tumour cell Line. Neuroendocrinology 2008;87(3):168–81.

104. Duran I, Kortmansky J, Singh D, et al. A phase II clinical and pharmacodynamic study of temsirolimus in advanced neuroendocrine carcinomas. Br J Cancer 2006;95(9):1148–54.

105. Yao JC, Phan AT, Chang DZ, et al. Efficacy of RAD001 (everolimus) and octreotide LAR in advanced low- to intermediate-grade neuroendocrine tumors: results of a phase II study [published correction appears in J Clin Oncol. 2008 Dec 1;26(34)5660.]. J Clin Oncol 2008;26(26):4311–8.

106. Yao JC, Lombard-Bohas C, Baudin E, et al. Daily oral everolimus activity in patients with metastatic pancreatic neuroendocrine tumors after failure of cytotoxic chemotherapy: a phase II trial. J Clin Oncol 2010;28(1):69–76.

107. Pavel ME, Hainsworth JD, Baudin E, et al. Everolimus plus octreotide long-acting repeatable for the treatment of advanced neuroendocrine tumours associated with carcinoid syndrome (RADIANT-2): a randomised, placebo-controlled, phase 3 study. Lancet 2011;378(9808):2005–12.

108. Yao JC, Shah MH, Ito T, et al. Everolimus for advanced pancreatic neuroendocrine tumors. N Engl J Med 2011;364(6):514–23.

109. Yao JC, Fazio N, Singh S, et al. Everolimus for the treatment of advanced, non-functional neuroendocrine tumours of the lung or gastrointestinal tract (RADIANT-4): a randomised, placebo-controlled, phase 3 study. Lancet 2016; 387(10022):968–77.

110. Bainbridge HE, Labri E, Middleton G. Symptomatic Control of Neuroendocrine Tumours with Everolimus. Horm Cancer 2015;6(5–6):254–9.

111. Capdevila J, Díez Miranda I, Obiols G, et al. Control of carcinoid syndrome with everolimus. Ann Oncol 2011;22(1):237–9.

112. Chan JA, Mayer RJ, Jackson N, et al. Phase I study of sorafenib in combination with everolimus (RAD001) in patients with advanced neuroendocrine tumors. Cancer Chemother Pharmacol 2013;71(5):1241–6.

113. Hobday TJ, Qin R, Reidy-Lagunes D, et al. Multicenter phase II trial of temsirolimus and bevacizumab in pancreatic neuroendocrine tumors. J Clin Oncol 2015;33(14):1551–6.

114. Castellano D, Capdevila J, Sastre J, et al. Sorafenib and bevacizumab combination targeted therapy in advanced neuroendocrine tumour: a phase II study of Spanish Neuroendocrine Tumour Group (GETNE0801). Eur J Cancer 2013; 49(18):3780–7.

115. Grande E, Capdevila J, Castellano D, et al. Pazopanib in pretreated advanced neuroendocrine tumors: a phase II, open-label trial of the Spanish Task Force Group for Neuroendocrine Tumors (GETNE). Ann Oncol 2015;26(9):1987–93.

116. Inzani F, Petrone G, Rindi G. The New World Health Organization Classification for Pancreatic Neuroendocrine Neoplasia. Endocrinol Metab Clin North Am 2018;47(3):463–70.
117. Sorbye H, Welin S, Langer SW, et al. Predictive and prognostic factors for treatment and survival in 305 patients with advanced gastrointestinal neuroendocrine carcinoma (WHO G3): the NORDIC NEC study. Ann Oncol 2013;24(1):152–60.
118. Dasari A, Mehta K, Byers LA, et al. Comparative study of lung and extrapulmonary poorly differentiated neuroendocrine carcinomas: a SEER database analysis of 162,983 cases. Cancer 2018;124(4):807–15.
119. Haugvik SP, Janson ET, Osterlung P, et al. Surgical treatment as a principle for patients with high-grade pancreatic neuroendocrine carcinoma: a nordic multicenter comparative study. Ann Surg Oncol 2016;23(5):1721–8.
120. Basturk O, Tang L, Hruban RH, et al. Poorly differentiated neuroendocrine carcinomas of the pancreas: a clinicopathologic analysis of 44 cases. Am J Surg Pathol 2014;38(4):437–47.
121. Horn L, Mansfied AS, Szczesna A, et al. First-Line Atezolizumab plus Chemotherapy in Extensive-Stage Small-Cell Lung Cancer. N Engl J Med 2018; 379(23):2220–9.
122. Patel SP, Othus M, Chae YK, et al. SWOG 1609(DART): A phase II basket trial of dual anti-CTLA-4 and anti-PD-1 blockade in rare tumors. Journal of Clinical Oncology 2019;37(15_suppl). TPS2658–TPS2658.
123. Vijayvergia N, Dasari A, ROss EA, et al. Pembrolizumab (P) monotherapy in patients with previously treated metastatic high grade neuroendocrine neoplasms(HG-NENs). Journal of Clinical Oncology 2018;36(15_suppl). 4104–4104.
124. Yao JC, Strosberg J, Fazio N, et al. Activity & safety of spartalizumab (PDR001) in patients (pts) with advanced neuroendocrine tumors (NET) of pancreatic (Pan), gastrointestinal (GI), or thoracic (T) origin, & gastroenteropancreatic neuroendocrine carcinoma (GEP NEC) who have progressed on prior treatment (Tx). Available at: https://academic.oup.com/annonc/article/29/suppl_8/mdy293.001/5140835.
125. Aristizabal Prada ET, Auernhammer CJ. Targeted therapy of gastroenteropancreatic neuroendocrine tumours: preclinical strategies and future targets. Endocr Connect 2018;7(1):R1–25.
126. Mita MM, Wolin EM, Meyer T, et al. Phase I expansion trial of an oral TORC1/TORC2 inhibitor (CC-223) in nonpancreatic neuroendocrine tumors (NET). J Clin Oncol 2013;31(15_suppl):e15004.
127. Pulido EG, Teule A, Alonso-Gordoa T, et al. A phase II trial of palbociclib in metastatic grade 1/2 pancreatic neuroendocrine tumors: the PALBONET study on behalf of the Spanish Taskforce Group of Neuroendocrine Tumors (GETNE). Ann Oncol 2017;28(suppl_5).
128. Dasari A, Halperin D M, Coya T, et al. A pilot study of the cyclin dependent kinases 4,6 inhibitor Ribociclib in patient with foregut neuroendocrine tumors. Abstract 2165. 15th Annual ENETS conference:Barcelona, Spain;7-8 March 2018.
129. Strosberg JR, Mizuno N, Doi T, et al. Pembrolizumab treatment of advanced neuroendocrine tumors: results from the phase II KEYNOTE-158 study. J Clin Oncol 2019;37(4_suppl):190.
130. Johnson ML, Meyer T, Halperin DM. First in human phase 1/2a study of PEN-221 somatostatin analog (SSA)-DM1 conjugate for patients (PTS) with advanced neuroendocrine tumor (NET) or small cell lung cancer (SCLC): phase 1 results. J Clin Oncol 2018;36(15_suppl):4097.

Overview and Current Status of Peptide Receptor Radionuclide Therapy

David L. Bushnell, MD[a,b,]*, Kellie L. Bodeker, MSHS, CCRC[c]

KEYWORDS

- PRRT • Lutathera • Dotatate • Radionuclide • Lu-177

KEY POINTS

- Peptide receptor radionuclide therapy (PRRT) improves progression-free survival in patients with nonoperable, progressive, somatostatin receptor–positive neuroendocrine tumors (NETs).
- PRRT is well tolerated, with rare clinically significant side effects related primarily to renal and bone marrow toxicity.
- Lutetium 177 (^{177}Lu)-DOTATATE is approved within the United States for the treatment of somatostatin receptor–positive gastroenteropancreatic NETs.
- The Food and Drug Administration approved standard treatment regimen for PRRT with ^{177}Lu-DOTATATE requires treatment cycles to be separated by 8 weeks to allow for bone marrow recovery.

BACKGROUND/CONCEPTS

The 2 most common radionuclides used for peptide receptor radionuclide therapy (PRRT) are yttrium 90 DOTA Phe1-Tyr3-Octreotide [^{90}Y-DOTATOC]) and lutetium 177 (^{177}Lu) (DOTA-phe1-Tyr3-Octreotate (^{177}Lu-DOTATATE, Lutathera(R) [Advanced Accelerator Applications, Milburn New Jersey). Both of these radioactive drugs target the subtype 2 somatostatin receptor (SSTR) with very high affinity (and to a lesser degree the subtype 5 receptor) present in high concentration on the surface of most types of neuroendocrine tumor (NET) cells. After binding to the cell surface SSTR, the complex becomes internalized with the radionuclide subsequently located in the cell cytoplasm. ^{177}Lu emits beta particles with each radioactive decay. The energy delivered to the tumor in the form of this beta radiation leads to cell death through

[a] Department of Radiology, University of Iowa Hospital and Clinics, 200 Hawkins Drive, Iowa City, IA, 52242, USA; [b] Iowa City Veterans Administration Health Care System, Iowa City, IA, USA; [c] Department of Radiation Oncology, University of Iowa Hospitals and Clinics, 200 Hawkins Drive, Iowa City, IA 52241, USA
* Corresponding author. University of Iowa Hospitals and Clinics, 200 Hawkins Drive, Iowa City, IA, 52242
E-mail address: david-bushnell@uiowa.edu

Surg Oncol Clin N Am 29 (2020) 317–326
https://doi.org/10.1016/j.soc.2019.11.005
1055-3207/20/Published by Elsevier Inc.

ionizations and free radical formation that damage DNA beyond the repair capabilities of the cell. The radiotherapies confer clinical benefit for patients with metastatic NETs, delivering modest objective response rates but significantly decreasing disease-related symptoms, thus improving quality of life.[1–5] Although both radiotherapies are recommended by European and North American NET societies for treatment of patients with nonoperable refractory disease, currently ^{90}Y-DOTATOC is available within the United States only through clinical trials.[6,7] In 2018, ^{177}Lu-DOTATATE (Lutathera) was approved by the US Food and Drug Administration (FDA) to treat adults with SSTR-positive gastroenteropancreatic (GEP) NETs, including foregut, midgut, and hindgut tumors. In 2018, based on high-level evidence, there was a uniform consensus from the National Comprehensive Cancer Network (NCCN) that ^{177}Lu-DOTATATE was a preferred treatment of patients with NETs who are progressing on octreotide/lanreotide therapy.[8] NCCN treatment guidelines recommend Lutathera be administered to low-grade or intermediate-grade NET (ie, Ki-67 $\leq$20%); this is not a requirement of the FDA-approved indication.[8]

TREATMENT PREPARATION AND PROCEDURE

Optimal patient selection for PRRT requires close collaboration and communication between referring clinicians and nuclear medicine physicians; ideally, patient evaluation occurs during a multidisciplinary tumor board review, consisting of expertise in multiple specialties. Adequate tumor targeting as a consequence of up-regulated SSTR tumor cell receptor expression is best demonstrated with gallium 68 DOTA-phe1-Tyr3-Octreotate (^{68}Ga-DOTATATE, Netspot, Advanced Accelerator Applications, Milburn, New Jersey) positron emission tomography (PET)/computed tomography (CT) imaging and represents a fundamental requirement for determining appropriateness of PRRT in a given patient. ^{68}Ga-DOTATATE PET/CT has now effectively replaced indium 111 (^{111}In)-pentetreotide (OctreoScan, Curium US LLC, Maryland Heights, Missouri) single photon emission computed tomography (SPECT) scan as the imaging examination of choice for this purpose. Although visual assessment of tumor uptake is considered reliable to select PRRT candidates, several studies indicate the tumor's maximum standardized uptake value (SUV), a measure commonly used with clinical fludeoxyglucose 18 (^{18}FDG) PET/CT examinations, from the Netspot PET images can help to predict response to this form of treatment.[9,10] Patients considered for PRRT should have adequate renal function, with a glomerular filtration rate (GFR) of greater than 60% of the age adjusted mean; however, patients on dialysis can be treated safely, provided forward-planning dosimetric measurements guide the amount of radioactivity to be administered.[11] Eligible patients should have sufficient bone marrow reserves; for the first PRRT cycle, recommended counts are platelets of at least 75,000 cells/μL and an absolute neutrophil count of at least 1000 cells/μL.[11]

Patients should receive PRRT approximately 3 weeks to 4 weeks after their last long-acting octreotide injection. Short-acting octreotide should be discontinued 12 hours to 24 hours prior and may be restarted 6 hours after infusion of Lutathera. Within the United States, PRRT typically is performed as an outpatient procedure, whether using the ^{90}Y-labeled or the ^{177}Lu-labeled radiopharmaceutical. This is allowed due to the low radiation exposure to the public from a patient who has just received treatment with ^{177}Lu or ^{90}Y. If a patient is using commercial travel shortly after treatment, however, the nuclear medicine physician should provide appropriate documentation to negate any travel security concerns stemming from activation of radiation detectors in airports.

Concurrent intravenous cationic amino acid administration (discussed later) is required to reduce the likelihood of long-term renal toxicity. The duration of the amino acid infusion is generally 4 hours, beginning 30 minutes prior to administration of Lutathera. The current FDA-approved dosing regimen consists of up to 4 individual treatment cycles of 200 mCi (7.4 GBq), each with an 8-week separation between cycles to allow for hematologic recovery. The radiotherapeutic infusion itself takes approximately 20 minutes to 30 minutes. In rare cases, patients may have side effects on the day of treatment, or in the ensuing few days, that can result in the need for hospitalization.[7] Infrequently, antiemetics, such as ondansetron, are needed to control nausea during the amino acid infusion and/or for several days after.

EFFICACY OF PEPTIDE RECEPTOR RADIONUCLIDE THERAPY IN GASTROENTEROPANCREATIC NEUROENDOCRINE TUMORS

The phase 3 NETTER-1 clinical trial (NCT01578239, A study comparing treatment with 177Lu-DOTA0-Tyr3-Octreotate to Octreotide LAR in patients with inoperable, progressive, somatostatin receptor positive midgut carcinoid tumours), which led in part to FDA approval of Lutathera, evaluated the efficacy of this treatment in patients with nonoperable, low-grade (1 or 2) midgut NETs with disease progression on high-dose Sandostatin LAR Depot (Novartis Pharmaceuticals Corporation, East Hanover, New Jersey).[3] At 20 months, progression-free survival (PFS) was 65% in the ^{177}Lu-DOTATATE treatment arm cohort compared with 11% in the control arm active comparator. Further data analysis from that study demonstrated that the median PFS for the ^{177}Lu-DOTATATE cohort was 28.4 months *versus* 8.5 months for the high-dose Sandostatin LAR Depot group.[12] In the same group of subjects, deterioration of quality of life occurred significantly sooner in control subjects compared with those receiving ^{177}Lu-DOTATATE therapy.[13] These results are consistent with several large retrospective studies published over the past decade evaluating ^{177}Lu-DOTA-TATE response and indicating survival advantages and excellent symptom control with PRRT.[5,14,15] Objective tumor response rates, however, are only modest, with reports indicating rare complete responses, with partial response rates of approximately 20% to 40%, depending somewhat on the specific treatment protocol.[4,16] **Fig. 1** shows an example of a patient with an excellent objective response after ^{177}Lu-DOTA-TATE PRRT. Perhaps as important, however, is the notable fraction of individuals with progressive disease at the time of therapy who demonstrate tumor stabilization after PRRT.[17]

It seems clear that in addition to grade 1 and grade 2 tumors, grade 3 GEP-NETs respond well to PRRT. In 1 moderate-sized study of patients with progressive grade 3 disease and adequate follow-up data, an impressive 47% of patients so treated demonstrated partial response after PRRT, with an additional 22% demonstrating stable disease.[18] The median estimated PFS was 36 months in this study, not unlike results reported for grade 1 or grade 2 disease. There is good reason to believe that other NET types can benefit from PRRT as well. Although not part of the NETTER-1 group, Typical/atypical lung carcinoids have been found to respond to this form of treatment with some investigators recommending treatment with Lutathera for these tumors when there is evidence of progression and good tumor targeting on pretherapy Netspot PET images.[19]

Both prospective and retrospective clinical studies have confirmed similar degrees of efficacy for PRRT with ^{90}Y-DOTATOC in patients with nonoperable low-grade GEP-NETs.[1,20] ^{90}Y-DOTATOC, however, currently is not FDA approved for routine clinical use. [90]Y may be more effective and appropriate for the treatment of larger tumors

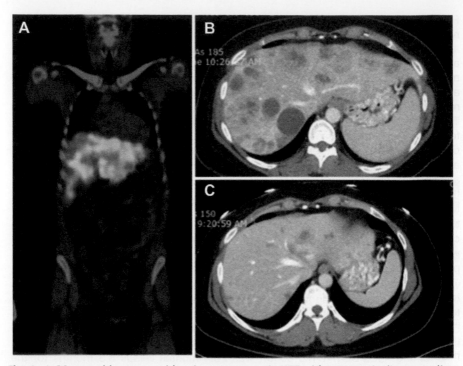

Fig. 1. A 36-year-old woman with primary pancreatic NET with metastatic disease to liver and Ki-67 12%. (*A*) Coronal ^{68}Ga-DOTATATE fused PET/CT image demonstrates widespread SSTR-positive metastatic disease in the liver. (*B*) Baseline axial contrast-enhanced CT prior to PRRT. (*C*) Contrast-enhanced CT image 6 months after 3 cycles of PRRT with ^{177}Lu-DOTA-TATE depicting substantial reduction in number and volume of metastatic lesions.

due to the long path length of the energetic 2.3 MeV (maximum) beta emission whereas the lower-energy beta particles from ^{177}Lu are advantageous when it comes to treating smaller tumor deposits less than 1 cm.[21] Evidence supporting this contention comes from both preclinical and clinical studies.[21–23] Some investigators have suggested a PRRT treatment paradigm in which both radionuclides are used.[21] Nevertheless, at this point, it is difficult to draw hard conclusions regarding the optimal use of ^{90}Y-labeled octreopeptides alone or in combination with ^{177}Lu-DOTATATE.

There are other categories of patients with nonoperable NETs who deserve PRRT consideration. Recent reports support excellent efficacy of Lutathera in certain individuals with higher-grade tumors. For example, in subjects with grade 3 tumors (Ki-67 between 20% to 55%) with progressive disease at time of PRRT therapy, an impressive 41% partial response rate was obtained after treatment with Lutathera. Median PFS was 16 months in this group.[24] Others report that there is a significant difference in PFS after PRRT when Ki-67 is less than 55% compared with greater than 55%, where PFS was 11 months *versus* 4 months, respectively.[25] Many of the subjects in this particular study had progressed despite chemotherapy prior to PRRT.[25] It also seems that salvage therapy is effective at controlling disease after recurrence or progression after an initial treatment regimen with either a ^{177}Lu-labeled or ^{90}Y-labeled octreopeptide. Although efficacy does not seem quite as good as with the initial treatment, retreatment nevertheless leads to overall disease stabilization in the majority of individuals who have progressed after good response to a first course of

PRRT.[26,27] PFS, however, is shorter after salvage PRRT compared with that after the first course of therapy.[26]

PRRT also has received attention as a potentially beneficial form of therapy in a neoadjuvant setting. One study reported, for example, that of 29 patients with nonresectable (due to vascular involvement by tumor), nonfunctional pancreatic NETs, 11 were eventually deemed surgical candidates after ^{177}Lu-DOTATATE PRRT. Of these 11, 1 refused surgery and 9 had what was considered a successful surgical outcome. The median PFS for these 9 individuals was 69 months compared with 49 months for those who remained nonsurgical candidates after ^{177}Lu-DOTATATE therapy.[28] Other investigators also have reported PRRT as a promising form of neoadjuvant therapy.[29] Most recently, PRRT was applied presurgery in individuals with primary pancreatic NETs where resection was already considered appropriate. The goal for PRRT in this study being somewhat more akin to adjuvant therapy with an interest in reducing tumor recurrence and/or development of future metastatic disease.[30] The investigators found that PFS was improved in patients undergoing PRRT (^{90}Y or ^{177}Lu) compared with those who did not receive PRRT, specifically for the group of subjects who underwent an R0 procedure. In addition, the risk of developing a postoperative pancreatic fistula was reduced in the PRRT group.

One of the appealing aspects of PRRT is the potential to utilize pretherapy imaging to predict response to treatment. This first was demonstrated some years ago with the use of an ^{111}In-labeled octreopeptide, which targets SSTRs.[31] PET/CT imaging with ^{68}Ga-DOTATATE is capable of identifying sub-centimeter NET deposits throughout the body that may not be seen with the ^{111}In-labeled agent. Tumor uptake levels of this ^{68}Ga imaging biomarker are used to help select appropriate candidates for PRRT, as discussed previously.[7] Tumor SUV measurements from ^{68}Ga-DOTATATE PET/CT images hold promise as a quantitative approach for identification of patients whose NETs are most likely to respond to PRRT.[9,10] For example, 1 recent study found that a tumor SUV cutoff of 16 was a good predictor of response to ^{177}Lu-DOTATATE.[9] Similar findings have been reported in other studies using tumor SUV for prediction of objective response.[10] Finally, on a related note, a recent study reported progress in identification of a blood genomic signature for predicting responders *versus* nonresponders to PRRT.[32]

SIDE EFFECTS

The side-effect/toxicity profile for PRRT is excellent. A large majority of patients are symptom-free during the administration phase of the ^{177}Lu-labeled or ^{90}Y-labeled octreopeptides and accompanying amino acid delivery. Fatigue and/or mild nausea may occur within the first few days after treatment and may last for up to a week. These early symptoms are related largely to the early general effects of whole-body radiation. In rare cases, approximately 1% to 2%, excessive vasoactive peptides and/or amines released from the tumor on the treatment day, or in the first day or 2 after treatment, may lead to severe symptomatology, such as flushing and diarrhea associated with hormonal/carcinoid crisis.[33,34] Hypotension also may occur. Patients experiencing hypotension typically respond to treatment with high dosages of subcutaneous or intravenous octreotide, fluids, histamine blockers, and supportive care. Depending on the secretory nature of the tumor, for example insulinoma, more specific treatment may be needed in this setting.[35] Patients with preexisting carcinoid syndrome or preexisting symptoms related to a specific hormone secretion pattern are at greater risk for an acute exacerbation with PRRT. Even more rare (<1%) are the reported cases of both clinical and biochemical tumor lysis syndrome early on after PRRT.[36]

Historically, renal toxicity after PRRT has been the primary concern with this form of therapy. [177]Lu and ^{90}Y octreopeptides are filtered by the glomerulus and then reabsorbed and concentrated in the proximal tubules of the kidney. The mechanism of this process involves membrane endocytosis and transport of the radioactive peptide molecule into the tubule cell cytoplasm. The emitted beta particles then may reach the glomerulus, where the radiation damage is most pronounced in the form of endothelial cell injury, leading to thrombotic microaniopathy.[37] Importantly, this process of small peptide tubular reabsorption can be reduced through substantially the use of positively charged amino acids, specifically lysine and arginine, delivered intravenously during the administration phase of PRRT, as described previously. Numerous studies have demonstrated reductions in the kidney concentration of radiolabeled octreopeptides of approximately 20% to 40%, depending on the individual, with appropriate coinfusion of these amino acid solutions.[38]

It is well established that although long-term renal impairment may occur, it is uncommon, particularly when ^{177}Lu-DOTATATE is delivered utilizing FDA-approved dosage guidelines for this agent. In this setting, grade 3 or grade 4 long-term renal toxicity has been reported to occur in approximately only 2% of patients.[3] Although changes in GFR may been seen in the subacute setting, in some instances toxicity may not be recognized for up to a year or more.[39,40] There remains a degree of uncertainty regarding the effect of risk factors for PRRT affecting the likelihood of associated kidney damage. For example, several studies have found that preexisting hypertension, kidney disease, and diabetes may increase the likelihood of developing renal toxicity whereas others have not.[39,41–43] It is probably prudent to give thought to these comorbidities, specifically depending on their duration and severity, when deciding whether an individual patient is appropriate for PRRT. It also is generally believed that ^{90}Y octreopeptide therapy is more likely to cause renal impairment than the corresponding ^{177}Lu-labeled agent although, even with ^{90}Y, the likelihood for clinically significant renal impairment remains quite low (approximately 5%).[41] The explanation for possible greater ^{90}Y-related renal toxicity lies in the higher energy of the beta particle emission, and thus longer path length, with a greater potential therefore for energy to be deposited in the more radiosensitive glomeruli.

Subacute hematologic toxicity involving platelets and neutrophils occurs in less than 10% of individuals, depending on the PRRT treatment protocol that is utilized.[44] For the FDA-approved clinical PRRT protocol, grade 3 or grade 4 thrombocytopenia or neutropenia is reported to occur in approximately 3% of patients. The nadir in counts typically is seen approximately 5 weeks to 6 weeks after administration.[3] It seems clear that baseline renal dysfunction is associated with increased hematologic toxicity probably due to reduced clearance of the radiopharmaceutical from the blood, with corresponding increase in radiation dose to marrow forming elements in the body.[45] In addition, prior treatment with alkylating chemotherapy drugs and older age (>70) are risk factors for acute/subacute myelotoxicity.[44]

Longer-term hematologic toxicity remains perhaps a greater concern. From the large number of subjects treated worldwide over the past 2 decades, it seems clear that the eventual likelihood of developing myelodysplastic syndrome or acute leukemia after PRRT is close to 2%.[46]

Salvage therapy is almost as well tolerated as an initial PRRT regimen. In 1 study where the overall median follow-up was 88.6 months, acute myeloid leukemia/myelodysplastic syndrome occurred in 2% of patients with repeat PRRT using ^{177}Lu-DOTA-TATE. In this series, 7% of patients so treated developed grade 3 or grade 4 acute/subacute hematologic toxicity. There were no cases of grade 3 or grade 4 radiation-related renal disease.[26] Toxicity after PRRT in patients with grade 3 tumors appears similar to that found in patients so treated who have lower-grade tumors.[18]

FUTURE PROSPECTS

There are many as yet unresolved questions and issues related to PRRT. For example, the current dosing paradigm for Lutathera may overtreat some patients whereas others may not require the full 4 cycles of therapy. Tumor uptake of Lutathera may decline notably after the second or third treatment cycle, raising a question about the value of a fourth treatment cycle. The promising use of PRRT with radiosensitizing chemotherapy needs to be evaluated further. The optimal sequencing of PRRT with drugs, such as everolimus (Afinitor, Novartis Pharmaceuticals Corporation, East Hanover, New Jersey) and sunitinib (Sutent, Pfizer Labs, New York), has yet to be determined. For patients with liver-dominant disease, delivery of therapeutic radiolabeled octreopeptides through the hepatic artery results in higher tumor radiation and needs further investigation. Perhaps as important as any of these, there is an urgency to understand how best to utilize normal organ and/or tumor dosimetry to personalize each regimen of PRRT as opposed to utilizing a 1-dosage-fits-all approach that has been approved for Lutathera.[47-51] There is good reason to believe that radiolabeled SSTR antagonists may be more effective than receptor agonists.[52,53] Finally, the potentially enormous therapeutic advantages of alpha particle emitters applied to PRRT may be seen in the not too distant future.[54,55]

REFERENCES

1. Bushnell DL Jr, O'Dorisio TM, O'Dorisio MS, et al. 90Y-edotreotide for metastatic carcinoid refractory to octreotide. J Clin Oncol 2010;28:1652–9.
2. Vinjamuri S, Gilbert TM, Banks M, et al. Peptide receptor radionuclide therapy with (90)Y-DOTATATE/(90)Y-DOTATOC in patients with progressive metastatic neuroendocrine tumours: assessment of response, survival and toxicity. Br J Cancer 2013;108:1440–8.
3. Strosberg J, El-Haddad G, Wolin E, et al. Phase 3 trial of 177Lu-Dotatate for midgut neuroendocrine tumors. N Engl J Med 2017;376:125–35.
4. Nicolas GP, Morgenstern A, Schottelius M, et al. New developments in peptide receptor radionuclide therapy. J Nucl Med 2019;60:167–71.
5. Brabander T, van der Zwan WA, Teunissen JJM, et al. Long-term efficacy, survival, and safety of [(177)Lu-DOTA(0),Tyr(3)]octreotate in patients with gastroenteropancreatic and bronchial neuroendocrine tumors. Clin Cancer Res 2017;23:4617–24.
6. Hicks RJ, Kwekkeboom DJ, Krenning E, et al. ENETS consensus guidelines for the standards of care in neuroendocrine neoplasms: peptide receptor radionuclide therapy with radiolabelled somatostatin analogues. Neuroendocrinology 2017;105:295–309.
7. Hope TA, Abbott A, Colucci K, et al. NANETS/SNMMI procedure standard for somatostatin receptor-based peptide receptor radionuclide therapy with (177)Lu-DOTATATE. J Nucl Med 2019;60:937–43.
8. Shah MH, Goldner WS, Halfdanarson TR, et al. NCCN guidelines insights: neuroendocrine and adrenal tumors, version 2.2018. J Natl Compr Canc Netw 2018;16:693–702.
9. Kratochwil C, Stefanova M, Mavriopoulou E, et al. SUV of [68Ga]DOTATOC-PET/CT predicts response probability of PRRT in neuroendocrine tumors. Mol Imaging Biol 2015;17:313–8.

10. Oksuz MO, Winter L, Pfannenberg C, et al. Peptide receptor radionuclide therapy of neuroendocrine tumors with (90)Y-DOTATOC: is treatment response predictable by pre-therapeutic uptake of (68)Ga-DOTATOC? Diagn Interv Imaging 2014;95:289–300.

11. Zaknun JJ, Bodei L, Mueller-Brand J, et al. The joint IAEA, EANM, and SNMMI practical guidance on peptide receptor radionuclide therapy (PRRNT) in neuroendocrine tumours. Eur J Nucl Med Mol Imaging 2013;40:800–16.

12. Strosberg J, Wolin E, Chasen BEA. Overall survival, progression-free survival, and quality of life updates from the NETTER-1 study: 177Lu-Dotatate vs. high dose octreotide in progressive midgut neuroendocrine tumors. Neuroendocrinology 2018;106.

13. Strosberg J, Wolin E, Chasen B, et al. Health-related quality of life in patients with progressive midgut neuroendocrine tumors treated with (177)Lu-Dotatate in the phase III NETTER-1 trial. J Clin Oncol 2018;36:2578–84.

14. Sansovini M, Severi S, Ambrosetti A, et al. Treatment with the radiolabelled somatostatin analog Lu-DOTATATE for advanced pancreatic neuroendocrine tumors. Neuroendocrinology 2013;97:347–54.

15. Kam BL, Teunissen JJ, Krenning EP, et al. Lutetium-labelled peptides for therapy of neuroendocrine tumours. Eur J Nucl Med Mol Imaging 2012;39(Suppl 1): S103–12.

16. Del Prete M, Buteau FA, Arsenault F, et al. Personalized (177)Lu-octreotate peptide receptor radionuclide therapy of neuroendocrine tumours: initial results from the P-PRRT trial. Eur J Nucl Med Mol Imaging 2019;46:728–42.

17. Garske-Roman U, Sandstrom M, Fross Baron K, et al. Prospective observational study of (177)Lu-DOTA-octreotate therapy in 200 patients with advanced metastasized neuroendocrine tumours (NETs): feasibility and impact of a dosimetry-guided study protocol on outcome and toxicity. Eur J Nucl Med Mol Imaging 2018;45:970–88.

18. Demirci E, Kabasakal L, Toklu T, et al. 177Lu-DOTATATE therapy in patients with neuroendocrine tumours including high-grade (WHO G3) neuroendocrine tumours: response to treatment and long-term survival update. Nucl Med Commun 2018;39:789–96.

19. Naraev BG, Ramirez RA, Kendi AT, et al. Peptide receptor radionuclide therapy for patients with advanced lung carcinoids. Clin Lung Cancer 2019;20:e376–92.

20. Bodei L, Cremonesi M, Grana CM, et al. Yttrium-labelled peptides for therapy of NET. Eur J Nucl Med Mol Imaging 2012;39(Suppl 1):S93–102.

21. Baum RP, Kulkarni HR, Carreras C. Peptides and receptors in image-guided therapy: theranostics for neuroendocrine neoplasms. Semin Nucl Med 2012;42: 190–207.

22. Hindie E, Zanotti-Fregonara P, Quinto MA, et al. Dose deposits from 90Y, 177Lu, 111In, and 161Tb in micrometastases of various sizes: implications for radiopharmaceutical therapy. J Nucl Med 2016;57:759–64.

23. Baum RP, Kulkarni HR, Singh A, et al. Results and adverse events of personalized peptide receptor radionuclide therapy with 90Yttrium and 177Lutetium in 1048 patients with neuroendocrine neoplasms. Oncotarget 2018;9:18.

24. Carlsen E, Fazio N, Granberg D, et al. Peptide receptor radionuclide therapy in gastroenteropancreatic NEN G3: a multicenter cohort study. Endocr Relat Cancer 2019;26:227–39.

25. Zhang J, Kulkarni HR, Singh A, et al. Peptide receptor radionuclide therapy in grade 3 neuroendocrine neoplasms: safety and survival analysis in 69 patients. J Nucl Med 2019;60:377–85.

26. van der Zwan WA, Brabander T, Kam BLR, et al. Salvage peptide receptor radio-nuclide therapy with [(177)Lu-DOTA,Tyr(3)]octreotate in patients with bronchial and gastroenteropancreatic neuroendocrine tumours. Eur J Nucl Med Mol Imaging 2019;46:704–17.

27. Sabet A, Haslerud T, Pape UF, et al. Outcome and toxicity of salvage therapy with 177Lu-octreotate in patients with metastatic gastroenteropancreatic neuroendo-crine tumours. Eur J Nucl Med Mol Imaging 2014;41:205–10.

28. van Vliet EI, van Eijck CH, de Krijger RR, et al. Neoadjuvant treatment of nonfunc-tioning pancreatic neuroendocrine tumors with [177Lu-DOTA0,Tyr3]Octreotate. J Nucl Med 2015;56:1647–53.

29. Sowa-Staszczak A, Hubalewska-Dydejczyk A, Tomaszuk M. PRRT as neoadju-vant treatment in NET. Recent Results Cancer Res 2013;194:479–85.

30. Partelli S, Bertani E, Bartolomei M, et al. Peptide receptor radionuclide therapy as neoadjuvant therapy for resectable or potentially resectable pancreatic neuroen-docrine neoplasms. Surgery 2018;163:761–7.

31. Kwekkeboom DJ, Teunissen JJ, Bakker WH, et al. Radiolabeled somatostatin analog [177Lu-DOTA0,Tyr3]octreotate in patients with endocrine gastroentero-pancreatic tumors. J Clin Oncol 2005;23:2754–62.

32. Bodei L, Kidd MS, Singh A, et al. PRRT genomic signature in blood for prediction of (177)Lu-octreotate efficacy. Eur J Nucl Med Mol Imaging 2018;45:1155–69.

33. Zandee WT, Brabander T, Blazevic A, et al. Symptomatic and radiological response to 177Lu-DOTATATE for the treatment of functioning pancreatic neuro-endocrine tumors. J Clin Endocrinol Metab 2019;104:1336–44.

34. de Keizer B, van Aken MO, Feelders RA, et al. Hormonal crises following receptor radionuclide therapy with the radiolabeled somatostatin analogue [177Lu-DO-TA0,Tyr3]octreotate. Eur J Nucl Med Mol Imaging 2008;35:749–55.

35. Tapia Rico G, Li M, Pavlakis N, et al. Prevention and management of carcinoid crises in patients with high-risk neuroendocrine tumours undergoing peptide re-ceptor radionuclide therapy (PRRT): literature review and case series from two Australian tertiary medical institutions. Cancer Treat Rev 2018;66:1–6.

36. Huang K, Brenner W, Prasad V. Tumor lysis syndrome: a rare but serious compli-cation of radioligand therapies. J Nucl Med 2019;60(6):752–5.

37. Moll S, Nickeleit V, Mueller-Brand J, et al. A new cause of renal thrombotic micro-angiopathy: Yttrium 90-DOTATOC internal radiotherapy. Am J Kidney Dis 2001; 37:847–51.

38. Rolleman EJ, Valkema R, de Jong M, et al. Safe and effective inhibition of renal uptake of radiolabelled octreotide by a combination of lysine and arginine. Eur J Nucl Med Mol Imaging 2003;30:9–15.

39. Bodei L, Cremonesi M, Ferrari M, et al. Long-term evaluation of renal toxicity after peptide receptor radionuclide therapy with 90Y-DOTATOC and 177Lu-DOTA-TATE: the role of associated risk factors. Eur J Nucl Med Mol Imaging 2008;35: 1847–56.

40. Barone R, Borson-Chazot F, Valkema R, et al. Patient-specific dosimetry in pre-dicting renal toxicity with (90)Y-DOTATOC: relevance of kidney volume and dose rate in finding a dose-effect relationship. J Nucl Med 2005;46(s):99–105.

41. Bodei L, Kidd M, Paganelli G, et al. Long-term tolerability of PRRT in 807 patients with neuroendocrine tumours: the value and limitations of clinical factors. Eur J Nucl Med Mol Imaging 2015;42:5–19.

42. Bergsma H, Konijnenberg MW, van der Zwan WA, et al. Nephrotoxicity after PRRT with (177)Lu-DOTA-octreotate. Eur J Nucl Med Mol Imaging 2016;43:1802–11.

43. Sabet A, Ezziddin K, Pape UF, et al. Accurate assessment of long-term nephro-toxicity after peptide receptor radionuclide therapy with (177)Lu-octreotate. Eur J Nucl Med Mol Imaging 2014;41(3):505–10.

44. Kesavan M, Turner JH. Myelotoxicity of peptide receptor radionuclide therapy of neuroendocrine tumors: a decade of experience. Cancer Biother Radiopharm 2016;31:189–98.

45. Svensson J, Berg G, Wangberg B, et al. Renal function affects absorbed dose to the kidneys and haematological toxicity during (1)(7)(7)Lu-DOTATATE treatment. Eur J Nucl Med Mol Imaging 2015;42:947–55.

46. Bergsma H, van Lom K, Raaijmakers M, et al. Persistent hematologic dysfunction after peptide receptor radionuclide therapy with (177)Lu-DOTATATE: incidence, course, and predicting factors in patients with gastroenteropancreatic neuroen-docrine tumors. J Nucl Med 2018;59:452–8.

47. Ilan E, Sandstrom M, Wassberg C, et al. Dose response of pancreatic neuroen-docrine tumors treated with peptide receptor radionuclide therapy using 177Lu-DOTATATE. J Nucl Med 2015;56:177–82.

48. Eberlein U, Cremonesi M, Lassmann M. Individualized dosimetry for theranostics: necessary, nice to have, or counterproductive? J Nucl Med 2017;58:97S–103S.

49. Sundlov A, Sjogreen-Gleisner K, Svensson J, et al. Individualised (177)Lu-DOTA-TATE treatment of neuroendocrine tumours based on kidney dosimetry. Eur J Nucl Med Mol Imaging 2017;44:1480–9.

50. Menda Y, Madsen MT, O'Dorisio TM, et al. (90)Y-DOTATOC dosimetry-based personalized peptide receptor radionuclide therapy. J Nucl Med 2018;59:1692–8.

51. Strigari L, Konijnenberg M, Chiesa C, et al. The evidence base for the use of in-ternal dosimetry in the clinical practice of molecular radiotherapy. Eur J Nucl Med Mol Imaging 2014;2014:1976–88.

52. Reubi JC, Waser B, Macke H, et al. Highly increased 125I-JR11 antagonist bind-ing in vitro reveals novel indications for sst2 targeting in human cancers. J Nucl Med 2017;58:300–6.

53. Bodei L, Weber WA. Somatostatin receptor imaging of neuroendocrine tumors: from agonists to antagonists. J Nucl Med 2018;59:907–8.

54. Haberkorn U, Giesel F, Morgenstern A, et al. The future of radioligand therapy: alpha, beta, or both? J Nucl Med 2017;58:1017–8.

55. Kratochwil C, Giesel FL, Bruchertseifer F, et al. (2)(1)(3)Bi-DOTATOC receptor-targeted alpha-radionuclide therapy induces remission in neuroendocrine tu-mours refractory to beta radiation: a first-in-human experience. Eur J Nucl Med Mol Imaging 2014;41:2106–19.

Moving?

Make sure your subscription moves with you!

To notify us of your new address, find your **Clinics Account Number** (located on your mailing label above your name), and contact customer service at:

Email: journalscustomerservice-usa@elsevier.com

800-654-2452 (subscribers in the U.S. & Canada)
314-447-8871 (subscribers outside of the U.S. & Canada)

Fax number: 314-447-8029

Elsevier Health Sciences Division
Subscription Customer Service
3251 Riverport Lane
Maryland Heights, MO 63043

*To ensure uninterrupted delivery of your subscription, please notify us at least 4 weeks in advance of move.

Printed and bound by CPI Group (UK) Ltd, Croydon, CR0 4YY

03/10/2024

01040406-0019